Restorative Dentistry

To Matthew, Charlotte and Christopher – the future

Restorative Dentistry

An Integrated Approach

Peter Jacobsen
MDS (Lond) FDSRCS (Eng)

Reader in Restorative Dentistry, Department of Adult Dental Health, University of Wales College of Medicine, Cardiff, UK
Honorary Consultant in Restorative Dentistry, University Dental Hospital NHS Trust, Cardiff, UK

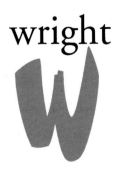

wright

OXFORD   BOSTON   JOHANNESBURG   MELBOURNE   NEW DELHI   SINGAPORE

Wright
An imprint of Butterworth-Heinemann
Linacre House, Jordan Hill, Oxford OX2 8DP
225 Wildwood Avenue, Woburn, MA 01801-2041
A division of Reed Educational and Professional Publishing Ltd

℞ A member of the Reed Elsevier plc group

First published 1998

British Library Cataloguing in Publication Data
Jacobsen, P. H. (Peter H.)
    Restorative dentistry: an integrated approach
    1. Dentistry, Operative
    I. Title
    617.6'05

ISBN 0 7236 1742 2

Library of Congress Cataloguing in Publication Data
Restorative dentistry: an integrated approach/[edited by]
    Peter Jacobsen.
    p.   cm.
    Rev. ed. of: Conservative dentistry. 1980.
    Includes bibliographical references and index.
    ISBN 0 7236 1742 2
    1. Dentistry, Operative.   I. Jacobsen, P. H. (Peter H.)
    II. Conservative dentistry.
    [DNLM: 1. Dental Restoration, Permanent.   WU 300 AR435]
    RK501.R473   98–15937
    617.6–dc21   CIP

Composition by Genesis Typesetting, Laser Quay, Rochester, Kent
Printed and bound in Great Britain by The Bath Press, Somerset

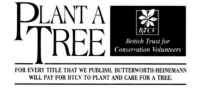

Contents

With contributions from

Periodontology

Martin Addy PhD MSc BDS (Wales) FDSRCS (Eng)
Professor of Periodontology, University of Bristol Dental School, Bristol
Honorary Consultant in Restorative Dentistry, United Bristol HealthCare NHS Trust, Bristol, UK

Removable prosthodontics

Alan Harrison TD QHDS PhD BDS (Wales) FDSRCS (Eng)
Professor of Dental Care for the Elderly, University of Bristol Dental School, Bristol
Honorary Consultant in Restorative Dentistry, United Bristol HealthCare NHS Trust, Bristol, UK

Dental biomaterials

Gavin J. Pearson PhD BDS (Lond) LDSRCS (Eng)
Professor of Biomaterials and Honorary Consultant in Restorative Dentistry, Eastman Dental Institute,
London, UK

Oral biology and pathology

David K. Whittaker PhD (Wales) BDS (Manc) FDSRCS (Eng)
Reader in Oral Biology, University of Wales College of Medicine, Cardiff
Honorary Consultant Dental Surgeon, University Dental Hospital NHS Trust, Cardiff, UK

Preface

This book began life as *Conservative Dentistry – An Integrated Approach*, published by Churchill Livingstone in 1990. The intention of that book was to distil the essentials of the subject and merge them with the appropriate aspects of the supporting sciences.

Since the late 1980s there has been a progressive loss of independent departments of conservative dentistry; most have merged with departments of periodontology and prosthetics to be all-embracing departments of restorative dentistry. Accompanying these changes has been the development of the specialist subjects of fixed and removable prosthodontics, periodontology and endodontics. Conservative dentistry, originally the largest subject in terms of United Kingdom dentistry, has been subsumed into this set of disciplines and has all but lost its status as a special subject.

The results of these changes could be the fragmentation of patient care and the compartmentalization of learning. As a concept, the total care of a patient receiving restorative dentistry must continue to be integrated; this book is intended to form a basis for such integration.

The challenge was to increase the scope of the original book and still retain a practical common-sense approach to clinical problems structured within the limitations imposed by the patient and the ability and facilities of the dentist. The integration means that there are not separate sections on the specialist subjects such as periodontology, dental biomaterials, occlusion, oral biology and so on but aspects of these topics are distributed throughout. These are *applied* sciences and to learn them in isolation can devalue their importance within the subject as a whole.

The book is intended to present the core of knowledge that forms the basis of clinical practice in restorative dentistry. It is not intended to be an encyclopaedic reference book and, of course, there may be the tendency to oversimplify; I hope I have not fallen into this trap. I have tried to include what is of fundamental importance and omit subtle variations in techniques and other aspects that will be learnt in practical classes.

The book assumes that a basic level of knowledge from technique courses has already been learnt and seeks to build on this. Some chapters are intended to revise and organize earlier learning and others are written to introduce more demanding subjects from a basic and practical viewpoint. There will always be a need to read extensive texts and a bibliography has been compiled to guide further reading.

I believe that undergraduates, in particular, have difficulty in organizing information into a logical sequence for learning and decision making. Flow charts, bulleted lists and tables have been included to help this problem and to show that no matter how complex a subject is, there is always a stepwise series of decisions involved, each decision inevitably excluding many other options. The undergraduate tends to present all the options (when he or she knows them!), rather than being selective and eliminating early those that are not applicable to that particular patient.

I have tried to eliminate the small print and esoteric techniques and concentrate on 'percentage dentistry' – the type of dentistry that brings success most often, for the satisfaction of both the patient *and* the dentist.

P. H. J.
Cardiff 1997

Acknowledgements

Many people, friends and colleagues have helped in the gestation, writing and production of this book.

The four specialist contributors, Martin Addy, Alan Harrison, Gavin Pearson and David Whittaker, worked magnificently to their deadlines and have borne with considerable fortitude the indignities of being 'integrated' within the overall style of the book. My especial thanks to them.

Three contributors to the original book, Dr John Lilley, Mr Richard Garn and the late Dr Robin Huggett, helped in creating the format of that book, the philosophy of which has continued here.

Mr Mel Davies and Dr Peter Staheli have read and criticized the draft and have made many helpful comments; Mrs Shelagh Thompson helped me update the sections on the management of the compromised patient.

Mr Frank Hartles and the staff of the Audiovisual Aids Unit at Cardiff have contributed greatly through the clinical photographs and much of the artwork – in particular Mr Rodney Doller, Mr Ron Lambert, Mr Mark Smith and Mrs Jo Griffiths all deserve a personal mention and thanks. The remainder of the artwork was done by Mr Peter Cox, freelance medical artist, and I thank him for his efforts.

Within the chapters on fixed prosthodontics, most of the illustrated cases are from my own clinical practice within the University Dental Hospital, Cardiff, and in this regard I would like to emphasize the need for such cases to be planned and treated by the efforts of an integrated team. Without the skills and support of Mr Jeff Lock, Chief Dental Technologist, and Mrs Helen Burrows and Mrs Michelle Davies, Dental Nurses, the quality of care that these patients received would have been considerably reduced.

The staff of the Medical Books Division of Butterworth-Heinemann, particularly Mary Seager, Hannah Tudge and Claire Hutchins, have assisted in the development and birth of the book.

Even bigger thanks are due to Mrs Karen Jacobsen who tolerated with considerable good grace and understanding the many hours of writing and editing that deprived her of her husband from family duties again – we're glad it's over!!

Finally, all my undergraduates and postgraduates provided the inspiration to put this thing together (again) – I hope they like it.

P. H. J.

SECTION I

THE PATIENT

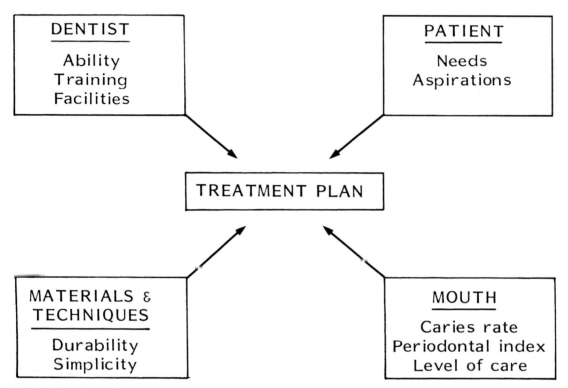

Fig. 1.1 Influences on the formulation of a treatment plan

1

The patient:
Limitations and expectations

> The provision of high quality restorative dentistry depends upon the dentist:
> - Making an accurate diagnosis
> - Devising a comprehensive and realistic treatment plan
> - Executing the treatment plan to a high technical standard
> - Providing subsequent continuing care

There is a very strong tendency, particularly in the field of fixed prosthodontics, for the dentist to become overinterested in the technical execution of treatment. There is a vast range of materials and equipment to stimulate this interest and compete for the dentist's attention. It is perhaps inevitable that dentists can become obsessive about types of bur or root canal file, the pros and cons of various materials and the precise techniques of restoration.

This is not to decry such interest because a high standard of technical execution is essential for the longevity of restorations. However, technical execution must be seen in the context of the four-point sequence listed above. Without a sound diagnosis and treatment plan, even the best technical execution will be doomed to failure.

A major influence on the formulation of the treatment plan is *the patient*. It is usually by their own volition that patients seek restorative advice and treatment, and they usually bring with them certain problems and limitations that influence treatment planning and the delivery of care.

Each patient also attends with strong preconceptions based on their previous experience of dentistry. These could be good or bad, with a single traumatic episode being able to reverse many years of co-operation. The patient will have some idea of what dentistry could or might do for them, and what they want from their dentist. Some of the patient's concepts could well be limited or unambitious, and education has a

major role to play here. Conversely, sometimes these concepts could be overambitious (complex bridgework for instance), and here re-education is often necessary to bring the patient down to the practical and feasible.

It might be that the dentist has the skills and technical facilities to perform advanced procedures, but before putting bur to tooth, the dentist must stop and ask whether this is really what *this* patient needs and wants. If the answer is no, then to proceed is an act of pure selfishness that might also be regarded as negligent!

Certainly the dentist may have certain treatment goals for all patients – no pain or caries, healthy periodontium, complete occlusion – but the way in which the dentist prescribes and delivers care has to be tempered by the patient's aspirations for their own mouth and their readiness to accept care. A prolonged treatment plan could be very inconvenient to a shift worker or to a mother with young children or to those with no personal transport. It might create restorations that would be beyond the maintenance capacity of the lazy or disinterested, or those with inadequate washing facilities. Perhaps the patient is a reluctant attender, extremely apprehensive of dental care and its possible discomforts, and would require some form of therapeutic help just to get the simple things done. The short, unambitious treatment plan is more likely to succeed here, and if the patient's confidence can be obtained, the more complex treatment could be provided later.

Advanced restorations require skill and facilities, and these have to be paid for, either by the state or by the patient. Both have limited resources and both deserve value for money. Committing resources to an ambitious treatment plan should involve judgement on the likely lifespan of the restorations in that particular mouth and its conditions, and whether the expense is justifiable – *cost benefit analysis*.

The intraoral conditions bring as much influence to bear. The caries rate, number of missing teeth, periodontal condition, presence of dentures and quality of previous restorative work all act as limitations to the scope of the treatment plan. All of us like to provide our best work for those who will appreciate it and look after it. Disinterest on the dentist's part is created by the appearance of large plaque deposits and evidence of little care.

The other side of the equation is what may be available and this relates to the dentist's skills and training, the materials and techniques at their disposal, and the facilities available for providing care (see *Fig. 1.1*). These, in turn, could well modify or even dictate the patient's aspirations – a clean, well equipped and efficient practice would indicate a good level of care to the average patient, whilst the reverse could well lower patient expectations.

The dentist should offer only what is realistically available and work within his or her own limitations. It is certainly no disgrace to say that certain options are beyond your capabilities and it is possible to consider referral to an appropriate specialist. It could also be that the options the patient has aspirations towards are those with a lower success rate, and it is sensible to tell the patient this frankly.

There is considerably more awareness of the cosmetic possibilities of modern dentistry and thus demand for new materials and techniques. Many of these are expensive and have not been fully evaluated over a sufficient period for total confidence in their durability. The patient deserves a proper explanation about the reservations regarding particular lines of treatment.

The provision of restorative treatment is a complex arrangement wherein the patient, the dentist, the technical support and the materials must be in harmony to produce a satisfactory result. The limitations of one element will inevitably change the effects of the others. It is important to remember that the treatment is only as good as its weakest link – don't let that be you!

The key to success throughout is communication – listen and learn from what the patient says, explain what can be done, and then decide jointly on what should be done. If you are not sure, do not commit yourself, but delay the decision and take advice from your colleagues or even your local consultant.

This book begins by talking about how to find out what's wrong with the patient and what does he or she want done about it, coupled with the limitations the patient brings to formulating a treatment plan, and then to executing it.

2

History and examination

It is very important to listen to what the patient has to say about his or her problems.

This aspect of care can be neglected in an obsession to 'get inside the mouth'.

The history is the basis for diagnosis and treatment planning – there is the potential of harm to the patient if it is neglected.

The history should provide a clear account of the patient's experience of health care prior to the current attendance. It should establish an organized body of knowledge about the patient's dental past and fitness to receive future treatment – it forms part of the rationale for his or her management.

The history, though, is very subjective and prone to differences in the perceptions and aspirations of the patient and the dentist. These differences may be reduced or exaggerated by the level of communication between the two, and the dentist must bear this problem in mind.

Clearly, it is the dentist's responsibility to create the right atmosphere for the patient to tell his or her story. The patient must be sitting comfortably in quiet surroundings and be confident in the dentist's sympathetic attention. The patient should be sitting upright, not supine and vulnerable, and facing the questioner with eyes at the same level. This avoids the 'operating' position, with its overtones of discomfort and interrogation.

The most limiting aspect of the history is that to a certain extent it is not strictly factual; it is the patient's perception of events or circumstances. Even items of medical history can be incorrectly remembered and misunderstood, and in difficult cases the patient's medical practitioner must be contacted for information. The dental aspects are often muddled, particularly in the identification of a troublesome tooth amongst thirty or so others.

The dentist has to sift this information and organize it, give it the weight it deserves, and then record it and draw conclusions from it. Inconsistencies in the story have to be picked up and a systematic approach used so as not to miss anything. However, the dentist must beware of the too precise patient with an obsessively detailed history, which can be just as misleading or unhelpful as that provided by the vague patient.

The history should be taken slowly, with pauses for writing in the notes; this helps the patient relax and lets further information come to mind.

Evaluation of dental pain

Of all the aspects of history taking, this is the one where a systematic approach is essential. The patient in pain can often be rambling and disjointed. The dentist must have a clear plan in mind and must bring the patient back to it by firm questioning.

The following questions are important:

- Where is the pain? (e.g. tooth, gum, face, ear)
- Does it change position, i.e. radiate elsewhere?
- Describe the pain (e.g. throbbing, sharp, dull)
- How long has the pain been there?
- How strong is it?
- How long does it last?
- What brings it on?
- What takes it away?
- Does it come at any particular time day or night?
- How often does it occur?
- Is it getting worse or getting better?
- Are there any associated symptoms? (e.g. swelling, bad taste)

It can be useful to have the patient scale the intensity of the pain from 1 to 10 and give some

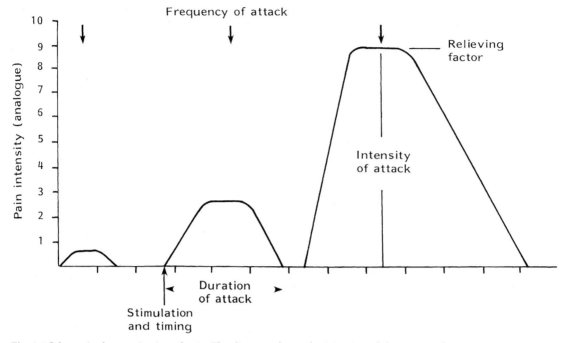

Fig. 2.1 Schematic characterization of pain. The diagram shows the initiation of the pain, its frequency, intensity, duration and the effect of any relieving factors

pictorial representation of the intensity, duration and frequency of each attack (*Fig. 2.1*).

Do not lead the patient; questions should be phrased so that a positive reply, rather than a plain 'yes' or 'no', is required.

Description of the pain will lead to certain provisional diagnoses and also allow exclusion of others.

Pulpal disorders

The correlation of symptoms with actual pulp state is very poor; it is possible for several grades of pathology to be present within the same pulp. For instance, a single pulp could have an area of necrosis, an area of chronic pulpitis and an area of acute pulpitis (Chapter 6), but in any given case it would almost certainly be the acute pulpitis that provoked the painful symptoms.

So, bearing in mind the pitfalls of the precise diagnosis, the following generalizations about symptoms can be made.

Physiological response

The pulp responds to extremes of temperature through a sound crown, but the pain is transient and stops as soon as the stimulus is removed.

When dentine is exposed by caries, trauma or simply gingival recession, then saliva and acid or alkali ions will reach the odontoblastic processes. The disturbance of the neutral pH causes symptoms, usually of a transient and mild nature.

Temperature changes may stimulate pain, either when larger areas of cervical dentine are exposed, or when caries has spread well into the tooth. However, the pain stops when the stimulus is removed, though in dentine hypersensitivity the pain can be quite unpleasant.

Once toxins or bacteria reach the pulp, the symptoms become more severe.

Acute pulpitis

The symptoms are classically an intense throbbing pain, initiated by heat, sometimes relieved by cold, well localized to one tooth, though sometimes radiating to the ear from the lower molar region. The patient is kept awake at night, and standard analgesics are not very effective. It is usually episodic, with increasing frequency and intensity of each episode, until it becomes continuous. It stops when the pulp dies or is removed.

Chronic pulpitis/slow dying (moribund) pulp

This condition often produces no symptoms, but may give rise to vague, dull and diffuse pain along a quadrant, i.e. it is poorly localized. Examination often reveals several teeth with deep restorations, any one of which could be the cause.

Apical infection

Chronic apical infection is usually symptomless – hence the need for continued radiographic review of root-treated teeth. Acute apical periodontitis usually creates an intense throbbing pain, not affected by temperature, fairly continuous, worse at night and initiated or made worse by biting or knocking the tooth. It is usually well localized, and percussing the teeth for diagnostic purposes is unnecessary (and cruel!). Routine analgesics are not very successful and the pain goes immediately when the pressure within the bone is relieved, usually when the infection has caused perforation of the cortical plate followed by a soft tissue abscess, or sinus formation. If pressure builds again in the soft tissues, then a throbbing pain is again likely, but not as intense as that produced by the rigidly confined infection.

In the latter case, swelling is an accompanying complaint.

Periodontal disease

General acute conditions give rise to generalized soreness of the mouth with perhaps 'bleeding gums', a 'bad taste' and 'painful eating' as accompanying symptoms.

Local conditions, such as pericoronitis or a lateral periodontal abscess, cause more localized pain and soreness, particularly on eating.

Chronic periodontal disease is usually painless, but symptoms of bleeding or a bad taste are good indicators. Mild acute exacerbations sometimes occur as a result of occlusal trauma, and these cause vague diffuse pain, similar to the moribund pulp.

Temporomandibular dysfunction and other facial pain

This is discussed in more detail in Chapter 26, but the clinician must be careful not to place difficult diagnostic pain problems into this category for want of any better ideas! Remember that the *most common cause of pain* around the jaws arises from pathology of the pulp and the periodontal ligament (*odontogenic pain*) and these must be investigated first.

Derangements and inflammation of the temporomandibular joint can lead to pain that is localized to the joint area, sometimes felt within the external auditory meatus, and often accompanied by clicking or crepitus in the joint.

The more common symptoms arise from the muscles of mastication and give rise to facial pain and headaches. The pain is usually in the area of the affected muscles, though occasionally retro-orbital pain is described. The character of the pain is typical of all acute muscular problems – soreness, tenderness, difficulty with movement – and sometimes a clear starting point is remembered, such as a wide yawn, removal of wisdom teeth, etc.

Pain described outside the muscle areas may not be from temporomandibular dysfunction; for instance the maxillary antrum sometimes produces overlapping anterior pain.

The most classic pain picture is that of *trigeminal neuralgia*, with its trigger zone and paroxysms of intense pain. However, this character can be modified into *atypical facial pain* that may be trigeminal in origin, psychotic or due to central nervous system lesions. Pain that crosses the midline is often psychotic in origin.

However, in all these cases, the purely dental causes must be eliminated first.

Diagnosis of pain – Summary

Obtain a full description of the pain; this will undoubtedly lead to an incomplete provisional diagnosis. However, an open mind is important until after the clinical examination, so beware of early categorization of pain.

Caries tends to affect several teeth in the same mouth, and so these teeth could exhibit different stages of the pathology. Symptoms of each could co-exist in the same quadrant, and confuse the pain picture completely. Here, each facet of the symptoms needs to be dissected out, and analysed separately.

Medical history

Information about the patient's general health is essential for the planning of his or her dental care. Some medical conditions will influence the component items of a treatment plan or change its whole direction, whilst others will influence the way in which 'normally' planned care is delivered; this is discussed in detail in Chapter 4.

Past and present disease experience should be questioned together with information about current drug therapy. A structured series of questions is the most reliable way of taking a medical history (*Table 2.1*), but the questioner must be careful not to miss anything because the patient misunderstands or mishears the questions. The series of questions needs to be expanded if particular problems are evident from the history. For example, if the patient

Table 2.1 Medical history taking

Have you suffered from:
    any serious disease?
    any heart or chest trouble?
    rheumatic fever, chorea, growing pains?
    pneumonia or bronchitis?
    jaundice, hepatitis?

Do you have
    bleeding disorders?
    diabetes?
    epilepsy?

Have you ever had a blood transfusion?
Have you ever given blood, or been turned down as a donor?
Are you allergic to any drugs or antibiotics?
Have you ever taken penicillin, and were you all right afterwards?
Have you ever been in hospital or had any operations?
Are you taking any tablets or medicines at the moment? (beware anticoagulants, steroids, drug abusers)
Have you been ill recently or consulted your doctor?

complains of soreness or ulceration of the mouth, then questioning on possible causative or modifying factors must be explored. If there is any doubt about the patient's general health it will be necessary to contact their general medical practitioner for information, particularly to ascertain whether the patient is suitable for the delivery of dental care without problems.

Previous experience of dentistry

The patient's previous experience will condition him or her to expect certain things of dentistry in general; these could be good or bad. The patient's attitude in turn is conveyed to the dentist, who may respond by tailoring the treatment plan according to perceptions of that attitude.

The patient may have high aspirations based upon previous experience, or vice versa. The dentist will judge the extent of the previous experience and may be influenced to continue the same basic pattern.

The important aspects to question are:

● Range of treatment experience
● Method of delivery of care, e.g. sedation
● Experience of analgesia/anaesthesia
● Prostheses: age, comfort, function
● General satisfaction with previous care
● Any particular problems

The answers will indicate any special needs, such as non-adrenaline containing local analgesic, use of sedation and so on.

The patient's opinion of his or her dentures will help the decision about possible replacement or relining (Chapter 24).

A patient dissatisfied with previous care could continue to be dissatisfied, even if the new dentist provides the best care possible. Unfortunately, dentistry and plastic surgery attract perfection seekers!

Family and social history

The general home and work environment may dictate how easy or difficult it is to carry out oral hygiene procedures or maintain a non-cariogenic diet. The home might also contain entrenched attitudes to dental care.

Work patterns – shift work, absences from home – or young children may reduce the ability to attend for prolonged courses of treatment.

Anxiety and emotional problems can be initiators of stress-related facial pain and muscle disorders (Chapter 26).

History taking   Summary

The efficiency of history taking is related to the confidence of the patient in the listening powers of his or her dentist, and the ability of both to communicate with each other.

History taking should not be a rigid system of checklists, though there must be a consistent basis for the dentist's questions. The programme of questioning must be flexible and adapted towards the individual patient – it is *the patient's* story.

Clinical examination

The clinical examination must establish the status of the oral tissues as a basis for diagnosis and treatment. It is important to observe and record health as well as disease, and to be as accurate as possible when doing it. These observations must be part of a continuing exercise that should be performed briefly at every visit, particularly over long courses of treatment – nothing remains static!

Comprehensive, sequential, up-to-date and easily read records are necessary to assess the progress of conditions, particularly when a preventive approach is being used, e.g. application of fluoride to early enamel caries. A brief scan of the records should re-inform the dentist of the patient's background at each visit. Many minutes spent thumbing back over old entries is wasteful, so updated summary sheets are essential. Reviewing the summary sheets provides the background for each visit and the decisions to be made as problems occur.

Extraoral examination not only gives clues about the patient's attitude to treatment, motivation or underlying medical condition, but may also indicate clinical/technical difficulties such as loss of vertical dimension or mandibular deviations. These problems may be identified during history taking by the observant clinician.

Palpation of the mandibular borders, temporomandibular joints and possible sites of lymph node involvement may reveal early pathology.

Intraoral examination should commence with the area of the main complaint, if the patient has one. This must be given priority over the completion of the full examination so that stabilization, particularly of pain, is achieved without delay (Chapter 3). Certainly if there is pain, which could have been prevented if time had been taken for a full examination first, then some form of stabilization will be necessary immediately (Chapter 3).

The examination of the teeth for caries and restoration defects should be done after a thorough *prophylaxis* to remove stains and debris which would otherwise obscure observation. A dry field and a good light are traditionally necessary, but a probe should be used with caution only.

The probe should not be used to test a 'sticky fissure' as the application of pressure will simply break it down further. Occlusal caries should be diagnosed principally by appearance – darkness

underlying the cuspal slopes – aided in the deeper lesions by radiography (see later). Additionally, transillumination is useful for unrestored teeth, and this technique can also reveal cracks in the enamel.

The margins of existing restorations are difficult to examine, particularly approximally, without using a probe, because such areas cannot be seen clearly and may be obscured by the restoration on radiographs. The probe must be used gently, though, to avoid creating a defect that did not exist previously (*Fig. 2.2*).

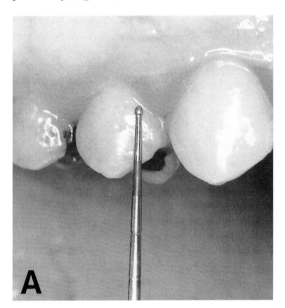

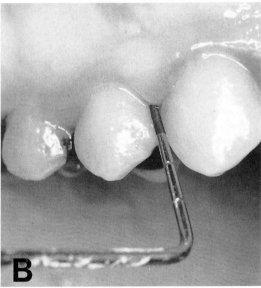

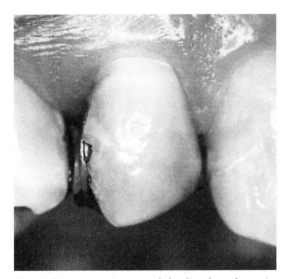

Fig. 2.2 Recurrent caries around the disto-buccal margin of the amalgam restoration in 5⌋. This is shown by the fracture of the enamel margin and the white zone around the bucco-cervical corner

Fig. 2.3 Community Periodontal Index of Treatment Needs (CPITN) probe in use. **A** Profile of the probe. **B** Probe inserted into a gingival crevice

The recording of caries and restorations is based on the use of the *dental chart*, which can easily become a static record. It is valuable as a record of the teeth and the planned restorations at the beginning of treatment, but as work proceeds it becomes out of date. Periodic re-charting should be done so that there is not just a chart of the teeth some years ago, when the patient joined the practice, with line upon line of restored holes at each course of treatment, but a single current chart.

Examination of the *periodontium* requires observation of gingival shape, size, texture and colour, and also crevice depth. Several indices have been developed for the assessment of the periodontium including measurement of plaque accumulation, gingival health, pocket depth, bleeding and treatment requirements.

A useful screening examination is the Community Periodontal Index of Treatment Needs (CPITN); this is also known as the Basic Periodontal Examination (BPE). The periodontium is examined with a World Health Organization CPITN probe to determine pocket depth, bleeding response and to detect calculus. The probe is light with a ball tip of 0.5 mm diameter that is designed to detect sub-gingival calculus without penetrating the floor of the pocket (*Fig. 2.3*).

The mouth is divided into sextants, the gingival crevice of each tooth is examined in at least four sites, and the worst clinical finding in that sextant is recorded as the code for that sextant. If the probing depth is more than 3 mm and the probing is accompanied by bleeding, this indicates *periodontitis*. The findings and clinical implications are shown in *Table 2.2*. Whilst this is a useful and easy system, it is limited in terms of overall treatment planning. It certainly records signs of existing pathology but the treatment plan can be completed only when the diagnosis is qualified by considera-

tion of modifying factors; this is discussed in detail in Chapter 13.

An *oral hygiene index* is also a useful way of monitoring the patient's cleaning efficiency, for use in both the surgery and the home. A simple scoring of the amount of plaque, following disclosing, on selected tooth surfaces is done and recorded in the notes. There are several oral hygiene or debris indices, but the simplest is that of Greene and Vermillion, that uses six teeth: an upper and lower molar on opposite sides, an upper and lower premolar on opposite sides and an upper and lower incisor on opposite sides. Both lingual and buccal surfaces are scored by:

0 = No plaque present
1 = Plaque present on cervical third
2 = Plaque present on both cervical third and middle third
3 = Plaque present on whole surface

The index is the total scored divided by the number of surfaces examined.

Precise examination and charting of the teeth and periodontium should be accompanied by the examination of the *oral mucosa* and *oro-pharynx*.

Examination of the *occlusion* is discussed in detail in Chapter 14 but, briefly, arch form, missing teeth and their effects, restoration of the occlusion by dentures, crowns and bridges should be assessed. Centric occlusion, centric relation and lateral and protrusive movements should be observed and noted and, where appropriate, a diagnostic articulated mounting should be used.

Special investigations

Pulp vitality testing

An indication of the condition of the pulp is of great diagnostic value, but the methods available fall very far short of the absolute. Most methods rely on nerve stimulation by electricity, thermal change or mechanical interference, but really the vitality of a pulp depends on its blood supply, which cannot be tested easily.

Complications also arise because of the varying state of the tissues in a single diseased pulp. Multi-rooted teeth can have one root containing vital pulp, and the other containing necrotic debris – a *false positive* could be recorded. Pus or inflammatory exudate in the root canal can conduct electricity and this is another reason for a false positive result.

False negative results can occur because the pulp is insulated by much secondary dentine, or where the enamel is unable to transmit the stimulus

Table 2.2 Community Periodontal Index of Treatment Needs (CPITN) analysis

Clinical finding	Code	Treatment indicated
No disease	0	No treatment
Gingival bleeding after probing	1	Oral hygiene
Supra- or sub-gingival calculus	2	Scaling and OHI
Pockets 4 or 5 mm deep	3	Scaling and OHI
Pockets 6 mm and deeper	4	Scaling, OHI and more complex treatment
No teeth in sextants	—	

OHI, oral hygiene instruction

because of its thickness or its proximity to large restorations.

Teeth restored with insulating materials, such as ceramics or polymers, are also difficult to test.

Electric pulp testing passes a low current at high potential through the tooth. The current must have a square wave form because it must pass through enamel and dentine, which are relatively poor conductors, and reach the other side at sufficient potential to stimulate the nerves of the pulp.

Unfortunately, numbers are ascribed to the patient's response, and this gives the test more apparent scientific validity than it actually possesses. It really is subjective with a 'yes' or a 'no' as the response. The patient's expectation of the test influences the result, particularly if the sensation from the first, control tooth is very painful. A preemptive response is very likely in the subsequent tests.

Because false positive and false negative results are possible with electric pulp testing it should be complemented with *thermal tests* to increase the information available. Ice sticks, or ice crystals made by evaporating ethyl chloride, can be used but the amount of ice applied must be substantial to create sufficient temperature differential to affect the pulp. Because the tooth crown is a good heat sink, a small pledget of cotton wool with ice crystals may have no effect.

Hot gutta percha or impression compound should be applied to a lubricated tooth surface to contrast with the cold results. Interestingly, the effect of heat is often less than that of cold since the temperature difference is larger when dropping from 37°C to 0°C, compared to the rise from 37°C to about 65°C.

The most reliable pulp test is the *test cavity*, and this can be done quite simply by starting a cavity in the tooth under test without local analgesia, having explained the purpose of this to the patient; the dentist stops as soon as there is a response.

Non-operative pulp tests must be interpreted with caution, but they produce one more piece of the diagnostic jigsaw to be placed alongside the clinical examination and the radiographic findings.

Blood tests

The oral tissues may be the first to reflect systemic disease and a full cell count and haemoglobin estimation may be indicated in cases of abnormal gingival inflammation to exclude blood dyscrasias such as leukaemia or anaemia.

Patients on anticoagulant therapy may require an International Normalised Ratio (INR) estimation prior to dental treatment that carries a risk of bleeding. Procedures such as scaling and polishing, root planing, inferior dental blocks and obviously extractions carry the most risk and the INR level needs to be less than 2.5 for these. Changes to anticoagulant therapy should be done in consultation with the responsible physician. This, of course, requires support from the local hospital, and if this is not forthcoming, the treatment plan has to be modified accordingly.

Radiography

Radiographs are essential for proper diagnosis and treatment planning in restorative dentistry.

Three views are important, the orthopantomogram (OPT/OPG), the bitewing and the periapical. The information they provide is:

OPT

- General but *imprecise* scan of the teeth and jaws
- Buried teeth, roots and cysts
- Apical infection
- Existence of root fillings
- Temporomandibular joint (sometimes)

Bitewing

- Caries: approximal and occlusal
- Depth of restorations
- Restoration integrity
- Interdental bone height
- Pulp chamber morphology

Periapical

- Apical infection
- Integrity of root fillings and posts
- Interdental bone
- Root fractures and perforations
- Resorption
- Root canal morphology

The OPT has some value as a routine scan for every *new* patient, particularly those who have had considerable dentistry; patients often cannot say what type of treatment has been performed. However, the value of a repeat OPT at any time must be questioned. As will be discussed below there are radiographs that give a better definition with lower exposure of the patient to ionizing radiation. If the posterior region of the body of the mandible needs to be seen, then a lateral oblique film will provide a better image.

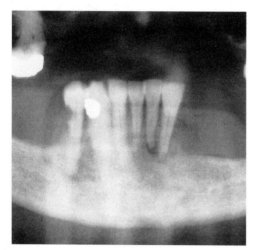

Fig. 2.4 Part of an orthopantomogram (OPT) showing an apparent apical radiolucency on ⌐1. Root canal therapy was started on the basis of this film

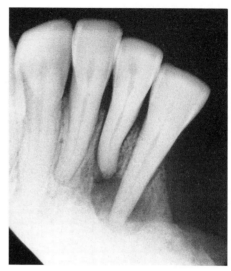

Fig. 2.5 Apical film of the suspicious area in *Figure 2.4*. The radiolucency is centred on the ⌐2, not arising from the apex, and turned out to be a lateral periodontal cyst

Only structures in the OPT *focal corridor* will be in focus and there may not be sufficient definition for the diagnosis of caries or for the accurate estimation of interdental bone height. In some areas, there may be masking of the root apices by overlapping structures, and occasionally apparent apical radiolucencies may be seen that are just artefacts. Overlap of the vertebral column in the midline is a particular problem.

In addition, because of variable image densities and the angulation of the beam in certain areas, dramatic misdiagnoses are possible. *Figure 2.4* shows part of an OPT that shows a very precise radiolucency, apparently associated with the lower left central incisor. Based on this film only, and without a vitality test, root canal therapy was started. The tooth was painful! An apical film was then ordered (*Fig. 2.5*), and suggests that the radiolucency is more associated with the lateral incisor than the central. The lateral incisor was vital to pulp testing.

The radiolucency is not 'right' for an apical area – it is round, not merging smoothly with periodontal space and is higher than it should be. A surgical exploration was undertaken and the radiolucency turned out to be a lateral periodontal cyst.

Clearly, then, bitewing and periapical films are required to investigate OPT observations and to show precise detail.

It must be remembered that the radiograph is a two-dimensional picture of a three-dimensional entity and is dependent on mineral densities for its image. The depth of a carious lesion can be

underestimated by as much as a third on a bitewing, and pulp horns can appear superimposed on the caries, whereas they are actually in a different plane.

Root concavities, particularly in the approximal cervical areas, may be shown as apparent areas of demineralization – 'burn out' (*Fig. 2.6*).

Angulation is critical for both films when assessing restoration integrity. Unless the X-ray beam is

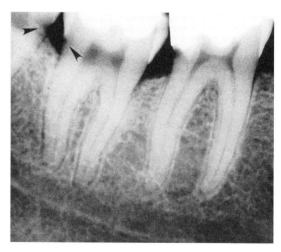

Fig. 2.6 Periapical radiograph of ⌐76 showing cervical radiolucencies (arrowed) mesially on 8⌐ and distally on 7⌐ that are artefacts caused by the curvature of the teeth. Contrast these with the more clearly defined recurrent caries under the distal margin of 6⌐

precisely aligned along a cervical margin, the restoration will obscure the margin and appear sound (*Fig. 2.7*). The periapical film taken using the long cone technique provides an image with minimal distortion, which is not the case if the bisecting angle technique is used. Bitewing films provide good definition of the crowns of the posterior teeth.

All radiographic findings should be confirmed wherever possible by repeating the clinical exam-ination with the films alongside. Thus cervical overhangs or apparent approximal caries should be confirmed by gentle probing.

Summary sheets for radiographs taken and their findings should be an integral part of the notes, allowing easy reference and review.

Of course, it almost goes without saying that the quality of radiographs – both in the taking and the processing – has to be of the highest order for accurate conclusions to be made.

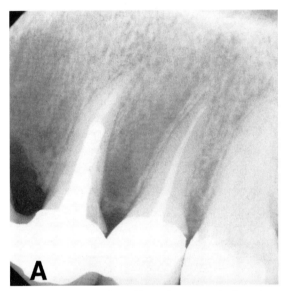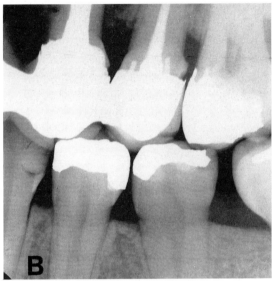

Fig. 2.7 A Periapical film of ⌊45 taken using the bisecting angle technique showing a bridge retainer with apparently good adaptation at the distal margin. **B** Bitewing film with its different angulation reveals a deficiency of the distal margin. A similar revealing film would be achieved using the long cone technique

---

History and examination – Summary

The meticulous collection and collation of all the information provided by the history, clinical examination, special tests and radiographs should provide the basis for the diagnosis and the treatment plan, and the continuing care of the patient. There can never be enough information, but be careful about guessing or taking things for granted. With clinical experience this might be acceptable, but for precision the information must be accumulated carefully and as fully as possible.

3

Diagnosis and stabilization

The diagnosis is the key to proper treatment planning and therefore of primary importance in the care of patients. In many simple conditions it is too easy to jump from examining the mouth to items of operative treatment. This avoids the discipline of:

● Diagnosis first
● Treatment plan second

Without this discipline, the management of the complex case becomes impossible. Decide what's wrong first *before* you decide what to do about it!

The diagnosis is the summation and conclusions drawn from the assembly of all the separate pieces of information gathered from the patient's story, clinical observations, special tests and radiography (*Fig. 3.1*). It is an intellectual jigsaw puzzle that is completed as a list of pathological conditions and simple restorative disorders. Each piece of the jigsaw must be placed in its correct position to make the diagnosis (*Fig. 3.2*). However, In distinction from the conventional jigsaw puzzle there is no picture for guidance and the incorrect interpretation of one or more pieces can create the wrong picture! (*Fig. 3.3*).

The *aetiology* of each condition should also be established so that this can be eliminated, if appropriate, to prevent recurrence of the problem.

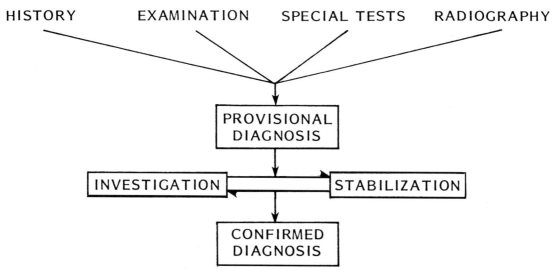

Fig. 3.1 The route to a confirmed diagnosis

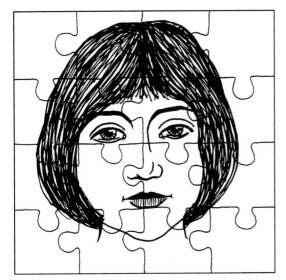

Fig. 3.2 The diagnostic jigsaw correctly completed

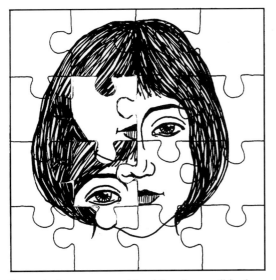

Fig.3.3 An incorrect assembly of the pieces will lead misidentification of the diagnosis

In some cases, it will be necessary to carry out some operative investigation, either to confirm a *provisional diagnosis*, or to determine the actual diagnosis. For example, a deep carious lesion will usually need to be opened and investigated to reveal its extent, and to detect the presence of a pulpal exposure. Planning the restoration of such a tooth before investigation would be premature.

Stabilization is a series of procedures designed to control actively progressing pathology rapidly, to achieve:

- Pain relief
- Arrest of tissue destruction
- Final diagnosis
- The basis to plan the definitive management

The operative phase is instituted immediately, sometimes before the history and examination has been completed, so that no time is wasted in relieving symptoms. The treatment should be planned to be completed as quickly as possible and the procedures will be short and sharp, e.g. pulp extirpation, extraction.

Diagnosis

Caries

Some conditions are obvious; cavitation of the enamel coupled with a brown base and whitened edges usually means caries. Indeed, the jump from what is seen to the diagnosis is so rapid that intermediate listing of physical signs is somewhat superfluous.

However, the aetiological factors may not be obvious. Is this one of many sites of primary caries, or an isolated recurrent carious lesion around a failing restoration? Is this the middle-aged onset of cervical caries with its problems of rapid spread, or just fissure caries that in some population groups would hardly qualify for a raised eyebrow?

So the *caries rate* is important, and the Decayed, Missing and Filled (DMF) score helps reflect this. But also the number of *active lesions* must be considered as an indication of the severity of the current pathology. *Diet analysis* would be appropriate for many patients with a high active caries rate, in order to determine the aetiology.

If it is an isolated recurrent lesion, this could be the result of operator error, and, if so, this must not be repeated on replacement of the restoration. Was it incorrectly sited margins, poorly finished enamel or the abuse of a matrix band? How deep has the caries spread around the restoration? Does the radiograph help, or is the lesion masked by the radio-opacity of the amalgam? Only removal of the restoration and the caries will answer this.

Restorations

The faults that can be diagnosed with long-standing restorations are numerous. There could be corrosion, ditching and fracture of amalgam, or discoloration, marginal staining and surface loss of

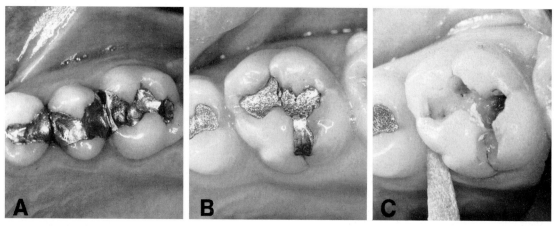

Fig. 3.4 A Ditched and corroded amalgams, but still satisfactory restorations. **B** A ditched and corroded occluso-palatal amalgam, but with a central fracture in it. This is much more suspicious. **C** Removal of the amalgam revealed deep caries in two sites occlusally, together with a mesial lesion. The bitewing of this tooth (6|) (*Figure 10.10*) was not very helpful

composite resin. There could be the technical faults of cervical overhangs, negative edges, incorrect occlusion, poor shade matching and perforations.

Having identified the fault, however, there is one very important question to be answered – has the fault induced any pathology? The reason for the question is that some faults are just minor technical errors or normal material behaviour, and to replace restorations purely for these reasons would be wrong.

Where pathology is associated with the fault, then clearly something must be done. *Figure 3.4A* shows ditched and corroded amalgams, that are technically less than pleasing, but in the absence of a positive diagnosis of associated pathology they should not be replaced. Contrast them with that in *Figures 3.4B* and *C*, with its suspicious fracture line and underlying caries.

Pulpal disorders

The history, pulp tests and radiography (Chapter 2) would have given some information about the possible state of the pulp. A deep carious lesion with no response to hot and cold and electric pulp testing, together with apical radiolucency on radiograph, would lead to a certain diagnosis of *pulp necrosis* and *apical periodontitis*.

However, what about the painless deep lesion with an ambivalent pulp testing response and normal apical anatomy on radiograph? Here it would be appropriate to make a provisional diagnosis of *chronic pulpitis* to be confirmed or refuted by operative investigation.

Episodes of intense pain localized to one tooth, with the pain lasting after the initiating stimulus has been removed, with normal apical radiographic appearance would suggest *acute pulpitis*.

Apical conditions

The diagnosis usually relies on the radiographic appearance of a radiolucent area at the root apex. For differential diagnostic purposes, a negative response to pulp testing is necessary to eliminate neoplasia such as cementoma, overlying fissural cysts, or simply an anatomical structure such as a foramen. If the tooth in question is already root filled, the diagnosis can be more difficult. Here, any symptoms and the history of the tooth would be important. Where the tooth is symptomless, an apical area may not be pathological, and serial radiographs are necessary to differentiate between a healing lesion and progressing pathology (*Fig. 3.5*). A static area may indicate healing by fibrous tissue without calcification that is not infected.

If the history is not clear then the dentist is left with his skill in radiographic interpretation to fall back upon. *Figure 3.6A* shows a central incisor that was apicected 18 months previously. The referring dentist thought that this was a recurrence of infection but there were no symptoms. The periodontal space should be traced around the tooth. Does the radiolucency have its origins there? Does it blend with the space? Can the periodontal space be seen 'through' the radiolucency, i.e. is there superimposition? The circular shape of the

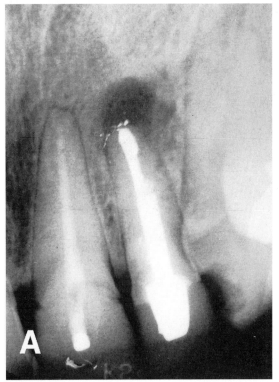
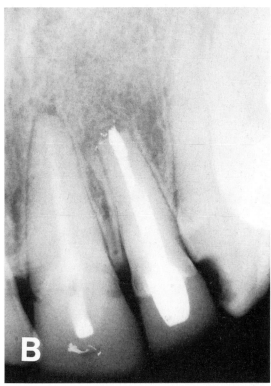

Fig. 3.5 A Periapical radiograph of |2 immediately after apicectomy and retrograde root filling. **B** Complete apical in-fill. This took 2 years and the decreasing area shown on films taken in the meantime had to be distinguished from apical pathology

radiolucency should raise suspicion that it is a foramen. The second film (*Fig. 3.6B*) confirms that it is the incisive canal.

If there are symptoms, and pain on percussion, then *acute apical periodontitis* is the diagnosis. A 'silent' apical area coupled with a negative pulp test indicates *chronic apical periodontitis*, an *apical granuloma*, or an *apical cyst*. The differential diagnosis between a granuloma and a cyst relies essentially on biopsy, as clinical and radiographic features do not distinguish them from each other.

Periodontal disease

The complaint of 'bleeding gums', the signs of reddened gingival margins with slight enlargement, and bleeding on probing with no pocket formation leads to the conclusion of the almost ubiquitous *chronic marginal gingivitis*.

But the severity of this, together with the amount of plaque and debris present, must accompany the diagnosis. Is there *hyperplasia* present as well, or just enlargement due to inflammatory oedema? Is the aetiology just *poor oral hygiene*, or are there other local factors such as faulty restoration margins that prevent the patient cleaning efficiently? Could there be systemic disorders such as blood dyscrasias present that modify the tissue response to the plaque?

Where soreness and even pain accompany the redness and bleeding, then an *acute gingivitis* may be present.

A plaque index is essential to accompany the diagnosis. Simple disclosing and the scoring of the extent of plaque coverage as described in Chapter 2 provides a good baseline against which to judge improvements.

The presence of a pathologically deepened gingival crevice, a *pocket*, accompanied by bleeding on probing, indicates *chronic marginal periodontitis*. Radiographs, particularly bitewings, may reveal vertical or horizontal bone loss caused by the inflammation. Vertical bone loss leads to the diagnosis of an *infra-bony pocket* (*Fig. 3.7*).

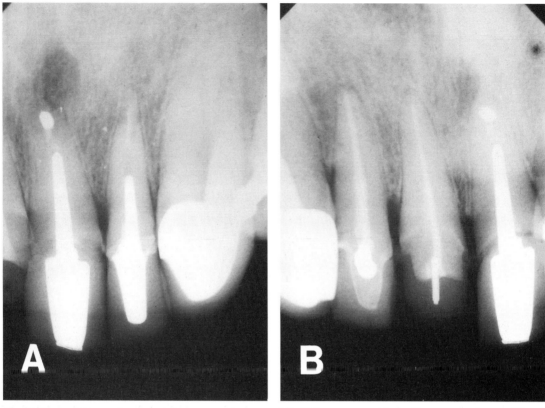

Fig. 3.6 The incisive canal masquerading as an apical area. **A** Radiolucency associated with a retrograde root filling. **B** Second film at a different angulation reveals the true nature of the radiolucency

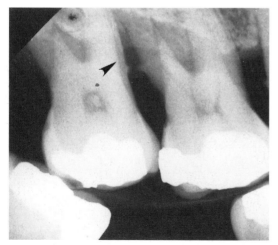

Fig. 3.7 Radiograph showing an infra-bony pocket (arrowed) at 7⌐

Occlusal disorders

Impacted and malpositioned teeth are obvious diagnoses here. But also, the signs of occlusal derangement following tooth loss should be diagnosed. These are tilting, drifting and over-eruption of adjacent teeth into the space that, in turn, may bring pathology such as caries of approximal root surfaces, and periodontal disease from food impaction and plaque accumulation (Chapter 18).

The inefficient restoration of the occlusion by dentures or crowns and bridges should be diagnosed, and the effects of occlusal interferences noted (Chapter 8).

Investigation of provisional diagnoses

The need for investigation in relation to the diagnosis of pulpal disorders has already been mentioned, but perhaps the most dramatic area where considerable investigation is necessary is the diagnosis of facial pain. Detailed descriptions of the various conditions is outside the scope of this book, but there is a considerable overlap of the symptoms of caries and pulpitis, and those of sinusitis, temporomandibular dysfunction, trigeminal neuralgia and atypical facial pain.

It is so important to remember that the most common cause of pain around the lower face and jaws is pathology of the teeth and periodontium. The dying or moribund pulp can produce the quite atypical symptoms of diffuse pain, unrelated to any stimulus, and radiating to areas served by the trigeminal nerve of the same side. The pulp will often be covered by a large, radio-opaque restoration, quite impervious to X-rays, and impossible to examine by non-invasive vitality tests. Worse still, because of the nature of caries, several of these restorations may exist together.

It is essential that all these restorations are investigated thoroughly before a committed diagnosis is made. It is very embarrassing to relieve long-standing facial pain by the extraction of a non-vital tooth when the patient has been taking carbamazepine for several months!

After careful clinical examination, pulp tests and radiographs, the next step is to remove individual restorations. Clinical experience will tend to suggest which teeth look suspicious, and which could be innocent.

The restoration removal can be started without local analgesia as a very reliable mechanical pulp test. Explain the purpose of this to the patient, and that an analgesic will be given as soon as any pain is felt. Inspect the pulpal aspects of the cavity carefully, and if no exposure is found and the tooth is vital, place a sedative dressing. If, on the other hand, an exposure is present then several different lines of treatment are possible. These are discussed in Chapter 11.

Stabilisation

Caries

Figure 3.8 illustrates a case of so-called acute caries. There is caries in most teeth, with some extensive loss of dentine. It would be quite wrong to approach the definitive restoration of $\overline{|6}$ first, find a carious exposure, root fill it, and then construct a pinned core and a full veneer crown. Whilst this was being done, the caries in the other teeth would be spreading ever onwards. Stabilization of the caries in the whole mouth is required.

The actual plan must be based on an overall assessment of the patient's expectations and the restorative possibilities. The extent of the caries does not reflect keen dental awareness! However, education is possible if interest is there.

First of all, make an estimate of how many teeth could be restored simply, how many would require root canal therapy and how many would require crowns. Present this estimate and the implications of time and effort to the patient, and await the reaction. A keen, motivated reaction would suggest opening, investigating and dressing all the lesions, stabilizing the pulp as appropriate (see later), and extracting only those that turn out to be absolutely unrestorable.

A disinterested reaction, on the other hand, would lead to extraction of those teeth whose prognosis was not assured after simple restoration, i.e. those with deep lesions.

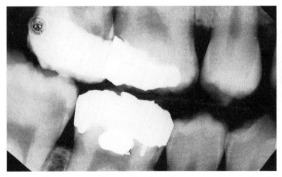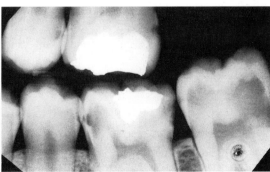

Fig. 3.8 Bitewing radiographs showing extensive caries that requires stabilization before definitive treatment is provided. There is deep primary caries in $\overline{7|67}$, recurrent caries cervically in $\underline{76|}$, and there are early lesions in almost all the other teeth

Acute pulpal and apical conditions

The most rapid and effective way of treating these is to extract the tooth. The pulp is removed, and drainage of an apical abscess is very clearly established by this procedure. However, if conservation of the tooth is indicated and root canal therapy is possible and it is restorable after such therapy, then rather different means must be used.

Acute pulpitis

This should be stabilized by pulp extirpation. However, this may not be straightforward, since local analgesia may be difficult to achieve sometimes. This difficulty may be related to the persistence of the pain stimulus altering the nerve impulse conduction and making blocking by analgesic more difficult.

The first alternative is to repeat the local analgesic injection, but use a different agent. For instance, if ligocaine was given first, repeat with prilocaine. The two agents potentiate each other. If this does not work, apply a topical corticosteroid paste to the exposed dentine. This will reduce inflammation and ease pain, and in 48 hours or so the patient should return for another attempt under local analgesia. Failing all these, the pulp will have to be extirpated under a general anaesthetic.

Ideally, the pulp should be extirpated from the full length of the root canal, so that remnants are not left behind to continue the pain. However, a diagnostic radiograph is necessary to assure this, and the duration of analgesia may not be long enough to allow it.

If only partial extirpation has been achieved, apply a topical corticosteroid as a root canal dressing and complete the extirpation at the preparation stage.

Total extirpation should be followed by root canal dressing with calcium hydroxide in propylene glycol.

Apical periodontitis and apical abscess

This diagnosis presumes pulp necrosis and the presence of infection or leakage of toxins beyond the root apex. The canal must be cleared of debris and drainage established for the apical exudate, whose accumulation causes the pain.

If an abscess has formed, then cutting an endodontic access cavity will be rewarded by pus leaking from the tooth. Pain relief can be instantaneous. If no pus or exudate appears, then a barbed broach should be used, well short of the apex, to clear any obstruction. If drainage is still not achieved, then passage of a fine (No. 8) file through the apical foramen must be considered. This

diameter will establish drainage, but will not create the later difficulties in root filling caused by larger apical perforations.

The use of local analgesic should be cautious in the presence of acute inflammation. Restriction of the blood supply to the area could result in spread of the infection. Also the local analgesic may not be effective.

It is better to use an air turbine as much as possible to reduce vibration, and support the tooth, perhaps with a composition splint at the same time. Use a conventional speed handpiece to break the final half-millimetre or so of dentine overlying the pulp.

If an abscess has pointed in the sulcus, this should be incised. Hot salt water mouthwashes should be used to apply heat to the alveolus and drainage should be maintained by the patient sucking the tooth to keep the access clear.

Systemic antibiotics. These should be restricted to cases where systemic involvement is apparent, i.e. raised temperature, malaise, tender regional lymph nodes or where there is some medical indication. In these circumstances, two high doses of oral amoxycillin are very effective: 3 g immediately and 2 g, 24 hours later. Systemic antibiotics should be avoided wherever possible for local 'mechanical' problems where the bacteria are within a root canal and sheltered from the blood and phagocytosis.

Review. Open drainage through the root canal should be restricted to 24–48 hours. After this, more will go up the canal than will come down. To complete the stabilization, the canal must be fully prepared (Chapter 12). The reason for this is that the walls of the root canal will be infected (in contra-distinction to the acute pulpitis case) and simply irrigating and sealing the canal will not remove the infection.

Traumatic injuries to the teeth

The immediate objective is the relief of pain and the procedure required will depend upon the site of any fracture and the state of the pulp. The pulp, however, can be concussed by a blow and may not provide a pulp test response for some weeks. Therefore, immediate stabilization must be followed by review for definitive diagnosis and management.

A complete history is essential in case of future litigation regarding the cause of the accident. All teeth in the area of the trauma should be pulp tested and radiographed, and if there are any soft tissue lacerations and missing tooth fragments, these soft tissues should be radiographed also.

Where there is any doubt on the whereabouts of fragments, the possibility of facial fractures or any general injury the patient should be referred to the local casualty department for complete investigation.

The treatment schemes for traumatized teeth are summarized below, but for more detailed consideration the reader is referred to a specialized text.

Enamel only fracture

Small fracture areas can be simply smoothed, whilst larger defects that may affect aesthetics or function should be restored with acid etch retained composite resin. The teeth should be reviewed in 4–6 weeks and the pulp tests and radiographs repeated. Negative pulp tests may indicate that root canal therapy is necessary.

Enamel/dentine fracture

Superficial. The tooth should be dressed with zinc oxide–eugenol cement in a temporary crown to aid pulp recovery. The crown must allow access to enamel for later pulp testing. If vital at review, then an acid etch retained composite resin restoration should be placed. Non-vitality would probably indicate root canal therapy.

Deep. This should be treated as if there were a pulp exposure.

Enamel/dentine/pulp fractures and deep enamel/dentine fractures

With these the pulp is unlikely to recover and the management depends on whether the root apex has closed or is still open.

Root formation complete. Conventional root canal therapy is indicated, plus semi-permanent restoration of the crown, usually by composite resin. A post crown should be avoided if at all possible, especially for young patients playing contact sports.

Root apex open. Root formation should be encouraged to finish. If the pulp is vital, pulpotomy is used to remove the coronal pulp, leaving radicular pulp to continue root formation.

If the pulp is non-vital, the canal should be carefully filed short of the apex, and filled with calcium hydroxide in propylene glycol. This material creates conditions favourable for root formation.

In both cases, when the apex has closed, the canal should be root filled.

If the apex does not close, then root canal therapy should be done – this is technically difficult (Chapter 12).

Root fractures

Apical third. If symptomless and vital, leave and review. Otherwise, root fill to the fracture line and review. Remove the apical fragment if there is evidence of pathology.

Middle third. If the coronal fragment is mobile, it should be splinted to the adjacent teeth. In the absence of symptoms or pathology, it may be possible to place a post through both fragments to increase stability. If the fragments are not in line, this will not be possible, and the tooth should be root filled to the fracture line, and reviewed. The fragment may need to be removed and it is possible to use a long post extending into the bone as an implant to increase the stability of the crown. The prognosis for the middle third root fracture is poor.

Coronal third. The prognosis depends on the extent to which the fracture goes beyond the epithelial attachment, usually palatally. A very oblique fracture is difficult to restore, and the tooth should be extracted.

A more shallow fracture would indicate root filling and the provision of a cast post and diaphragm to prevent root splitting later. The immediate stabilization is to extirpate the pulp and provide a temporary crown. The easiest way to do the crown is to use the tooth fragment and to acid etch it to the adjacent teeth, over the sealed root access.

Dislocation and avulsion

The dislocated tooth can be repositioned and splinted for about a week. Pulp recovery is unlikely and the root canal treatment should be done whilst the splint is in place.

The avulsed tooth can be replanted, but the success of this depends on the length of time it has been out of the mouth and how it was stored during that time. Milk is probably the best storage medium, though a parent could keep the tooth in his or her own buccal sulcus to be kept moist by saliva.

Before replanting, the tooth should be washed in normal saline, but no other cleaning should be done. Splint the tooth in place and carry out root canal therapy whilst the splint is on. It is unwise to leave the root canal empty.

Calcium hydroxide has been shown to inhibit external resorption, and this can be left in the canal for some time, with periodic replacement. The splint should be removed after a week.

Review

A traumatized tooth will require regular review by radiography, and if vital at the outset, pulp tests. Slow dentine formation can be induced by trauma, leading to the obliteration of the canal and difficult root canal therapy. If this is seen, the tooth should be root filled immediately whilst it is still possible. Late loss of vitality is also possible.

The other main complication of trauma is root resorption, either internal or external. Internal resorption is treated by removal of the pulp and root filling.

External resorption can sometimes be arrested by calcium hydroxide being placed in the canal. Hydroxyl ions diffuse to the outside of the root and raise the pH there. This seems to inhibit cell activity. As a sequel to the resorption, the periodontal ligament is replaced by ankylosis of the tooth to bone, and the tooth can remain firm for many years even though it has little root. If infection supervenes, the tooth will require extraction.

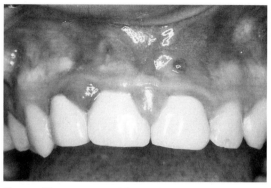

Fig. 3.9 Chronic marginal hyperplastic gingivitis associated with crowns on 21|1. The crowns must be corrected before the gingivae will resolve

Acute gingival conditions and severe chronic periodontal disease

Acute gingival conditions should be treated by mouthwash and systemic antibiotics appropriate to the causative organism.

In the presence of severe chronic periodontal disease, most restorative work is impossible because of gingival bleeding or exudate, or incorrect level of the gingival margin. Scaling and polishing, and instruction in oral hygiene is required first, followed by review. However, if the standard of the existing restorations is contributing to plaque retention, then the faulty ones should be removed and well fitting provisionals placed, pending resolution of the gingival problems (*Fig. 3.9*).

Intracoronal cavities can be provisionally restored with polycarboxylate cement, placed with the aid of a matrix, or even amalgam. This provides better gingival and contact area contour. Replacement of the temporary amalgams should be done after resolution of the soft tissue inflammation.

Diagnosis and stabilization – Summary

Draw conclusions from the history and examination – the diagnosis

If the data are inconclusive, make a provisional diagnosis

Investigate to confirm the diagnosis

Control active pathology as rapidly as possible

When stable, draft the definitive treatment plan

4

General principles of treatment planning

> Whilst making a diagnosis is an intellectual challenge, the formulation of the treatment plan has to combine experience, ability and common sense.
>
> There is absolutely no use in compiling an elaborate and technically demanding series of procedures that is inappropriate to this particular patient, with this particular pathology in these particular circumstances.
>
> Once the diagnosis is made, there may be two or three equally 'correct' treatments for the condition.
>
> Making the decision as to which treatment is appropriate is the skill of treatment planning.

Treatment plan

The treatment plan is the basic blueprint for the delivery of care. It combines priorities for therapy with the organization and management of that therapy. It must combine *prevention* of disease with the eradication and repair of pathology.

The treatment plan must fit the profiles of both the patient and the dentist (*Fig. 4.1*) As discussed in Chapter 1, the patient will have some ideas about his or her dental future, and the dentist will have some resources and technical skills at his or her disposal to fulfil treatment objectives.

Basically, the resources available, governed by the dentist and the dentist's techniques, should, through the medium of the treatment plan, match the resource consumption of the patient, governed by the patient's expectations and pathology.

Figure 4.2 projects the patient from diagnosis, through agreement and formal *consent* to the treatment and its delivery, to oral health and the very important concept of continuing care.

To a large extent, the left side of *Figure 4.1* is dealt with in succeeding chapters, and problems created by the patient are considered here.

Patient's influence on treatment planning

Motivation, expectations and availability

These go hand in hand – a well motivated patient will almost always find a way to make him- or herself available for treatment. A string of failed appointments belies initial protestations of interest and desire for treatment!

If there are doubts about the patient's commitment, then this should be reflected in a cautious start to the treatment plan. One or two visits to the hygienist, followed by a short appointment with the dentist for a simple restoration and review of oral hygiene, would be appropriate. Provided active pathology has been stabilized, then the weaker patient might well benefit from a repeated oral hygiene lesson, together with the message that unless oral hygiene improves, restorative work will not be started. Certainly, this must be the case prior to advanced restorations.

As was discussed earlier, the extraction of a tooth may fit a patient's expectations more than attendance for four or five visits for root canal therapy and a crown. It may be that the

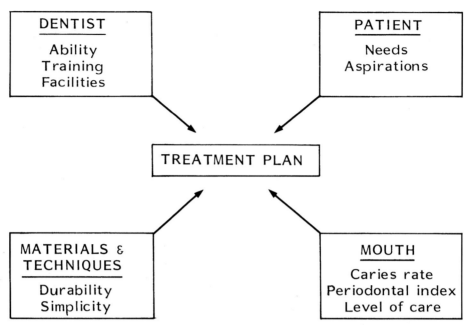

Fig. 4.1 Factors influencing a treatment plan

restorative treatment is well within the dentist's capabilities, but it will be somewhat wasted if the patient loses interest after the first hour, when the root canals were being identified. Of course, this is not to suggest that the dentist should not try to educate and inform about restorative possibilities. It could be that the

patient never realized the scope of modern dentistry. However, initial enthusiasm must be maintained so that it is not just the product of the dentist's ambitions.

Apprehension

No one likes visiting the dentist, mainly in view of the prospect of minor surgery to a very tender area of the anatomy, but also because of the folklore surrounding the profession.

The majority of those who actually come for treatment are able to control their apprehension successfully, but a minority have tremendous difficulty. Often, apprehension stems from a single unpleasant experience, perhaps as a child, and frequently pain from poor analgesia is remembered vividly. Many of these will respond to sympathetic listening, careful explanations about treatment, an unhurried, relaxed chairside manner and a great deal of patience – *tender loving care* (TLC).

Simple procedures with complete analgesia should be done first to establish confidence, and then more complex work may be possible. The more intractable cases may be candidates for:

- Oral sedation
- Inhalation sedation

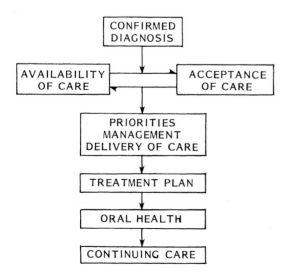

Fig. 4.2 Route to oral health and continuing care

- Intravenous sedation
- General anaesthesia

Oral sedation

The use of a low dose of an anxiolytic drug may reduce mild apprehension so that dental care can be delivered normally. Diazepam is probably the most used and 5–10 mg the night before the appointment and repeated 1 hour before, having arranged the appointment to be in the early morning, is a suitable dosage. However, this must only be a short-term measure; the use of such drugs should be limited to the lowest possible dose for the shortest possible time.

Inhalation sedation

This technique involves the administration of between 20–40% nitrous oxide together with a minimum of 30% oxygen. The level of nitrous oxide is set by observing the patient's response. Appropriate training and facilities are required and these are listed in the national guidelines cited in the bibliography.

The operator must encourage and reassure the patient during induction and treatment. There is certainly an element of hypnosis in the procedure. Local analgesia must be used for painful procedures.

It is not possible to use inhalation sedation if the nasal airway is obstructed, the patient cannot lie supine or the patient is in the first trimester of pregnancy.

Intravenous sedation

A few patients are not able to respond to inhalation sedation, and for these the administration of a sedative intravenously is usually successful. Modern, short acting benzodiazepines, such as midazolam, are very suitable for outpatient sedation. Midazolam has a very short half-life and therefore a short recovery period. It also induces amnesia, which can be very helpful.

The patient should not have eaten for 4–6 hours before the sedation is begun, but may drink small quantities after that. No alcohol should be taken, but regular medication should be taken as usual. Any anxiolytics will probably reduce the dose of sedation required.

The patient should be supine and the drug should be administered through an in-dwelling venous cannula in the antecubital fossa, hand or forearm. The drug is injected slowly and carefully titrated against the patient's response; oversedation, particularly with the elderly, is a potential risk. Oximetry is essential to detect hypoxaemia that may result from respiratory depression. Again the reader is referred to national guidelines for further information.

Communication is important as the patient will respond slowly to command. Local analgesia is also necessary. If sedation becomes less, then a further increment titrated against response should be given.

After treatment is completed, recovery should be observed and the patient can go home escorted, when lucid and capable of walking unaided. The patient must avoid driving, sport and alcohol for 12 hours.

General anaesthesia

Intubated general anaesthesia in day stay facilities should be reserved for those who cannot be treated in any other way. It may also be appropriate for stabilizing urgent cases who will subsequently have definitive treatment under inhalation sedation.

It is really the last resort and is a compromise because of the limited time available – say, about an hour – and the difficult working conditions of an operating theatre. Only very basic conservation should be planned and any teeth of dubious prognosis should be extracted.

The patient should be screened by urinalysis and blood pressure determination to ensure fitness for anaesthesia. Haemoglobin estimation and blood count has been discontinued by most anaesthetists except where a general indication exists. The patient must be starved and not have any acute respiratory infections. Patients with medical problems should be admitted for observation before and after the anaesthetic.

Care must be taken during treatment not to flood the pharynx with water and to ensure all pieces of tooth, amalgam, etc. are removed from the mouth.

The patient must be accompanied home and looked after for 24 hours. He or she should return for a normal outpatient appointment for review and occlusal adjustment of restorations, which is not possible in theatre.

This review visit should also begin an acclimatization programme to help the patient accept normal dental care. Many patients dislike the experience so much that they are very susceptible to conversion to less traumatic techniques.

Age

Age *per se* has a limited effect on treatment planning. The young patient with an immature dentition would probably be unsuitable for conventional bridgework due to large pulps and a developing gingival margin. Playing contact sports also hazards anterior crowns and bridges, but such activity is not necessarily age related.

In the older patient it is the combination of age with infirmity that limits the delivery of care. A fit 70-year-old could well have the same treatment as a fit 50-year-old. However, an unwell 50-year-old could well be more disadvantaged.

Having established this, there are changes in dentition that affect incidence of certain pathologies and make some aspects of dental care more difficult. These changes are discussed in Chapter 5. Gingival recession, a predisposition to root caries and sclerosis of root canals are all problems that may influence the technical aspects of restorative dentistry. These will be compounded if the patient has already had a high experience of dental disease. It is more difficult to maintain an ageing dentition of complex restorations than one with no restorations at all!

An elderly patient may have more difficulty in performing oral hygiene procedures and this difficulty could be compounded by the presence of complex restorations provided in the past. He or she might not be able to tolerate long periods in the dental chair for complex care and will certainly have more difficulty in adapting to dentures (Chapter 24).

Influence of medical history on treatment planning and management

The taking of the medical history and its importance was outlined in Chapter 2. Medical conditions may influence:

● The content of the treatment plan and/or
● The way in which care is delivered

For example, some conditions may indicate the extraction of a tooth rather than its restoration, whilst others may indicate that restorations, planned normally, are carried out under special conditions.

Cardiovascular conditions

Probably the most confusion arises from the influence of a history of *rheumatic heart disease*. Transient *bacteraemias* may lead to bacteria colonizing scarred areas of the endocardium, usually the valve edges, causing *bacterial endocarditis*. Bacteraemias occur every day from chewing or defaecation, and certain dental procedures may cause them.

The precise relationship between dental procedures and the development of bacterial endocarditis is still the subject of considerable debate. There are many patients who have had no antibiotic cover for many years of dentistry, including extractions, with no apparent ill effects.

The reader is advised to follow the nationally agreed recommendations, which are to provide antibiotic cover for susceptible patients for dental procedures which carry a <u>high</u> risk of major bacteraemia. These procedures are:

● Extractions
● Scaling and polishing, pocket probing, root planing
● Surgery involving the gingival margin

There is currently no incontrovertible evidence that endodontic procedures are incriminated in the aetiology of endocarditis, though care must be taken to remain within the confines of the root canal (this is true for all root canal therapy anyway). Suggestions that minor procedures, such as pulp extirpation, gingival retraction, or placing a matrix band, are incriminated in the aetiology have been made. Supporting evidence for this is patchy and provision of an appropriate antibiotic regime for multiple visits for routine dentistry is difficult. Such suggestions will encourage the continued misuse of antibiotics. In all cases, the gingival margins should be cleaned with an antiseptic such as chlorhexidine prior to treatment.

The definition of the susceptible patient is more difficult. Not all patients who give a history of rheumatic fever will have scarred endocardia, revealed by the presence of a murmur. To prescribe antibiotics for these patients would appear wasteful, if not a further misuse of antibiotics. It is safer to request an opinion from a medical practitioner, preferably a cardiologist, as to whether cover is indicated.

Other cases where cover is definitely indicated are patients with:

● A previous history of endocarditis
● A prosthetic heart valve
● Congenital cardiac defects

These patients are at a *high risk* from endocarditis.

The regime for prophylaxis is based on the degree of risk and the patient's previous recent therapy with antibiotics. The current recommendations can be found in the British National Formulary (BNF).

All patients in the at-risk groups should be informed of the need to maintain good oral hygiene and those patients who are candidates for cardiac surgery should be well restored first.

Treatment planning

The healthy patient with a history of rheumatic fever should be treatment planned as normal. The higher risk patient, particularly if there is a history of endocarditis, should be planned more radically, because the risks are that much higher. A tooth requiring a possibly difficult root filling should be extracted and any areas of chronic infection should be regarded with suspicion and the teeth not given the benefit of the doubt.

Other cardiovascular conditions may make prolonged courses of treatment risky or difficult. This group includes stroke and cardiac infarction. Full recovery from such an episode, of course, should bring no problems, though the dentist ought to be prepared for a recurrence in the chair and revise his management of collapse.

For those patients with incomplete recovery, treatment should be planned to be simple and provided in short appointments. Blood pressure measurement before, during and after treatment is useful for the assessment of patient stability. Trauma from extraction should be avoided if at all possible.

Stroke patients with residual paralysis may need advice on oral hygiene aids, such as electric toothbrushes, to assist them. It will be sometimes necessary to train the patient's carer to perform oral hygiene procedures for the patient.

Blood-borne viruses and prevention of cross-infection

The two most important blood-borne viruses in dentistry are hepatitis B virus (HBV) and human immunodeficiency virus (HIV).

Patients who are ill with hepatitis B or AIDS should receive dental treatment under hospital conditions. Those people who are known to be infectious, but are well, may be treated in normal dental practice and should be treatment planned as 'normal'.

Many carriers are unidentified, and these are treated unknowingly as normal patients. These and the known ones constitute a combined hazard to the dentist and his staff, and to the patients following them in the surgery. The basic routine for the *prevention of cross-infection* should be applied to all patients – *universal precautions* – and the recommendations are referred to in the bibliography.

In brief, the key recommendations are:

- Protection of the operator and close-support dental nurse by gloves, masks and glasses
- Decontamination and sterilization of all instruments and equipment that have touched the patient or have been handled by 'contaminated' staff
- Use disposable equipment wherever possible
- Use precise surgery routines to avoid contaminating areas, such as inside drawers or the stock of temporary crowns, that will be difficult to sterilize later
- Clean contaminated surgery surfaces and protect them by using tray systems, towels and cling film
- Decontaminate all items before they are sent to the laboratory
- Decontaminate laboratory work before it reaches the chairside

Other medical conditions

General infirmity or *terminal illness* would indicate a minimum of complex work being attempted. The plan should be to stabilize sources of pain and discomfort as simply as possible.

Blood dyscrasias and *diabetes* may give rise to gingival problems because of the reduced resistance to infection and these will preclude anything but stabilization being carried out. The medical condition should be resolved prior to definitive conservation.

The operator would wish to conserve teeth wherever possible in *epileptics* to avoid dentures, in *haemophiliacs* to avoid extractions, and in cases with irradiated bone where post-extraction healing can be prolonged and difficult.

It is important to see patients before *radiotherapy,* whenever possible, to remove any teeth of dubious prognosis. There should be no exposed bone in the mouth prior to radiotherapy. After radiotherapy the dentist may have a role in advising on the care and management of mucositis, xerostomia and radiation-induced caries.

The management of *xerostomia* involves advice on elimination of anything that impairs salivation (such as alcohol consumption and smoking), use of sugar free chewing gum and use of saliva substitutes containing fluoride.

Altered management of a normal treatment plan would be appropriate for a controlled diabetic, where treatment is best carried out immediately after a meal when the blood sugar is higher.

Patients having *orthopaedic joint prostheses* or *indwelling catheters* do not require antibiotic prophylaxis for dental treatment provided there is no other indication for prophylaxis.

Restorative dentistry for pregnant patients requires some minor modifications. The generally held view is that invasive procedures are best avoided in the first and third trimesters, and radiography avoided totally throughout. However, where urgent treatment including radiography is

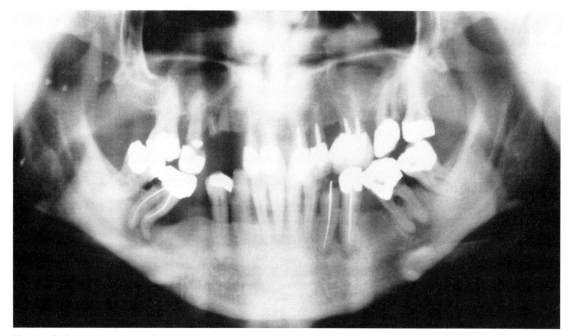

Fig. 4.3 Orthopantomogram of a patient who has experienced extensive restorative dentistry. There is now gross caries and periodontal disease. The chances of success for future work are small and, in any case, the volume of work required is daunting. The patient was treatment planned for a clearance and complete dentures

required, this should be done in any event. It is also important to complete treatment and reach stability in the second trimester, so that treatment is not required later when the patient is uncomfortable, or immediately after the baby is born, when the mother has other priorities.

Level of previous care

The well restored and cared-for mouth encourages more of the same. It indicates the patient's desire for continuing care and his or her ability to maintain restorations in plaque-free and caries-free conditions.

Unfortunately, the quality of the previous restorative care, rather than its volume, can also modify a treatment plan. If the restorative work has not been provided to a high standard then, even though the patient has been a regular attender, the sheer volume of replacement work required may inhibit a totally restorative approach (*Fig. 4.3*).

Several missing teeth and a partial denture might well lead to extraction of a difficult restorative problem and its addition to the denture.

Oral hygiene and periodontal disease

A high active caries rate may dictate extractions and simple restorations only, and generalized periodontal disease might indicate the same. Oral hygiene must be effective before advanced restorations are contemplated and the use of fluoride and chlorhexidine mouthwashes or gels may be of assistance.

Occlusion

Evidence of deterioration in occlusal relationships following tooth loss would indicate bridges or partial dentures (Section IV). Inadequate occlusion on bridges or dentures might indicate their replacement.

Radiographic findings

The major use of radiography is in diagnosis (Chapter 2). However, it is absolutely essential in the planning of endodontics. The presence of patent root canals, and absence of obstruction by secondary dentine, pulp stones or curvature, can only be decided by good radiographs.

Having diagnosed acute pulpitis clinically, the radiograph will lead the planner to contemplate root canal therapy, or to recommend extraction. It might be very desirable to save the tooth, but it might be technically impossible.

General structure of a treatment plan

Priorities

The simple treatment plan designed to treat chronic gingivitis, caries and failed restorations would begin by preparing the supporting tissues for restorative work – scaling and polishing, and preventing the recurrence of gingivitis – instruction in oral hygiene. This phase is better carried out by the dental hygienist, leaving the dentist free to perform more complex functions.

The priorities for simple restorations would relate to size, doing the largest first, unless the periodontium was being influenced by a poor contact area or overhanging margin.

Oral hygiene should be reviewed continually during treatment with encouragement, or further reminders if necessary. If advanced work – crowns or endodontics – is planned, this should be placed at the end of the plan after gingival resolution and the completion of simple restorations. Oral hygiene review should also be satisfactory.

Extractions are best regarded within the framework of stabilization, since the affected teeth could give rise to pain whilst other work is being done. Also there is the possibility of damaging new restorations during surgery, particularly of impacted teeth. If the patient is to be referred for oral surgery, then this should be arranged early, but almost certainly the work will not be carried out until after the general practitioner has completed other treatment. At the time the referral is made, it is important to include information on proposed treatment of other teeth so that the referring practitioner's responsibilities are established.

Any surgery involving the gingival margin, e.g. apicectomy, should be done well in advance of crowns or veneers proposed for the affected teeth.

Partial denture planning should be built-in alongside the planning of restorations, since the design may require rest seats or specially modified crowns.

Structure

A schematic arrangement for a treatment plan could be:

1. Prepare supporting tissues – scale and polish
2. Preventive measures – topical fluoride, fissure sealing, oral hygiene instruction, dietary advice
3. Design bridges or partial dentures
4. Simple restorations
5. Pinned restorations
6. Root canal therapy
7. Review oral hygiene and periodontal condition
8. Periodontal therapy, if necessary – root planing, surgery
9. Crowns
10. Construct dentures/bridges
11. Recall and continuing care

Review and recall

The simple treatment plan has within its structure the review of oral hygiene procedures, but some other procedures would require formal review prior to progress in treatment.

For example, apical surgery should not be followed immediately by crowns on the affected teeth. Two or three months should elapse whilst the gingival tissues stabilize and the margins reach a constant level, and an indication of apical healing is apparent.

Extractions and alveolar remodelling should be followed by review, perhaps six months later, before permanent bridges are considered.

The listing of a formal *recall* as part of the treatment plan is essential to indicate the responsibility for *continuing care*. The actual recall interval can be decided as appropriate to the patient's condition.

Six months would be routine for most patients to monitor plaque control and caries status, and to check for other oral pathology. Shorter intervals would be necessary for those having difficulties, whilst the well-maintained patient could be left to his or her own devices for as long as a year.

Radiographic review of crowns and endodontics is essential. Symptomless loss of vitality under a crown preparation must be detected by the apical condition changing. Progressing healing of an apical lesion following root canal therapy should be monitored. The intervals could get progressively longer: begin at six months, then a year later and two–three years regularly after that.

Treatment planning – Summary

Decide on items for prevention and treatment
Order these according to priority in the patient as a whole
Consider the treatment methods that are appropriate:

- For this patient
- At this time
- In this practice
- With this dentist

Review oral hygiene and prevention
Recall to commit the patient to continuing care

RESTORATIONS AND THEIR ENVIRONMENT

5

Applied biology of the teeth

Techniques for the restoration of tooth structure require a detailed knowledge of the tissues against which the material is to be placed. The purpose of this chapter is to describe the hard tissues of the human tooth and their relationship with their environment. The implications for restorative dentistry of enamel and dentine structure and pulp physiology are discussed.

Introduction

Caries is a microbially initiated disease causing localized destruction of mineralized tissues in the body, including bone. For the purpose of this book only caries of the teeth will be considered and the signs of presence of the disease will be described as the localized destruction of enamel, dentine and, more briefly, of cementum. As is the case with other pathological conditions, a clear understanding depends upon a knowledge of the basic structure of the tissues involved.

Enamel structure and chemistry

Enamel is the outer protective covering of the crown of the tooth and is an extremely hard, brittle, white, shiny substance. It is composed basically of billions of crystals of hydroxyapatite which are roughly octagonal in cross section with a diameter of about 360 nm. The length of the crystals has proved difficult to determine but they are thought to be long and ribbon-like, extending for some distance through the enamel. The crystals are tightly packed together so that organic matrix lying between them is minimal, constituting only about 2 per cent by weight of the enamel but much more than this by volume. Therefore between the crystals are micropores or pores, the size of which can be measured with some accuracy, and changes in these spaces is one of the methods of indicating the presence of carious attack. Under these conditions the enamel is said to have developed *increased porosity*. The

methods available for such studies are discussed in Chapter 6.

Prisms

The crystals of enamel are not randomly arranged but are grouped together to form rods or *prisms* of material, extending from the enamel–dentine junction to the surface of the tooth. In the original English scientific literature the preferred term is that of 'prisms' whereas in more recent writings the term 'rod' is preferred and in fact induces a clearer image of the structure in the mind of the reader. Because the remainder of this book will use the word 'prism', the old-fashioned term will be used here.

Each prism has a mean cross-sectional diameter of about 5 microns but because the surface area of the outer enamel is greater than that of the enamel–dentine junction the prisms tend to increase in diameter from the junction to the outer surface. The cross-sectional shape of the prisms has been variously described as octagonal to fish scale or keyhole shaped, but this depends to some extent on the angle of section through the prisms. The keyhole concept is the classical construction in human enamel and is shown diagramatically in *Figure 5.1*. The broad part of the keyhole is often referred to as the head, and the narrow part as the tail. There is controversy as to what constitutes the boundary of each prism. Current research suggests that prism boundaries may be formed by both sudden changes in hydroxyapatite crystal orientation and an increased concentration of *organic matrix*.

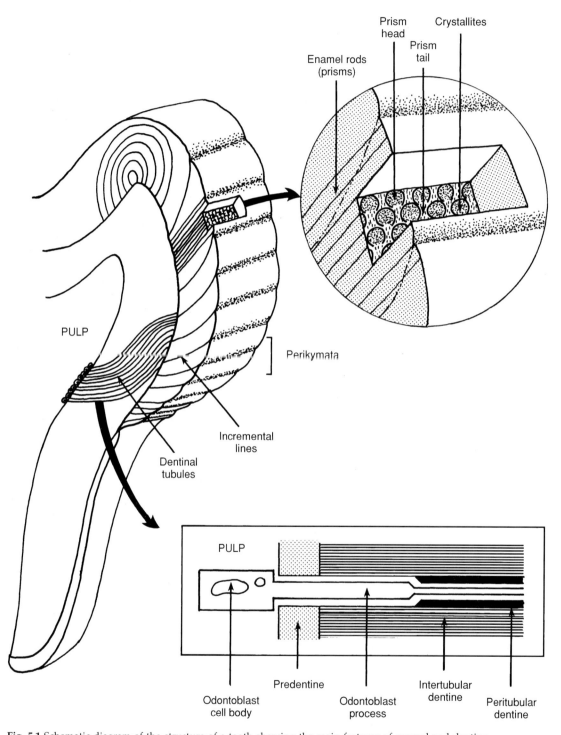

Fig. 5.1 Schematic diagram of the structure of a tooth showing the main features of enamel and dentine

Matrix

The nature of the organic matrix has received much attention, but because of its small amount has proved difficult to analyse with certainty. In the immature tooth the matrix consists of two distinct proteins, amelogenin and enamelin, and during maturation much of the amelogenin is removed. The cells responsible for secreting and maturing the enamel during development are the *ameloblasts* and they migrate outwards from the putative enamel–dentine junction for a distance equal to the thickness of the enamel at that point on the tooth.

When the ameloblasts have completed their secretory activity, the final thickness of the enamel is determined and this cannot be altered throughout life, since the ameloblasts then degenerate. In principle enamel is a dead tissue which cannot repair itself. However, we will see later that chemically speaking some repair or re-structuring of enamel is possible.

Incremental nature

The enamel is laid down by the ameloblasts in increments, arranged rather like the layers in an onion over each cusp of the tooth. In cross-section these appear as concentric rings through the enamel and are known as *incremental lines* or brown striae of Retzius (*Fig. 5.1*). Each line represents the point which the ameloblasts had reached at a particular time in their functional activity. The incremental line is not pigmented, as the name brown striae would suggest, but is probably caused by a slight change in direction and diameter of the enamel prisms. These incremental lines reach the surface of the tooth at an acute angle and there is evidence that they modify the progression of caries in the natural lesion.

Surface structure

Although the enamel prisms have been depicted as extending from the junction out to the surface, in practice this is often not the case. Many of the prisms in certain parts of the tooth and in certain teeth stop short of the surface. The surface layers of the tooth are therefore made up of *aprismatic enamel* that may have been produced because the activity of the ameloblasts changes before they cease secretory activity. Too little attention has been paid to this outer layer on the teeth and it is conceivable that it may be related to caries susceptibility and is certainly of importance when etching and bonding techniques are under consideration.

Ionic exchange

Once the teeth have erupted, ionic interchange is possible between the crystals of the enamel and ions in the surrounding environment. For example, the calcium ions may be exchanged for strontium and the hydroxyl part of the molecule may be replaced by fluoride, which appears to protect the tooth against carious attack. Epidemiological studies have shown that newly erupted teeth may be more susceptible to caries than teeth in more mature individuals, so that great efforts are now made by restorative dentists to prevent so far as possible the commencement of carious attack, which becomes much less likely in the older individual.

Morphology of teeth

The overall shape and detailed morphology of the teeth varies considerably between teeth and even within tooth types. Thus the incisors are quite different in shape to the canines, premolars and molars and in different individuals premolars may themselves vary somewhat in shape. These factors are important in restorative dental procedures and should be studied in greater depth in standard texts of tooth morphology. It is usual in current dental practice to distinguish to some extent between restorative procedures in deciduous teeth and permanent teeth; this is because there are structural differences between them, the most important being relative size of the teeth, the thickness of the enamel and underlying dentine, the relative size of the pulp chambers (which are larger in deciduous teeth) and the bulbosity of the enamel of deciduous teeth at the cervical margin. However, there is evidence accruing recently that the structure of the enamel of deciduous and permanent teeth may differ and this may affect the rate of progression of caries. For instance, it has recently been shown using micro-radiographic techniques that deciduous teeth are somewhat less well mineralized than their permanent counterparts. This may account for their whiter appearance, since more porous enamel tends to be less translucent so that the yellowness of the underlying dentine does not show through so clearly.

Dentine structure, chemistry and sensitivity

Dentine

The bulk of the structure of the tooth, both crown and root, is made up of a less well mineralized but more flexible tissue known as dentine. This also is composed of hydroxyapatite crystals, but in a less concentrated form than in enamel. The majority of the crystals are arranged more or less parallel to the enamel–dentine junction, but in the three-dimensional sense are much more random than those in enamel. They are laid down in a matrix composed of *glycosaminoglycans*, in which have been laid down *collagen fibrils* secreted by the odontoblast cells in their movement inwards from the enamel–dentine junction towards the future pulp. The matrix of dentine, therefore, consists of a rather dense, flexible material, the general shape of which is retained even after removal by acids of all of the mineral component. Whilst caries of enamel results in cavitation and loss of the material, at least initially in dentine a rubbery, stained matrix may be retained for some time.

Odontoblast processes

As the odontoblasts migrate inwards from the junction towards the pulp, they leave behind them a cell process which becomes enclosed in a tubule incorporated into the matrix. The dentine is therefore permeated by millions of cell processes radiating out from the odontoblasts through the whole thickness of the dentine, at least in the younger tooth. These processes may have side communicating branches so that a syncitium of cells is formed. When the dentine mineralizes, crystals are laid down in the ground substance and fibres of the matrix, but are not laid down in the cell processes. In the mature dentine, therefore, the cell processes are contained in mineralized tubules running through the dentine. With increasing age these tubules narrow by the deposition of mineralized material in their walls (intra-tubular dentine), and there is still disagreement as to whether mature dentine possesses viable cell processes throughout the length of its tubules.

Dentinal tubules

Although these tubules radiate from the pulp to the enamel–dentine junction they do not travel in straight lines. In the longitudinal plane they tend to follow a sigmoid curve from the outer dentine towards the pulp, so that the cell body is placed more apically than the periphery of the process (*Fig. 5.1*). This arrangement has some clinical significance which will be discussed later.

Mineralization

Unlike enamel, dentine matrix does not mineralize as soon as it is produced. There is a delay between laying down the matrix and its mineralization in the form of calcospherites, which finally coalesce to produce a more or less homogeneously mineralized tissue. In some parts of the tooth a failure in this fusion of calcospherites seems to occur. Firstly, in the coronal portion large non-mineralized, star-shaped spaces are left in many teeth following an incremental line below the enamel–dentine junction. These defects are known as *interglobular spaces* and the cell processes of the odontoblasts run straight through them. Their significance in relation to spread of caries is not known. At the periphery of the root just below the cementum, much smaller defects in mineralization are observed, known as the *granular layer of Tomes*. No clinical significance has been ascribed to this structure.

Secondary dentine

As the odontoblasts migrate pulpally they lay down the adult form of the tooth, completing the root some two-and-a-half to three-and-a-half years after eruption of the tooth. If they were to continue at this rate of production of dentine then clearly the pulp chamber would be obliterated within a few years of establishment of the dentition. Once the mature outline of the tooth has been completed the odontoblasts slow down and, although continuing to migrate inwards, do so at a rate enabling the pulp chamber to survive into old age. The dentine laid down in the initial stages of tooth development is known as *primary dentine* and that laid down after the odontoblasts have slowed is known as *regular secondary dentine*. As can be seen in Chapter 6, the odontoblasts may change their rate of production of dentine and its type under the influence of carious attack.

Dentine sensitivity

In order to enable dentine to react in this manner it must be responsive to outside stimuli and many patients who have suffered cavity preparation under inadequate anaesthesia will testify that this is the case. The exact mechanism is still not clear, largely because technical problems of fixation and examination of tissue remain unsolved. The pulp is well supplied by nerves, both non-medullated (controlling blood vessel tone) and medullated (capable of transmitting common sensation and pain). These latter nerves have endings in a plexus close to the odontoblast cell bodies and also have nerve endings on the cell bodies themselves. There is clear evidence that some of these nerve fibres extend some distance into the dentine and have presumably been incorporated into it during its formation. About 1 in 2000 tubules appear to contain nerve fibres but only for quite short distances. It is interesting to consider that this so-called sparse innervation is probably greater than that found in the fingertips!

As has been already stated, there is some doubt as to whether living odontoblastic cell processes extend throughout the thickness of the dentine in the mature tooth. If they do, then loss of enamel may result in osmotic changes at the peripheral end of the tubules, thus resulting in fluid exchange and distortion of the processes. This event may be transmitted along the process and then converted by transduction into nerve impulses, either at the inner third of the processes themselves or at the cell body region. If the cell processes do not extend throughout the thickness of the dentine then it is conceivable that fluid balance changes in the outer part of the tubules may initiate distortion of the processes, resulting in impulses eventually to the nerve plexus.

Enamel–dentine junction

The junction between the enamel and dentine lies on the original basement membrane separating the enamel organ on the outside from the papilla or mesodermal tissue on the inside at an early stage of tooth development. In most human teeth it is not a flat sheet but is deformed into a crater-like appearance, producing on section the appearance of scallops. The concavities of these scallops face towards the enamel and the convexities towards the dentine. That is to say the outer surface of the dentine, if the enamel were to be removed, appears like the surface of the moon with irregularly shaped craters. The inner surface of the enamel is composed of convexities fitting into these craters. This has the effect of increasing the surface area between the two tissues. In some parts of the human tooth, particularly near to the neck of the tooth, the enamel–dentine junction may be more or less flat.

Smear layer

During restorative procedures, removal of decayed enamel and dentine and extension of the cavity for prevention, retention and access may be carried out using hand instruments such as chisels and hatchets, but is also commonly done using rotary instruments of various types and speeds. Rotating instruments may result in smearing of the crystal and organic content of both enamel and dentine over the cut surface. This smearing may be a purely physical effect or may be engendered by heat at the point of cutting and grinding. Hand instruments,

however sharp, may also cause heavy smearing on the enamel surface, especially on the floor of an approximal box. The clinical implications of the smear layer are discussed below.

Pulp

The pulp and the dentine cannot be separated either anatomically or functionally. Anatomically, the cell bodies of the dentinal processes lie in the peripheral region of the pulp, and the *odontoblast cells* and their processes are therefore intimately associated with both dentine and pulp tissue. Functionally, the reactions of both dentine and pulp to external stimuli are dependent upon both the cell processes and bodies of the odontoblasts and, therefore, reaction is a combined function of both tissues. The three dimensional shape of the *pulp chamber* varies in different teeth. Thus, in an upper incisor the coronal part of the pulp chamber is somewhat flattened buccolingually and broad mesiodistally, and the radicular portion of the pulp chamber is roughly triangular in shape and conical in length. In multirooted teeth such as the molars, the form of the pulp chamber is obviously much more complex. It is important for the restorative dentist to appreciate the general form of the pulp chamber in each tooth type, although variations exist even between teeth of similar notation. A standard text on tooth morphology would provide this information. It has already been stated that the relative size and shape of pulp chambers in deciduous teeth are larger than in permanent teeth and therefore exposure of the pulp chamber is considered by many to be a greater hazard in deciduous dentitions.

The healthy pulp is of a jelly-like consistency, having a ground substance of glycosaminoglycans in which is interspersed a loose and sparse network of collagen fibres. These collagen fibres are produced and maintained by fibroblasts, which are the commonest cell type in the healthy pulp. There are also macrophages, pluripotential histiocytes and occasional monocytes. There is a complicated vascular supply consisting of arteries entering the apical foramen and dividing into an extensive network of arterioles, particularly in the peripheral parts of the pulp. These arterioles connect directly with venules so that arterio-venous shunts exist. There is an extensive capillary plexus, particularly in the region of the odontoblast cell bodies at the periphery of the pulp. Although difficult to demonstrate, there is an adequate lymphatic drainage from the pulp, and veins and lymphatics leave together through the apical foramina. Innervation of the pulp has already been discussed in relation to sensitivity of the dentine.

Periodontium

The tooth is supported in its bony socket by a specialized connective tissue – the *periodontal ligament*. At the cervical margin or neck of the tooth it is continuous with the connective tissue underlying the *gingivae*. At the apex, it is continuous with the tooth pulp. It bridges the gap between the root cementum and the alveolar bone and is approximately 0.2 mm in width. It is composed of fibres in a gel-like ground substance that contains nerves, blood vessels and cells.

Fibres

Most of the fibres in the ligament are type I collagen, although some type II collagen and specialized oxytalan and elastin fibres are present in small amounts. The collagen fibres are arranged in bundles which pursue a complex wavy course. At their cementum end the bundles are smaller in diameter than at their alveolar bone end. They form branching networks around the neurovascular bundles but no single fibre bundles appear to traverse the whole distance from tooth to bone. The collagen bundles are incorporated into bone and cementum in the same way as are tendons, that is to say, in the form of mineralized Sharpey's fibres. The fibre bundles are 'crimped' along their course and the fibre bundles overlap each other; it has been suggested that this allows response to loading under occlusal forces. The functional activity of the ligament will be described later. The fibre bundles are arranged in specific named groups associated with the gingival, crestal, radicular, apical and inter-radicular portions of the tooth. Their arrangement is shown diagrammatically in *Figure 5.2*.

The oxytalan fibres lie parallel to the length of the tooth root and are attached to cementum at one end. They have been implicated in both tooth eruption and support and may be involved in support of blood vessels.

Ground substance

The major components are hyaluronic acid, glyco-proteins and proteoglycans. Hyaluronic acid and the polysaccharide components of proteoglycans are glycosaminoglycans. Water content is about 70%.

Vasculature

The periodontal ligament is well supplied with blood vessels that are mainly derived from the superior alveolar branches of the maxillary artery or from the inferior alveolar artery in the mandible.

There may be other sources deriving from the buccal, masseteric or lingual arteries in the mandible or from the palatal or facial arteries in the maxilla. The veins drain into larger veins in the inter-alveolar bone and usually do not follow the route of the arteries. Within the ligament itself the blood supply is most extensive in the cervical part and least extensive in the middle third. Most of the vessels enter the ligament as perforating arteries from the intra-bony vessels and they run parallel to the long axis of the tooth, passing between the principal fibre bundles of the ligament. Many branches arise from these vessels and they form a capillary plexus that is more complex at the bone surface than at the cementum surface of the ligament. There appear to be arterio-venous shunts in the cervical part of the ligament and these resemble renal glomeruli. There is some evidence that, in older patients, the vascularized spaces are larger and encroach upon areas previously occupied by fibres and bone.

The actual rate of blood flow has not yet been reliably determined but is controlled by both α and β adrenoreceptors, allowing both constriction and dilatation of vessels.

There are lymphatics present, although not in great numbers, and they tend to follow the venous drainage.

Nerves

These are derived from either the superior or inferior dental nerves. Some of the bundles of nerve fibres run from the apical region of the periodontium towards the cervical margin of the tooth. They are joined by nerves passing through foramina in the bone to enter the ligament horizontally. Large fibres are myelinated and terminate in specialized nerve endings that are associated with mechanoreceptor activity. These monitor forces on teeth and may be involved in reflex jaw opening and masticatory control. Small fibres terminate as free nerve endings associated with appreciation of pain. Autonomic nerves are present and they control regional blood flow in the ligament.

Cells

Most of the cells of the ligament are fibroblasts. They are responsible for the unusually high 'turn-over' rate in this tissue resulting in the fibres being constantly synthesized, removed and replaced. The fibroblasts are spindle shaped, large cells and they align themselves along the length of the fibre bundles. They are able to produce *and* remove collagen fibres, thus diseases affecting their function can seriously damage the ligament.

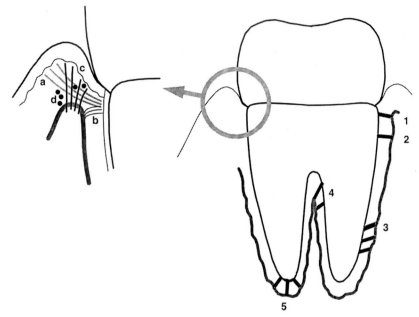

Fig. 5.2 Schematic diagram of the structure of the periodontium. Principal fibre groups: 1, alveolar crest; 2, horizontal; 3, oblique; 4, inter-radicular; 5, apical. Gingival ligament groups: a, dentogingival; b, dentoperiosteal; c, alveogingival; d, circular

Some of the epithelial cells (Hertwig's sheath) responsible for mapping out the shape of the tooth root remain in the ligament as cell 'rests' and they may subsequently proliferate to produce periodontal cysts.

There are undifferentiated cells of mesodermal origin and it is probable that they can differentiate into any type of mesodermal cell in the ligament.

As the ligament is bounded on the tooth surface by cementum and the outer surface by alveolar bone, there are cementoblasts and osteoblasts present. Bone remodels readily, so osteoclasts are seen in the ligament. Cementum is much more stable, thus in adult (but not deciduous) teeth cementoclasts are rarely seen.

Response to movement and load

Clearly, the ligament is responsible for the support of the teeth and attaches the tooth to the bone. There is still debate, however, as to how the ligament functions during normal physiological activities such as eruption or response to loading in an axial or tangential direction. It has been suggested that the ligament may contract during eruption, that migration or contraction of fibroblasts may occur, or that pressure may be exerted by vascular or fluid elements. The evidence is complex and largely derived from experiments on rodent teeth. It seems that the vascular theories are the most probable.

Mesial drift or movement of erupted teeth towards the mid-line has been attributed to activity in the periodontal tissues. At present there is conflicting evidence, and physiological mesial movements in response to tooth loss or wear cannot be fully explained.

In respect of functional loading on the teeth, there is also controversy. The weight of evidence suggests that the ligament does not behave purely as a suspensory ligament but that it behaves in a visco-elastic manner. It is now thought that all the components act together like a hydraulic shock absorber. In this case the fibres, ground substance, blood in the vessels and tissue fluids are all important. The system is very complex and is as yet imperfectly understood.

Age changes in teeth

It is sometimes difficult to distinguish between changes occurring in tissues due to age and changes occasioned usually in the older person because of increased exposure to external stimulation. This is particularly so in the case of the hard tissues of the teeth.

Enamel

In the case of enamel, although it is in principle a non-reactive tissue, most of the changes that occur as age progresses are due to ionic exchange between the external environment and the tooth. These have been described earlier. They may result in an enamel with a slightly changed refractive index, so that the colour of a person's tooth may change somewhat with age, usually becoming rather darker. The small but important organic content of the teeth, especially in relation to lamellae, may also take up staining as life progresses, contributing to this change in colour. Because enamel is non-replaceable in bulk, certain parts of the tooth tend to become worn as age progresses. Whilst not a true age change, this phenomenon of surface loss is often used by anthropologists to age individuals, although considerable information is required as to the diet responsible for the wear pattern.

Dentine

In the case of dentine there do seem to be changes more directly associated with age. There is evidence that the amount of intra-tubular mineralization increases with age and this occurs from the periphery of the odontoblast tubules working inwards towards the pulp. The effect of this is to produce sclerotic dentine where the refractive index and homogeneity of the tissue is more uniform. This phenomenon occurs particularly under regions of surface wear or caries in the crown, but is strikingly evident in the apical part of the tooth, spreading upwards from the apex to, in old age, two thirds or more of the way along the root. On tooth section this *sclerotic dentine* gives a transparent appearance to the root dentine and its extent provides a standard method of ageing dead bodies in forensic investigations. Its clinical significance will be discussed later.

Pulp

The pulp, although reducing in size as age progresses, may also change in consistency. It is reported that the fibrous content of the pulp increases relatively with age and there is evidence that the number of viable odontoblasts reduces.

Cementum

Cementum was a tissue of lesser interest to restorative dentists in the past but, with the advent of interest in root caries, may assume a greater importance in the future. It is for this reason that the tissue structure has not been discussed in detail. It has been reported recently that incremental lines in cementum may be related to seasonal changes and therefore may be used to age an individual. Whilst this seems a possibility in hibernating animals, the prospect seems unlikely in the human tooth.

Micro-environment of the tooth

When the tooth erupts into the mouth any cellular remnants on its surface are quickly lost. This brings the enamel surface in direct contact with the saliva, some of the proteins of which are instantaneously deposited on the enamel surface.

Saliva

Flow rates of saliva are at a maximum during masticatory activity and there is also a diurnal rhythm. It is not clear whether salivary flow rates are reduced to zero during sleep but they are certainly very low. Saliva contains anti-bacterial agents and is also of some importance in the initial digestion of food. This is brought about by its content of amylase. It is also functionally necessary for the sense of taste since substances can only affect the taste buds when in solution. To the restorative dentist, apart from the physical problems of dealing with it clinically, saliva is largely viewed as a protective medium for the teeth. It contains mucus mainly secreted by the submandibular and sublingual glands and it is this mucus which forms the protein coating on newly erupted teeth. It is a self-cleansing material since it washes the teeth following meals and, as already mentioned, it has some anti-bacterial and possibly antiviral activity (secretory IgA).

Two features of saliva, however, are of great interest to the restorative dentist. Firstly, saliva is an excellent buffer, largely due to its content of bicarbonates and to some extent its proteins. A buffer is a substance which tends to prevent changes in pH. During meal-times when perhaps acid substances are ingested or when the products of breakdown of food produce acid, the buffers in saliva tend to neutralize this acid. The increased flow of saliva at meal-times produces increased buffering activity. Secondly, saliva is supersaturated with calcium and phosphate ions. It is therefore largely the source of ionic interchange between the micro-environment of the mouth and the tooth itself. Fluorides may be contained in saliva and may be concentrated by plaque forming on the surface of teeth.

Dental plaque

Plaque is a bacterial deposit on the protein pellicle of the tooth and its ecology is complex and variable. In most people it consists of a basic bacterial flora of the *Streptococcus mutans* type perhaps along with lactobacilli. In older plaque filamentous organisms of the *actinomyces* type become apparent. Many of these organisms, particularly *Streptococcus mutans*, break down refined carbohydrates, producing extracellular glycans and large amounts of acid. As will be seen below, the relationship of the numbers and types of various micro-organisms to the prevalence of caries is an extremely difficult problem and it must be remembered that caries is a multifactorial disease and studies of any one factor may be unrewarding. As an illustration of this point, it is known that plaque on the surface of teeth is capable of concentrating fluorides, so that in an external environment of one part per million there may be eight to ten parts per million in the plaque. This concentration of fluoride may be toxic to some bacteria, although there is evidence that many bacteria combine the fluoride and remain metabolically active. The suggestion has been made that the presence of some young plaque capable of concentrating fluoride may be useful to the tooth surface, in that interchange with the surface hydroxyapatite crystals may be aided. Most clinicians, of course, would recommend removal of plaque, thereby denying the production of low pH and the formation of carious lesions.

Restorative implications

In our descriptions of enamel, dentine, saliva and plaque, the reader will have detected that the information is rarely academic but is necessary for a full understanding of the process of carious attack and of the dentist's ability to prevent or repair it. Important aspects of basic dental science and clinical restorative dentistry are emphasized by a few examples.

Enamel prisms

The reader will have appreciated that the detailed orientation of the enamel prisms is complex since it varies in different parts of the tooth. In the cuspal region the prisms follow a wavy and complex course, probably adding to the strength of this part of the enamel. In the cervical region they may slope towards the cervical margins and, in deciduous teeth, may be more horizontal in this part of the tooth.

Surface preparation

It is important that unsupported prisms are not left, since these may be extremely friable and the restorative dentist seeks to ensure that the periphery of his or her preparation lies along the general direction of the prisms. This produces maximum strength and reduces the likelihood of future fracture at the periphery of the restoration. Clinical practice must be tempered with common sense, and it is recognized by most restorative dentists that sometimes the load on a particular part of a restoration part is minimal and it may not be necessary to follow these guidelines. The same principles apply to the preparation of the surface of a cavity and attempts are often made to avoid leaving loose enamel crystals present even though these are invisible to the operator. Thus some operators advocate the cleaning and disinfection of a cavity before placing a restoration. It is probably less important in relation to enamel than to dentine unless bonding techniques are anticipated, in which case the prisms of the enamel must be exposed in order to produce a good key for the resin bond. This latter consideration may be important not only in relation to finishing cavity margins but in preparing surfaces of enamel where bonding to unprepared enamel is required.

Remineralization

It is clear from the description of enamel that in biological terms it is a non-healing tissue. This is why most approaches to dental caries in the past have been not so much treatment as repair of an untreatable defect. This is now changing and it is becoming apparent that at least in the early stages of carious attack demineralization or increased pore spacing in enamel may be repaired to some extent by removing the attacking medium and allowing the super-saturated nature of saliva to take its effect or, if necessary, by applying super-saturated remineralization solutions to the early carious lesion. It is now well recognized that caries is not a continuous process but is a start–stop phenomenon. It seems logical to assume, therefore, that the condition in its early stages is reversible and this fact forms the basis for most restorative, preventive and early treatment regimes.

Saliva and plaque

The importance of saliva and its consequent plaque formation on teeth has already been touched upon. Current opinion holds that removal of plaque by adequate oral hygiene procedures, especially during the first two decades of life, will prevent or markedly reduce the prevalence of caries. Extensive restorative procedures are therefore contra-indicated in patients unable to control their plaque formation, and initially the prevention of caries in children and eventually the management of established caries in adults depends as much upon oral hygiene procedures, diet and fluoride application as upon excellent technical restorative procedures.

Secondary dentine

Odontoblastic processes in their tubules follow a sigmoid course as they traverse towards the pulp. This is especially the case in the radicular part of the tooth. This means that the cell bodies associated with a particular tubule are much more apically placed than the carious attack at the periphery of the tubule. Therefore, any reactive secondary dentine will not be developed directly at the base of the cavity but will be placed more apically. This is important to recognize since the protective effect of secondary dentine distancing the attack from the pulp is useful in the apical portion of the cavity, but exposure of the pulp is much more likely more cervically.

Progress of caries

The rate of progression of caries through enamel and dentine is not known with precision but it appears to take 3–4 years for an early lesion to progress through enamel. It is then believed that the rate of progression through dentine is much more rapid. Clinically, it is obvious that when the lesion reaches dentine it spreads laterally along the enamel–dentine junction and this may be a reflection of the lower mineral content of the dentine and also of the inter-connecting lateral processes of the odontoblastic processes. The importance clinically is that caries has to be followed laterally at the enamel–dentine junction, thereby producing undermined enamel which will need to be removed subsequently.

Dentine sensitivity

The question of reaction of dentine to external stimuli is one of the most important factors in aiding the dentist in his or her control of carious attack. We have already noted that progress of caries through dentine is more rapid than through enamel but this situation is limited by the fact that the dentine will react to attack, producing irregular secondary dentine, sometimes known as tertiary dentine. Perhaps the interesting question concerning the sensitivity of dentine is not how it is brought about but why it is necessary in the first place. Sensation in most parts of the body is a defence mechanism, allowing the organism to withdraw from noxious stimuli. People cannot readily withdraw the teeth, although they might conceivably seek to place unpleasant foods in another portion of the mouth. It may be that the sensitivity of dentine is concerned more with trophic mechanisms controlling the health of the pulpal tissue and may be associated in some way with the response of the odontoblast and its processes to outside stimuli. A major difference between dentine and enamel is that the former is capable of responding to carious attack or wear or fracture of the tooth and has a potential for healing. This will be discussed in greater depth in Chapter 6, but the living nature of the odontoblastic processes, cell bodies of the odontoblasts, and the continuing ability of the tissue to lay down pre-dentine mineralizing into dentine enables the tissue to respond to loss of tooth substance by walling off the vulnerable pulp tissue.

Pulpal involvement

Some dentinal lesions approaching the pulp may have sterile but cariously affected dentine at their base and a micro-exposure in this region could easily be contaminated from bacteria in the saliva. For this reason it is advisable for the operator to use rubber dam when excavating deep cavities of this nature. If pulpal involvement occurs on a small scale, the tooth should be made caries-free at the enamel–dentine junction and in a symptomless tooth calcium hydroxide can be used as an indirect pulp capping agent which will encourage the laying down of reparative dentine, walling off the lesion. If there is frank exposure of the pulp with bacterial invasion then eventually endodontic treatment will be necessary, but in the short term and to produce comfort for the patient, anti-inflammatory drugs may be placed over the carious exposure. It is very important in the initial stages of treatment planning to investigate all teeth with carious lesions, to excavate active caries and to dress temporarily the cavities by one or other of these methods. This not only allows the patient to remain in comfort whilst a lengthy treatment plan is carried out, but also allows the teeth to respond to sedative dressings, thereby making future cavity preparation less hazardous.

Because of the sigmoid nature of the dentinal tubules particularly in the root, the response to stimuli will be more apically placed than the stimulus itself, and this should be remembered during cavity preparation because the gingival base of the cavity will be better protected than the coronal portion, which is more easily exposed into the pulp.

6

Pathology of caries and pulpal disorders

An understanding of the pathology of caries and the way it affects the pulp is fundamental to much of restorative dentistry. This chapter considers the scientific evidence associated with the aetiology of caries, the ways in which enamel and dentine are destroyed and the effects on pulp. The clinical implications of these processes are discussed.

Introduction

Caries is essentially an attack on the mineralized tissues of the body, resulting in demineralization and in some cases in destruction of the matrix. In principle it may occur in all of the hard tissues including bone but for the purposes of this book discussion will be restricted largely to enamel and dentine. In the young, healthy human the dentine of the tooth is entirely protected by enamel or by the gingivae and periodontal tissues in the root area. Caries therefore must commence at the enamel surface. In older individuals where gingival recession and loss of periodontal and bone support has occurred the root of the tooth may be exposed to the mouth and caries may then occur *de novo* on the cementum and dentine.

Factors influencing caries

The crown of the tooth is in a micro-environment of its own, mainly that of the saliva, microbial deposits derived from the saliva and other sources, food debris and other dietary constituents. Whether caries commences or not seems to depend upon the quality of this environment, the ability of the tooth to resist demineralization, immunological reactions by the host and the length of time for which all these factors are in operation. The disease therefore has been described as *multifactorial* and in some texts as many as fifty factors have been

described in relation to carious attack. It is more profitable to group the factors into three: firstly, those associated with the host including the quality of the saliva and the bacterial flora therein; secondly, outside factors associated with diet and the substrate on which these bacteria act; and finally, the tooth itself and those features which either predispose to or resist carious attack (*Fig. 6.1*).

Host factors

When a tooth is developing within the alveolar process its enamel surface is protected by means of an *organic pellicle* and cellular covering. As it erupts into the oral cavity much of this protection is lost, but immediately on contact with the saliva a secondary organic pellicle is laid on the enamel surface and it is to this that organisms within the oral cavity attach themselves.

Microorganisms

Initially most of the organisms are streptococcal in nature, producing an immature plaque on the surface of the tooth. If this is allowed to be maintained other organisms of filamentous nature such as actinomyces will also be involved and the plaque is said to be mature. The organisms colonizing the plaque will depend upon those present in the oral cavity and may therefore vary from individual to individual. However, it has recently been shown that breast fed children may acquire

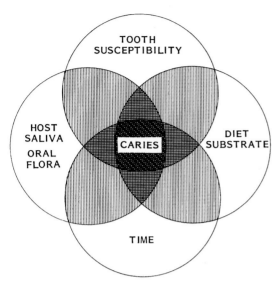

Fig. 6.1 Factors influencing the onset and spread of dental caries. Microbial breakdown products of dietary components may produce an adverse local environment that, if operative for sufficient time, may result in caries in a susceptible tooth

Streptococcus mutans from their mother, so that in this sense caries may be thought of as an infectious disease.

There has been a great deal of research to establish the nature of organisms associated with dental caries, much of which lies outside the scope of this chapter. Some of this work has been carried out on gnotobiotic animals, where it was shown that the difference between animals which were caries active and those which were caries resistant lay in the fact that the latter lacked particular microorganisms. In human enamel caries large numbers of organisms have been described on the enamel surface but in caries-susceptible individuals it seems that the most obvious organisms are lactobacilli and *Streptococcus mutans*. In older plaques, *Actinomyces* species are present but most studies have not implicated these particularly in the development of the early lesion. In the case of root caries the most commonly isolated organisms are of the actinomyces type followed by lacto-bacillie, *Streptococcus mutans* and *streptococcus sanguis*.

Saliva

Not only is the saliva responsible for the micro-environment of plaque organisms, but is in itself important in the development of early carious lesions. This is because caries is essentially a demineralizing disease requiring a fall in pH at the surface of the tooth. If the saliva is capable of resisting this change in pH because of *buffering capacity* then caries is less likely to ensue. It is known that high flow rates of saliva improve its buffering capacity so that caries is dependent not only on the quality of the saliva but also upon its quantity. It is, for instance, well known that caries increases in patients with xerostomia following irradiation of tumours in the oral region but there may also be changes of diet associated with these problems. Saliva is a supersaturated solution of calcium, phosphate, hydroxyl and fluoride ions and these may reduce the solubility of enamel and promote remineralization of early lesions. In addition, the saliva contains non-specific antibacterial agents such as lysozyme, lactoperoxidase and lactoferin and in addition contains immunoglobulin (Ig) A molecules. In those patients with inflammation of the periodontal tissues, IgC may be present in the serum exudate. It has been suggested that it may be possible to immunize patients against caries, but in Western society where caries prevalence seems to be falling it seems unlikely that this will be an acceptable procedure.

Oral hygiene

The final host factor of importance in caries is the ability to improve oral hygiene thereby removing the plaque from the surface of the teeth and preventing the production of acids initiating caries. Oral hygiene is usually considered to be mechanical using toothbrushes, toothpastes, floss and similar methods, but it must be remembered that oral hygiene is also a natural phenomenon which some individuals do well and others do not. The use of the tongue as a means of oral hygiene has received relatively little study but may well be a factor in reducing caries.

Diet

The second main group of factors associated with caries of the teeth is that of diet. Microbial plaque on the surface of teeth is only disastrous if there is sufficient substrate for these bacteria to work upon. Fermentable carbohydrates need to be present for acid to be formed. The problem is that in the presence of fermentable carbohydrates, the plaque bacteria produce acid rapidly, so that the pH in relation to the plaque falls precipitously very quickly. The recovery from this position to normal pH levels is an extended process. The major part of our dietary fermentable carbohydrate is sucrose, but lactose is present in milk and maltose is derived from the hydrolysis of starch. It seems that it is the frequency of fall in pH which is important and this information enables dentists to plan dietary advice for their patients. Attempts have been made to replace these fermentable carbohydrates by other types of sugar such as xylitol, which is a sugar alcohol but is not metabolized to acid by the plaque organisms. There are however difficulties in changing habits of a lifetime.

Tooth susceptibility

The third factor related to caries incidence appears to be the structure of the teeth themselves.

Morphology

Caries tends to occur at certain points on the teeth, such as the depth of the fissures and below the contact areas and cervical margins, and this suggests that the shape and morphology of the tooth is important, along with its ability or otherwise to shed food debris or to be cleansed by the patient's musculature or salivary flow. Packing of food between teeth which are malaligned may also constitute a problem. Fissures which are deep and difficult to cleanse may well be more liable to caries than shallow, cleanable fissures but the details of tooth morphology are best studied in texts related to that subject.

Chemistry

Using techniques of micro-probe analysis and micro-biopsy it has been possible to show that tooth structure varies chemically between different individuals. For example fluoride levels vary between individuals and this in itself may have an influence on their caries resistance.

Surface structure

It has become clear that the outer surface structure of enamel is extremely variable, and indeed in many patients in some of their teeth and at certain sites, the prisms of the enamel may in fact not reach the surface. The surface of the tooth in contact with the micro-environment is therefore said to be *aprismatic* but the relationship of this structural variation to their caries resistance is not clear.

Research methods

Most of the modern techniques of scientific investigation have been applied to caries over the decades. These have included epidemiological studies on the incidence of the disease and biochemical studies on the environment of the mouth and of the teeth themselves. It is beyond the scope of this book to discuss these in any detail. However, in order to understand the principles of restorative dentistry it is necessary to have a working knowledge of the pathology of the lesion itself.

Ground sections in polarized light

Most of the early work in this area consisted of the production of ground sections through teeth containing natural early lesions and much of it was directed towards the technology of producing sufficiently thin sections to be of use in these studies. Sections between 50 and 100 microns in thickness have now been achieved and these may be examined either in the light microscope or, more profitably and commonly, in the polarized light microscope. Polarized light is vibrating in one plane and this plane may be rotated by suitable crystalline materials. Enamel is such a material, as is dentine by nature of its hydroxyapatite content and its collagen matrix. When polarized light is passed through enamel it is rotated both by the crystals themselves and by the arrangement of the crystals in the form of prisms; the former is said to be *intrinsic* birefringence and the latter *form* birefringence. In the case of dentine the light is rotated by the crystals of hydroxyapatite and also by the repeat pattern of the collagen. Carious attack affects both the size and shape of the crystals and the spaces between them and the overall outline of the enamel prisms. In the case of dentine it may alter the collagen component as well. For these reasons carious lesions exhibit altered birefringence, the direction and extent of which not only indicates the extent of the lesion but may be used quantitatively to deduce the degree of demineralization.

Transmission electron microscopy

The availability of the transmission electron microscope (TEM) in the early 1960s held promise of detailed investigation both of normal and carious enamel, but it proved almost impossible to produce sections of sufficient thinness for this technique to be fully exploited. Thin sectioning is possible in partially demineralized enamel but there is doubt as to whether the sectioning procedure may alter the crystalline structure of the material being examined. Attempts were made to solve this problem by cutting thick sections through the lesions and taking carbon replicas which themselves could be examined in the TEM, and considerable progress was made using this technique.

Scanning electron microscopy

A decade later the scanning electron microscope became available and, since this records information from a cut surface by excitation of secondary electrons, thin sectioning was no longer needed. Although the method has been exploited to some extent in studies of caries, interpretation of the images and particularly the formation of smear layers during sectioning has proved difficult. Methods of removal of the smear layer using either chemical or preferably ion etching techniques are now in progress and back scatter electron imaging, which provides information from beneath the cut surface, is a recent promising advance. Modern SEMs allow analysis of emitted X-rays from the specimen being studied and electron microprobe analysis of this nature allows chemical analysis to be made in various parts of the lesion. X-ray and electron crystallography have also featured in studies of caries.

Microradiography

Since carious lesions in both enamel and dentine are characterized by loss of mineral, microradiographs can be used to demonstrate changes of mineral density within the lesions. It is necessary to use a graduated step wedge in order that a standard may be compared with the radiographic image and plane or parallel sections of known thickness are required in order to make the necessary calculations of mineral loss.

Microbiopsy

Recently, microbiopsy techniques have been evolved so that small portions of a carious lesion from a known position can be excised and analysed using some of the methods previously described. These biopsies are also available for biochemical study. Using such techniques the distribution, for instance, of fluoride ion within a lesion may be determined.

All of these methods have now been applied to natural human lesions and to artificially induced lesions in human and in animal teeth, so that the process of caries in mineralized tissues is now more fully (but still incompletely) understood.

Caries of enamel

When mineral is removed from the enamel by carious attack, the individual crystals making up the prisms diminish in size and the enamel is said to become more porous.

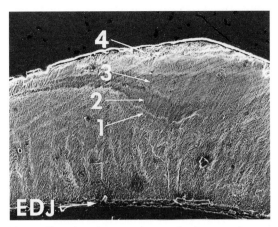

Fig. 6.2 Scanning electron micrograph of a ground section of an early 'white spot' carious lesion. It consists of four zones: 1, Translucent zone; 2, Dark zone; 3, Body of the lesion; 4, Surface zone. EDJ = Enamel–dentine junction

White spot lesion

Even a slight increase in porosity of the enamel changes its optical characteristics and in the initial stages it becomes less translucent, so that the earliest evidence of caries is known as a white spot lesion. At this stage the surface of the enamel is still intact and the lesion may be difficult to detect clinically. Histological studies using polarized light have shown that the lesion at this stage is not continuously progressive but may *remineralize*, so that processes of both destruction and repair are occurring simultaneously. When examined under the polarizing microscope in water, the lesion is described as cone shaped with its base just below an intact surface zone. The body of the lesion appears to be dark in colour and the incremental lines are accentuated. The use of quinoline as an inhibition medium of different refractive index allows further details of the early lesion to be described. Four zones may be seen in an early white spot lesion (*Fig. 6.2*).

Advancing front

Zone 1 is a translucent zone present at the advancing front of the lesion and is usually only seen in sections examined in quinoline. This zone is more porous than sound enamel, having a pore volume of about 1% compared with 0.1% in intact enamel.

Dark zone

Zone 2 is known as the dark zone and lies superficial to the translucent zone. It appears dark when examined in quinoline. Polarized light studies have shown that the pore volume is increased to 2–4% in this region. It is thought that the dark appearance is occasioned because some of the pores are too small to allow quinoline to enter, so that they retain air following sectioning. It has been speculated that some remineralization may be occurring here, reducing some of the pore sizes.

Lesion body

Zone 3 is the body of the lesion and since more than 5% of the enamel is porous and the size of the pores are large enough to allow water to enter, the body appears dark when examined under polarized light in water but translucent when examined in quinoline. In some parts of the body the pore volume may increase to 25%.

Surface zone

The fourth zone is known as the surface zone and is best seen in sections examined in water. It is an intact surface layer with a pore volume of less than 1% and is usually between 20 and 50 microns in thickness. Thus the early lesion is more demineralized in its depth than at its surface, and although it was first thought that the surface zone was caused by a hypermineralized zone at the surface of the tooth, it may be reproduced following removal of this surface layer. It is now thought that it may be caused by re-crystallization of dissolved mineral elements from deeper in the lesion.

Fissure caries

The foregoing description is that of an early lesion on the smooth surface of a tooth, and in the case of early fissure caries similar appearances are noted around the fissure wall. It should be noted that in many fissures examined in sections there is an enamel defect at the base, so that the lesion spreads very quickly into dentine. This may explain the recently described phenomenon of 'bomb' caries in teeth that have been subjected to fluoride ions during development or subsequently. The enamel around the sides of the fissure is resistant to carious attack by reason of its fluoride content, but the lesion spreads rapidly into dentine, spreading along the enamel–dentine, junction and cavitating the dentine although the fissure may appear clinically intact.

Electron microscopy

Electron microscope studies on early carious lesions have provided conflicting evidence. In most cases the interprismatic regions seem to be preferentially dissolved, but larger, unusually shaped crystals may be seen in this region and these may represent a remineralization phenomenon. The biopsy techniques previously described have shown that in the translucent zone the cross section diameters of the crystals are 25–30 nm compared with 30–40 nm in sound enamel. In the dark zone of the lesion crystal diameters may be 50–100 nm, whereas in the main body of the lesion they may be only 10 nm in diameter. These findings again support the view that remineralization of crystals is occurring in various parts of the early carious lesion.

Microradiography

Microradiographs of sections through the early lesion are sufficiently sensitive to demonstrate loss of mineral if this is more than about 5%. The body of the lesion therefore shows up well using this technique and the intact surface zone is also readily seen. In high resolution microradiography the outline of the incremental lines may be visible within the body of the lesion.

Biochemical studies using biopsies of the lesion or electron probe micro-analysis have confirmed these changes in enamel caries and have also shown that fluoride levels are high in this artificially porous material.

Progress of the lesion

As the lesion progresses through the enamel its apex may reach the enamel–dentine junction before collapse of the intact surface zone occurs, so lesions may be quite deep before they are easily detectable clinically. The enamel lesion, however, is extremely porous by this stage, so acids are able to diffuse easily across the junction and into the dentine. The implication is that dentine may be involved even when lesions appear to be restricted to enamel on standard clinical radiographs.

Caries in dentine

Caries spreading to dentine may be either subsequent to enamel caries having reached the enamel–dentine junction or in certain circumstances, that is exposure of the root of the tooth, it may commence *de novo* in the cementum and spread to the dentine directly.

Coronal caries

Involvement of dentine in the crown of the tooth may be either underneath smooth surface caries, usually at the contact area or immediately below it, or may be an extension of caries in an occlusal fissure. When the carious process reaches the enamel–dentine junction, it tends to spread laterally, involving the dentine on a wider front. In this way the enamel is undermined, so the resultant cavity preparation requires removal of sound enamel in order to approach infected dentine and to remove unsupported enamel prisms which, under areas of stress, will tend to fracture. Lesions of the occlusal fissures may directly involve dentine, since in many cases enamel is deficient at the base of the fissure.

Root caries

In patients where the root surfaces have become exposed, usually due to chronic inflammatory periodontal disease, but also in continuing eruption to compensate for occlusal wear, the root becomes directly exposed to plaque and carious attack. Chronic infective periodontal disease and continuing eruption due to occlusal wear are both commonly seen in older people, so that root caries tends to be a disease of old age. Root caries may extend from lesions at the cervical margin of the enamel or may attack dentine exposed directly by the aforementioned means. Root caries can be of two types. Active root caries is soft and pale in colour, whereas arrested lesions, possibly caused by good oral hygiene techniques, tend to stain and be hard and dark brown.

Dentine is a living reactive tissue and must be considered in association with the living pulp tissue beneath. Reactions to dentine caries therefore involve consideration of both the dentine itself and the underlying pulp tissue. The reaction and response of the pulp are considered below.

Microorganisms

Once the enamel has been penetrated, bacteria can gain access directly to the dentinal tubules and so the tissue becomes infected. The initial invasion of dentine appears to be mainly acidogenic, the acid presumably diffusing ahead of any microorganisms. The first organisms to invade the dentine appear to be lactobacilli and also cariogenic streptococci, notably *Streptococcus mutans*. Underneath the enamel–dentine junction, the microbiological population is mixed and organisms producing proteolytic hydrolytic enzymes may be found. At the advancing edge of the dentinal lesion is a zone

of demineralized dentine that bacteria have not yet penetrated. This is because the tubules are smaller than the diameter of most bacteria and only when the tubules have become laterally enlarged by dissolution of the intertubular matrix do bacteria enter. Superficial to the demineralized dentine is a zone of penetration in which bacteria are present in the tubules. Superficial to that again is a zone of complete destruction where the mineral content and organic matrix of the dentine have both been destroyed.

Effect on dentinal tubules

Once the dentine is infected it may react in several different ways. Those tubules directly located in the centre of the demineralized zone may appear to be empty because the cell processes of the odontoblasts have withdrawn. During section preparation these empty tubules may be filled with air, producing a dark colour under the light microscope, often referred to as a dead tract. Odontoblastic cell processes less acutely involved in the carious process, that is usually those at the periphery of the lesion, may react by laying down calcified material as the cell processes withdraw, thereby equalizing the refractive index of the dentine and producing a transparent or translucent sclerotic zone. The crystals in these tubules, when examined in the electron microscope, may have larger and more irregular crystals than in the normal dentine. They are considered to represent the result of remineralization. Sclerotic dentine may be considered as an extension of the normal process of production of peritubular dentine. The sclerotic dentine may consist initially of fine crystals of whitlockite and, at later stages of mineralization, a mixture of whitlockite and hydroxyapatite. The final obliteration of the tubule appears to be by hydroxyapatite crystals.

Secondary and tertiary dentine

The lesion eventually spreads towards the pulp of the tooth and the stimulus may cause reactionary tertiary dentine to be laid down in the pulp at the depth of the lesion in an attempt to wall off the advancing caries from the pulp. It may be a relatively well-formed tissue containing dentinal tubules and may be similar in structure to normal secondary dentine. It may also be an abnormal tissue with very few tubules and numerous interglobular zones. Reactionary dentine is most frequently formed when the stimulus is mild and the blood supply to the pulp is good, so it is more likely to be seen in younger teeth. If the stimulus is overwhelming, the odontoblast cells lining the pulp may be killed, and then of course no reactionary dentine can be produced. Under these circumstances the carious lesion will directly involve the pulp and this is discussed in the next section.

Response of the pulp

In the early stages of infection, the pulp reacts as would any other healthy tissue.

Hyperaemia

An inflammatory reaction occurs and in its initial stages this is characterized by hyperaemia. The pulpal blood vessels dilate, become more permeable, and fluid and defence cells pass out into the surrounding pulp tissue. This increases the pressure within the pulp and this pressure, unlike in soft tissues, cannot be relieved because of the enclosed nature of the pulpal tissue. The pressure therefore rises and the patient suffers pain. Initially this may be the case when transient stimuli, such as very hot liquids, or very cold liquids, are placed in contact with a carious lesion. The pain may last only as long as the stimulus is applied. Once the carious lesion has approached closely to the pulp, the stimulus may be continuous and the reaction of the pulp will depend upon the duration and intensity of this stimulus.

Chronic inflammation

If the lesion is progressing slowly towards the pulp, then toxins and thermal stimulation may be of a low grade nature and the result is chronic inflammation. Lymphocytes, plasma cells, macrophages and monocytes can be seen in the pulpal tissue and the tissue may survive. There may be no increase in intrapulpal pressure and therefore no symptoms.

Acute inflammation

If the stimuli reaching the pulp are stronger, then the blood vessels dilate, fluid passes out into the tissues and the pressure builds up to such an extent that the arterioles entering through the apical foramina may be occluded. Polymorphonuclear leucocytes are the main cells involved in acute inflammation. The increase in intrapulpal pressure leads, usually, to severe pain.

Pulpal necrosis

The rise in intrapulpal pressure may occlude the pulp's blood supply. This may be accompanied by an overwhelming bacterial infection from the carious lesion. The result of both of these is pulp death and the ceasing of any pain.

It is possible for a necrosed pulp to remain quiescent for many years with no evidence of such pathology. The apical foramen may become blocked with calcific deposits – a natural root filling.

On the other hand, the apical foramen may remain patent and there will be pathological effects in the periapical region.

Periapical involvement

The first effects of the pulpal infection are leaking of bacterial toxins and tissue breakdown products through the apical foramina to the periapical tissues. The response of these tissues may be either acute or chronic in nature, depending upon the severity of the stimulus. Later, bacteria may pass out into the tissues.

Acute periapical infection

The acute inflammatory reaction at the apex is also enclosed, this time by bone. The fluid exudate and the presence of oedema tends to force the tooth out of the socket and it is painful to bite on and there is a continuous throbbing pain. If left untreated there is continued pressure built up and the pain becomes intense. The pressure of the exudate and pus so formed leads to bone resorption and the fluid tracks through the bone along the line of least resistance. Eventually the periosteum may be penetrated, resulting in a release of pus and consequent reduction or relief of pain. A symptomless, progressively enlarging swelling is a common finding.

Chronic periapical infection

This is the more common sequel to pulp death and may arise from low grade irritation from the root canal, i.e. bacterial by-products leaking out into the apical tissues, or from the partial resolution of an acute response.

The precise pathology is again related to the virulence of the organisms and the host tissue reaction. The lower grade activity results in a more gradual removal of bone and the formation of granulation tissue. It is usually symptomless and often discovered only by diagnostic radiography.

Alternatively, the chronic response may, if the balance changes in the lesion, exacerbate into an acute one with the symptoms described above appearing.

The apical response is usually induced by toxins and tissue breakdown products only. The bacteria remain within the pulp chamber undisturbed by phagocytes. If any do pass beyond the apical foramen, they are usually killed by inflammatory cells. If, on the other hand, the bacteria leave the root canal in sufficient numbers and/or the inflammatory response loses its potency, then infection of the apical tissues, as opposed to irritation, will follow. The lesion may remain chronic though, with no evidence of the different circumstances.

The apical tissue response in a chronic lesion is usually granulomatous and may be accompanied by proliferation of epithelium. The epithelium originates from the cell rests of Malassez, which are the remnants of the epithelial root sheath of Hertwig. The inflammatory process appears to stimulate the growth of the cells. The *chronic apical granuloma* is a mass of chronic inflammatory cells, variable amounts of strands or sheets of epithelium and perhaps some pus, all surrounded by a fibrous tissue capsule.

In certain circumstances the epithelium forms a *periapical cyst*. Various theories of cyst formation have been proposed. These are:

- The block of proliferating cells enlarges and the central cells break down to form a cavity

- Cavities in the granuloma due to pus formation allow the epithelium to proliferate along the surface to form a continuous lining

- Strands and sheets of epithelium join up into a shell by chance

Once the epithelium lines a cavity, osmosis occurs. Fluid passes through the cell layer and the osmotic pressure causes slow expansion. For all this to happen and be seen takes some time – probably two years.

In the chronic periapical lesion, therefore, there may be a cyst or small cysts within a granuloma or a lesion that is essentially a cyst surrounded by a fibrous capsule, with no granulation tissue outside it. The cyst may become infected, depending upon the movement of bacteria from the root canal.

Relationship to clinical management

It should be clear from this description of the pathology of the carious lesion that in its earliest stages, i.e. the white spot lesion, there may be considerable difficulties in clinical diagnosis.

Early caries

The surface of the enamel is still intact and therefore the lesions can only be diagnosed either visually or radiographically. The use of a mirror and strong lighting may indicate a slight change in optical density below the contact area, and high intensity transillumination with a small fibreoptic probe may be more useful. Bitewing radiographs are unlikely to pick up the very early lesion, and it is said that by the time a lesion is visible using this means, it may well have progressed towards the enamel–dentine junction. All is not lost, however, since changes in oral hygiene practice, removal of plaque, administration of fluorides and good dietary control may cause such lesions to remineralize even though they were never diagnosed.

Remineralization

As these early lesions are cycling between destruction and repair, the clinician aims to tip the balance towards repair. There is some evidence that such remineralized lesions may resist further attack better than normal enamel. It may be that many patients diagnosed as caries free, have in fact remineralized early lesions from their own saliva.

Once cavitation of the surface has occurred, remineralization will not replace the normal contour of the tooth. For this reason probing should not be used in diagnosis of early lesions, since cavitation may be produced by the clinician. The early diagnosis of carious lesions is discussed in Chapter 2.

Very early caries is perhaps best diagnosed by a study of the risk factors to which the patient is subjected. Therefore, a good dietary history will be needed and it is clear that the younger patient is at greater risk than the older. The adequate secretion of saliva and its buffering capacity should be investigated and it may be useful to look at the types of organisms present in the saliva so that the high risk lactobacilli and *Strep. mutans* may be discerned.

Excavation of caries

Once the caries has involved the dentine, it will be necessary to remove softened and infected necrotic material. It is clear from the progression of the lesion that this may involve a larger cavity than at first appreciated, since the lesion will have extended along the enamel–dentine junction. It is currently believed necessary to remove all of the infected dentine at the junction. When the softened dentine in the bulk of the lesion has been removed, the decision has to be made on how to deal with the infected area of dentine overlying the pulp. A current approach is to excavate the infected dentine, leaving the attacked translucent zone over the pulp intact. The determination of this zone has largely relied on clinical experience, but dyes have been produced which may stain the infected dentine but not the translucent zone (Chapter 11). Providing the tooth has been symptomless and appears to be vital, the translucent area of dentine covering the pulp may be capped with a calcium hydroxide paste, the rationale here being to protect the pulp and induce the formation of reparative dentine. If there is clinical evidence of acute or chronic inflammation of the pulp usually by symptoms, then the inevitable sequel may be death of the pulp requiring eventual root canal therapy. Decisions as to how to stabilize and treat the initial carious lesions should be made in the early appointments before planning the detailed restorative treatment. Thus it is far better to treat temporarily all the lesions in the mouth at an early stage rather than going ahead with definitive restorative treatment of a few.

Reactions of the pulp underlying carious lesions may give some clinical information to the dentist as to the health or otherwise of the tissues. Thus a patient who complains of transient pain following hot and cold drinks, the pain lasting for the duration of the stimulus, may well have pulpal hyperaemia which may be reversible if stabilization of the cavity is achieved using the methods described. Once the pulp has become infected it may, if the inflammation is chronic, produce no symptoms. Under these circumstances the patient may complain of no pain and the pulp may eventually recover. However, it may slowly die without symptoms and the dentist should be aware of this possibility and keep future checks on the health and vitality of that particular tooth. If the patient complains of continuous lancing pain then the tooth pulp is almost certainly acutely inflamed and a vital removal of the pulp or the tooth is probably indicated. In patients where this has not occurred, the acute continuous pain may eventually resolve for a time as the inflammation expands through the apical foramen and the pressure is released. During hyperaemia the patient may be able to localize the intermittent sharp pain to a particular tooth, but when acute pulpitis intervenes the pain may radiate over a larger area. As the inflammation extends into the periapical tissues and in the absence of the satisfactory response by the patient it may eventually involve alveolar bone. The pain then may become deep-seated and throbbing and may be localizable because the tooth is tender to percussion or biting. If the infection extends through the bone, producing a localized osteitis, it may track through the bone, reducing the pressure somewhat and therefore the pain, but then raise the periosteum either buccally or lingually to produce again severe pain and the presence of an apical abscess. If this abscess discharges into the buccal or lingual sulci the pain may again cease because of reduction of pressure. However, it may spread above the level of attachment of the muscles of the mandible and maxilla and the final sequel is a *cellulitis* or facial swelling over the area. Patients are likely to seek emergency dental treatment at any point where the pressure is high either in the pulp, the periapical tissues, the bone or the facial tissues. Reduction of pressure at certain stages of the advance of the infection explains why patients frequently sit in the dental chair saying, 'The pain was acute but it stopped as soon as I came to see the dentist.'

7

The periodontium in health and disease

This chapter and Chapter 13 will summarize those areas of periodontology that are of clinical relevance to an understanding of the disease, its treatment and restorative dentistry. The text is devoted almost entirely to gingivitis and chronic adult periodontitis. The space available does not allow for an exhaustive text on periodontology and readers are referred to the bibliography for additional reading.

Introduction

Periodontal disease, which encompasses gingivitis and periodontitis, is highly prevalent in all populations. The development of gingivitis is due to the accumulation and maturation of supragingival plaque and subgingival plaque is associated with the advancing lesions of periodontitis. As periodontitis progresses, bone loss will compromise the integrity of teeth resulting in looseness and/or drifting out of their normal alignment. In planning restorative dental procedures the periodontal status of the individual must be considered and rectified, if unhealthy, before commencing restoration of the dentition. As importantly, the consequences of particular restorative procedures to periodontal health should be evaluated, particularly in the treated periodontal patient who clearly has a susceptibility to the disease.

Healthy periodontium

The periodontium comprises the tissues investing and supporting the teeth, namely the *gingiva, alveolar bone, periodontal ligament* and *cementum.*

Gingiva

The gingiva is the only tissue of the periodontium that is visible and comprises the marginal and attached gingiva, that are separated from each other by the free gingival groove and from the alveolar mucosa by the mucogingival junction. The tissue is pink in colour and may be stippled to produce an 'orange peel' appearance. The colour may be modified by different degrees of melanin pigmentation and keratinization

The structure consists of keratinizing stratified squamous epithelium attached to the alveolar bone by connective tissue. There are collagen fibres embedded in an extracellular matrix that are arranged in groups by virtue of their orientation and named:

- Circular (around the teeth)
- Transeptal (joining teeth)
- Dentogingival (cementum to free gingiva)
- Dentoperiosteal (cementum to attached gingiva)
- Crestal (alveolar crest to attached gingiva)

The *marginal gingiva* forms a cuff 1–2 mm wide around the tooth and fills the interdental space as a labial and lingual papillae joined by a *gingival col* between the tooth and below the contact point. It forms the gingival crevice (0–2 mm deep) and here is lined by crevicular epithelium that is non-keratinizing stratified squamous epithelium.

The marginal gingiva is joined to the tooth at or just above the cemento-enamel junction by the junctional epithelium, that has cells arranged parallel to the tooth surface with wide intercellular spaces, and contains small numbers of neutrophils.

The *attached gingiva* is a mucoperiosteum tightly bound to the alveolar bone and has a variable width that does not correlate with health. The absence of attached gingiva is not necessarily pathological, providing plaque control is adequate.

Alveolar bone

Alveolar bone consists of cancellous bone covered by a thin layer of compact bone that supports the teeth and is tooth dependent; it resorbs to a variable degree when teeth are lost. The bone adjacent to the tooth root is perforated (the *cribriform plate*) and receives the insertion of the periodontal ligament fibres. The alveolar crest maintains a relatively constant distance of 1–2 mm from the cemento-enamel junction (*biologic width*).

Periodontal ligament

The periodontal ligament suspends the tooth in the socket and acts like a visco-elastic shock absorber, permitting small movements of the teeth when under load. It consists of principal collagen fibre bundles (*Sharpey's fibres*), namely *alveolar crest*, *horizontal*, *oblique* and *apical*, all of which extend from the cementum to the alveolus. It has a very high connective tissue turnover.

Cementum

Cementum is the usually thin layer of calcified connective tissue covering the whole of the root surface and into which the periodontal ligament fibres are inserted. There are two types, *acellular* (cervical area) and *cellular* (mid and apical area), depending on the presence of cementocytes within the structure.

Periodontal disease

This section considers *gingivitis* and *periodontitis* as essentially separate entities. At present, there is insufficient evidence to permit the conclusion that factors relevant to gingivitis are relevant to periodontitis. The concept that plaque causes gingivitis and, in time, gingivitis inextricably progresses to periodontitis that in turn, left untreated, leads to tooth loss, is no longer held.

Nevertheless, gingivitis and periodontitis are not mutually exclusive nor unrelated; indeed gingivitis is one aspect of periodontitis (see definition of periodontitis). Data indicate that not all gingivitis

progresses to periodontitis and populations with poor oral hygiene and severe gingivitis have incidences of periodontitis little different from those populations with less plaque and gingivitis.

Gingivitis is thus a poor predictor of future periodontitis in the as yet unaffected individual or tooth site. Even in individuals treated for periodontitis and therefore, by definition, susceptible to the condition, the recurrence of gingivitis is a poor predictor (30%) of recurrence of periodontitis.

Conversely, and most importantly, the absence of gingivitis is highly predictive (99%) of no recurrence of periodontitis. Taken together, the evidence supports the concept that periodontitis is always preceded by gingivitis, and the prevention of gingivitis through supragingival plaque control will prevent the occurrence or recurrence of periodontitis. This concept has widespread implications for public health preventive programmes for periodontal disease and is also of major relevance to the total care and long-term management of the restorative patient. A high standard of supragingival plaque control must be practised by all patients, particularly those who already exhibit a susceptibility to periodontitis.

Gingivitis

Definition

Gingivitis is inflammation of the marginal gingiva without loss of attachment.

Clinical features

Inflamed gingiva exhibits redness, variable swelling, bleeding, usually in response to minor trauma such as toothbrushing, and increased flow of the crevicular fluid. Pain is not usually present, although vague sensory symptoms may be reported by some individuals (wedging, tingling, itching).

Aetiology

Epidemiological data have shown a strong correlation between plaque and gingivitis (correlation coefficient ≈ 0.8).

Controlled clinical trials have proved a direct cause and effect relationship between plaque and gingivitis. This forms the basis for the prevention of gingivitis and logically, therefore, periodontitis through the control of supragingival plaque.

Plaque formation

Enamel in the mouth is always covered by a salivary pellicle of glycoprotein that increases in thickness with time to several micrometres. Even if removed by polishing, pellicle re-forms in minutes. Primary plaque-forming bacteria, Gram positive facultative streptococci such as *Streptococcus sanguis* and some Gram-negative *Actinomyces* species, attach to this pellicle. These primary plaque formers are essential for the attachment of other bacteria.

The adsorption mechanism is complex and involves a number of forces and physical interactions between the bacteria and oral surfaces. Compatible surface free energies, hydrophobicities and specific attachment sites are important factors in bacterial adherence. Bacterial seeding is slow and the plaque mass increases mainly by bacterial division.

Over a period of a few days increased proportions of anaerobic Gram negative cocci attach and proliferate. These are followed by rods and filamentous bacteria such as fusiforms, and finally spirochaetes and other motile rods can be found. Supragingival plaque thus develops in thickness and complexity and these are almost certainly mutually dependent processes. It is in association with the later stages of plaque development that the clinical features of gingivitis appear.

Pathogenesis of gingivitis

Bacteria are not thought to penetrate crevicular epithelium, but induce an inflammatory response in the gingiva by chemical byproducts. Bacteria release a range of enzymes capable of damaging all cellular and supporting tissues of the gingiva, and these also allow the penetration of high molecular weight bacterial endotoxins through crevicular epithelium. The net result is an inflammatory response with elements akin to both acute and chronic inflammation. Neutrophils and macrophages accumulate in the connective tissue and pass into the gingival crevice. Vascular dilatation and vascularity increases, with fluid extravasation, and lymphocytes and plasma cells appear within the tissues.

Epidemiological considerations

Gingivitis is considerably less prevalent and less severe in the primary dentition, whilst periodontitis affecting deciduous teeth is rare and usually a feature of an underlying systemic disease affecting host defence, e.g. cyclical neutropaenia.

Gingivitis is highly prevalent (100%) in the permanent dentition from a young age whilst the severity and number of sites affected varies at the extreme in individuals. The most important factors influencing the severity of gingivitis relate to those that influence the oral hygiene practices of individuals, by either directly or indirectly affecting compliance and dexterity.

In general, oral hygiene and gingival health are worse in :

- Low social classes
- Males compared to females
- Pre-teenage years compared to teenage (further increase in age has little affect on oral hygiene)
- Individuals who toothbrush less than twice daily (further increases in toothbrush frequency do not improve oral hygiene)
- Smokers
- Physically and mentally handicapped individuals
- Right buccal quadrants of the dental arches in right-handed toothbrushers
- Individuals wearing removable dental prostheses or fixed or removable orthodontic appliances

Oral hygiene and gingival health are little affected by:

- Tooth crowding
- Mucogingival anomalies – high fraenal attachments, shallow sulci
- Narrow zones or absence of attached gingivae

Gingival health is *always* compromised by restorations that encroach upon the gingival crevice.

Modifying factors

The gingival response to supragingival plaque appears to be exaggerated or changed by certain local and systemic factors including:

- Incompetent lips and mouth breathing, particularly during adolescence
- Puberty
- Pregnancy
- Contraceptive pill
- Drugs – notably Epanutin, cyclosporin A, nifedipine and other calcium channel blockers, notably amlodipine, felodipine and lacidipine, that possibly result in gingival hyperplasia
- HIV infection
- Neutropaenias, notably cyclical neutropaenia
- Leukaemias, particularly acute leukaemias where marked swelling may occur due to gingival infiltration with large numbers of leukaemic cells
- Nutritional deficiency, notably of ascorbic acid

NB. Most of the modifying factors listed above for gingivitis do not appear or have not been proven to modify periodontitis (see section on periodontitis below).

Strategies for prevention of gingivitis

The basis for the control of gingivitis is supragingival plaque control. Two aspects are important:

- Prevention of development of a mature pathogenic plaque (*primary control*)
- Removal or modification of factors which facilitate plaque formation and retention (*secondary control*)

Primary control can be achieved by mechanical and chemical approaches, namely:

- Prevention of bacterial attachment (*antiadhesive approach*)
- Prevention of bacterial proliferation (*antimicrobial approach*)
- Regular removal of accumulated plaque (*mechanical and chemical cleaning approach*).

All of these approaches are possible and have been achieved in other environmental and industrial areas where microbial plaques pose problems. In the oral cavity, success to date has only been realistically achieved with the antimicrobial and mechanical cleaning approaches (see Chapter 13).

Secondary control has preventive and therapeutic implications for restorative treatment that involves:

- The preparation and placement of restorations
- Positioning of margins in relation to the gingiva
- The design and precision of fixed and removable prostheses construction

Therapeutic considerations concern the replacement or removal of fixed or removable restorative plaque traps, treatment of carious cavities and removal of supragingival calculus.

Periodontitis

Definition

Periodontitis may be defined as gingivitis with loss of attachment typically producing a periodontal pocket. This is a useful definition since it describes the histological lesion of periodontitis and suggests an approach to management that is based on preventive and therapeutic strategies.

Clinical features

Loss of attachment whereby the junctional epithelium migrates along the root surface results in the typical lesion of periodontitis, namely a *pocket*. The true pocket is measured from the cemento-enamel junction to the base of the attachment, whereas pocket depth is the distance from the gingival margin of the base of the pocket. Pocket depth may therefore be greater than the loss of attachment when the gingival height is above the cemento-enamel junction, or be less when the gingival margin is below the cemento-enamel junction (recession).

Colour change is variable in periodontitis. Thus, the gingival margins may exhibit all the features of gingivitis or appear perfectly normal. Usually, however, there is bleeding on probing when the probe is inserted to the base of the pocket and a purulent exudate may also be seen at the pocket orifice. Pain is not a feature of periodontitis although vague sensory symptoms may be reported, such as awareness of the teeth.

Aetiology

Subgingival plaque, derived from supragingival plaque, is always associated with the advancing lesions of periodontitis. The progression of gingivitis to periodontitis is thought to occur when *periodontal pathogenic microorganisms* act upon a *susceptible host*.

Periodontal pathogens   In excess of 400 species of microorganism have been found in periodontal pockets, of which about a third have yet to be identified. To date, approximately 20 are considered putative pathogens and most of these are obligate anaerobes.

Strong evidence exists for the following organisms to be considered actual pathogens:

- *Actinobacillus actinomycetemcomitans* (facultative anaerobe)
- *Porphyromonas gingivalis*
- *Bacteriodes forsythus*

Less strong evidence supports *Campylobacter, Eubacterium, Fusobacterium, Prevotella, Peptostreptococcus* and *Eikenella* species as periodontal pathogens. The mere presence of these organisms in periodontal lesions is not necessarily indicative of progressing disease.

Microbiological diagnosis is therefore of little or no value in the diagnosis and management of periodontal disease; this includes the decision to use and the choice of antimicrobial therapy.

The micro-organisms associated with periodontitis can be found at several sites:

- Periodontal sites:

    Root surface
    Pocket lumen
    Pocket epithelium
    Dentinal tubules

- Oral sites:

    Tongue
    Tonsil

- Extra-oral sites:

    Spouse/partner
    Family pet

Susceptibility There is some evidence for a major gene effect in *early onset forms* of periodontitis that dictates susceptibility. However, in adult periodontitis, there is no evidence for a major gene effect.

Neutrophil defects are associated with increased or rapid periodontal breakdown that even affect the deciduous dentition. These include cyclical and other neutropaenias, leukaemias, Chediak–Higashi syndrome, Down's syndrome and Papillon–Lefèvre syndrome.

Smoking is a risk factor, probably due to adverse effects on host defence mechanisms, and the response to treatment in smokers appears compromised.

Limited evidence suggests diabetes mellitus is a risk factor for periodontitis. Conversely periodontitis may be a risk factor for arteriosclerosis and low birthweight and may compromise diabetic control.

Stress is suspected as a risk factor for periodontal breakdown but evidence is lacking. Part of the increased susceptibility with smoking, diabetes and stress may be adverse effects on polymorph function.

Excessive occlusal loading and food packing appear to be co-destructive factors in periodontitis.

Pathogenesis Periodontal lesions typically develop as loss of epithelial attachment at the cemento-enamel junction. Associated with this is widening of epithelial spaces, ulceration of the sulcular epithelium, breakdown of collagen and ground substance, and bone resorption.

For this process to occur, pathogenic factors must overcome or exceed protective mechanisms. The latter are derived from the intact nature of the sulcular epithelium, gingival crevicular fluid, rapid tissue turnover and non-specific and specific defence and immune systems. The major pathogenic factors are the bacterial enzymes and toxins that can have direct destructive effects and/or initiate adverse host immune responses. These adverse host immune responses include the production of cytokines and host enzymes such as collagenase, and are probably initiated by bacterial lipopolysaccharide.

Epidemiological considerations

Chronic adult periodontitis shows a very low incidence in the second decade of life but increases progressively in succeeding decades. Approximately 60% of 60–70 year olds will have chronic adult periodontitis affecting one or more teeth. The average rate of progression of periodontitis, measured by radiographic bone loss or loss of attachment, is approximately 0.1 mm/year.

In any population only a small proportion (8–10%) exhibit advanced periodontitis (loss of attachment >6 mm) at one or more sites. A relatively small proportion of individuals and percentage of sites in those individuals account for most of the advanced periodontitis in any population.

Periodontium and restorations

The relationship between the periodontium and the provision of restorations involves certain key areas:

- Prevention
- Treatment planning
- Technical execution
- Maintenance

Whilst gingivitis is almost universal, the accurate prediction of susceptibility of individuals and particular intra-oral sites to periodontitis is not possible. Even in those patients who are known to be susceptible, the site specificity for rapid breakdown cannot be predicted. Therefore, *prevention* of gingivitis or recurrence of periodontitis must be a high priority for all restorative dentistry patients.

The provision of restorations for most patients must be viewed as having the potential to influence adversely their susceptibility to gingivitis and possibly periodontitis. Virtually all restorations compromise plaque control and the procedures used to place them may be harmful too. The more complex the restoration the higher the risk. *Treatment plans* should therefore be based on providing the minimum number of restorations of the simplest and least plaque-retaining type.

When considering the design of bridgework (Section IV), whilst direct masticatory loads are modified by biofeedback where the periodontium is reduced, excessive twisting or tilting forces widen the periodontal membrane space and can cause tooth movement and/or physiological mobility but not loss of attachment. The viscoelastic nature of the periodontal ligament has to be considered when restorations are linked between teeth, as in fixed bridgework, or when teeth are linked to osseo-integrated implants, which have no mobility.

Technical aspects of restorations of importance in prevention or initiation of periodontal disease relate particularly to the effects on the gingival sulcus. Mechanical instrumentation and restoration margin placement in the gingival sulcus may directly produce loss of attachment, particularly if there is encroachment on the biologic width. The gingival sulcus limits the subgingival extent of restorations and may therefore introduce aesthetic restrictions, particularly in the anterior region. Subgingival restoration margins always result in a variable degree of bacterial-associated gingival inflammation, but this may not necessarily progress to periodontitis. However, overhanging subgingival restorations cause loss of attachment and alveolar bone loss.

Lost interdental papillae can also have implications for aesthetics, and surgical mucogingival techniques to rebuild papillae are difficult and unreliable. Once gingival recession occurs, loss of cementum rapidly results, thereby predisposing sites to dentine hypersensitivity.

Operative treatment may be required to remove aetiological or co-destructive influences on periodontitis, such as marginal overhangs, negative edges or incorrect restoration contour.

For the maintenance of periodontal health, restorative dentistry must be of the highest quality both in design and execution. In addition, patients have an equal role to play in performing regular and efficient plaque control. The dentist must ensure that appropriate oral hygiene measures are taught and periodically reinforced as part of the continuing care programme.

8

Functional anatomy of the occlusion

Occlusion is probably the most daunting and confusing subject within restorative dentistry. Much of this confusion arises because there is little scientific evidence to support clinical practice, and terminology is often random. There is considerable work on the anatomy and physiology of occlusal function but the establishment of generally agreed principles for occlusal restoration and therapy remains elusive.

This book tries to take a pragmatic approach and considers:

- What constitutes 'normal' occlusal anatomy and physiology (this chapter)
- The basic requirements for restoration of the occlusion (Chapter 14)
- The causes and management of 'occlusal dysfunction' (Chapter 26)

Whilst the word 'Occlusion' refers strictly to the act of closing the teeth together, it has come to include the way in which:

- The mandible moves in relation to the skull
- The teeth are aligned in each jaw
- Teeth contact each other during the complicated movements of chewing or speaking
- The dentition should be restored
- Disorders of the masticatory apparatus should be managed

The study of occlusion in a functional sense therefore includes the temporomandibular joints and the neuromuscular control of mandibular movement, as well as the teeth themselves.

The masticatory apparatus is unique in the whole body because of the close interactions between differing structural entities. Malfunctions in the joints themselves, the muscles operating them, the neuromuscular reflexes controlling them or imperfections in the interdigitation of up to 32 teeth may all result in dysfunction of the masticatory apparatus as a whole.

Temporomandibular joints

Articulation between the fused right and left portions of the maxilla and mandible is by the temporomandibular joints (TMJ). Each is unique in the body in terms of function since it is the only place in which left and right joints are linked via a relatively inflexible bone, the mandible. This means that movements of each joint may not take place independently of the other, therefore it is possible that undue stresses on one joint may be transmitted to the other. The joints are also unique in that their pattern of movement and the forces transmitted to them are modified by the teeth.

Anatomy

The upper part of the TMJ is composed of the *glenoid fossa* that is an oval depression in the base of the temporal bone. This depression is bounded anteriorly by the *articular eminence*, a bony swelling down which the head of the *mandibular condyle* moves during function.

The glenoid fossa lies immediately in front of the external auditory meatus, and its posterior border is limited by the squamo-tympanic fissure and the postglenoid tubercle. The tubercle is a small, conical eminence separating the articular surface from the anterior margin of the tympanic part of the bone.

The roof of the glenoid fossa is sufficiently thin to be transparent if transilluminated in a dried skull, which suggests that the joint is not adapted to bear much stress.

The other half of the joint is the *condylar process* of the mandible, a rounded structure about 15–20 mm in the mesiolateral dimension and 8–10 mm anteroposteriorly. The long axis of each condyle is angulated so that lines drawn through them will meet at a point posterior to the mandible itself. This is because the condyles appear to be set at right angles to the main body of the mandible on each side.

In the adult, the articulating bony surfaces of both condyle and glenoid fossa are composed of dense cortical bone that is covered by dense fibrous connective tissue.

Ligaments

The ligaments probably do not support the joint during normal function, but restrict the *border movements* of the mandible, and therefore define the *envelope* within which all movements occur. There are four ligaments associated with the joint.

The *temporomandibular ligament* extends from the base of the zygomatic process of the temporal bone and the articular tubercle, and runs downwards and backwards to be inserted into the neck of the condyle. It appears to be separate from, and lateral to, the *capsular ligament* that forms a kind of collar around the neck of the condyle and runs upwards to be attached around the periphery of the glenoid fossa.

The capsular ligament completely surrounds the joint cavity to form a synovial capsule.

During opening of the jaw, the temporomandibular ligament restricts hinge movement, but when wider opening occurs, the head of the condyle moves forward on to the articular eminence. This relaxes the temporomandibular ligament, and causes the third ligament, the *sphenomandibular*, to become taut. This ligament is situated some distance from the joint itself, and arises from the spinous process of the sphenoid bone, passing downwards and forwards to be inserted into the lingula on the lingual side of the ramus of the mandible.

The fourth ligament is the *stylomandibular*, that extends from the styloid process to the posterior border of the angle. This also limits the anterior movement of the mandible.

Temporomandibular disc

The joint cavity is divided into upper and lower compartments by a biconcave, oval shaped disc of fibrous tissue that is sandwiched between the head of the condyle and the bone of the glenoid fossa. Its inferior surface is concave and its superior surface convex, and it has the appearance of a baseball cap placed over the head of the condyle with the peak arranged anteriorly.

The crown of the cap is thickened by a posterior band of dense connective tissue and, at the junction of the crown and the peak of the cap, there is a second thickening, the anterior fibrous band. Between these bands is a less dense intermediate zone, and behind the posterior band is the bilaminar region, consisting of an upper part attached to the posterior wall of the glenoid fossa and a lower part attached to the back of the condyle (*Fig. 8.1*).

The borders of the disc are attached to the fibrous capsule of the joint, except anteriorly, where the peak of the disc is attached to fibres of the lateral pterygoid muscle. There may be some attachment of the disc laterally to fibres of the masseter and temporal muscles.

Posteriorly, the disc is attached to a thick layer of vascularized connective tissue, and in this region the disc contains elastic fibres. The part of the capsule inserted into the disc from above, and that is attached to the glenoid fossa, is loose and therefore permits extensive sliding movements of the upper joint compartment.

The lower part of the capsule that attaches the disc to the neck of the condyle is much denser, allowing only hinge movement in the lower joint compartment. A synovial membrane, composed of connective tissue with many capillaries, lines the peripheral parts of the disc and the capsule but does not cover the articulating surfaces. It secretes synovial fluid into the joint spaces. This fluid has a jelly-like consistency and is composed largely of hyaluronic acid. The amount of synovial fluid present in normal function is very small and it is assumed that the joint spaces are normally collapsed.

Microscopic anatomy of the joint

Bones

The articular surfaces consist of fibrous connective tissue overlying undifferentiated mesoderm that itself overlies a thin layer of hyaline cartilage. This cartilage is most predominant in younger joints, and is a growth cartilage taking part in the normal development of the joint, and may be involved in remodelling processes in adulthood.

Below the layer of cartilage is compact bone covering the cancellous bone of the internal structure of the mandible. In old age, not only may the cartilage zone be lost, but so may the fibrous tissue covering at least some areas, resulting in denuding of the compact bone layer.

Articular disc

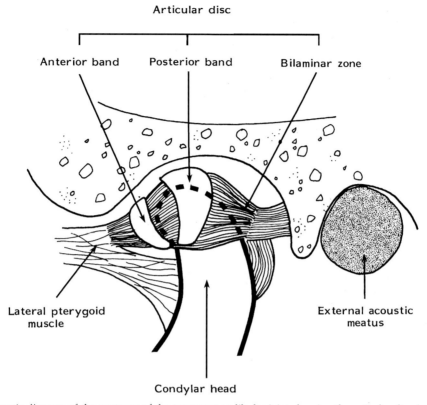

Anterior band   Posterior band   Bilaminar zone

Lateral pterygoid
muscle

External acoustic
meatus

Condylar head

Fig. 8.1 Schematic diagram of the anatomy of the temporomandibular joint showing the articular disc (meniscus) as the shape of a 'baseball cap' lying over the condylar head, and dividing the joint space into upper and lower compartments

Disc

The central part of the disc consists of dense connective tissue, but peripherally it has a looser texture, rich in vessels and nerves, particularly posteriorly in the bilaminar region. The capsule and parts of the disc are enervated by branches of the auriculo-temporal nerve that are arranged so that they are not compressed during movements of the joint.

The blood supply to the temporomandibular joint is from the superficial branch of the external carotid artery.

Muscles of mastication

These may be divided simplistically into closing and opening muscles. However, it must be remembered that relaxation of the closing muscles is necessary to allow the opening muscles to operate,

so that all the muscles are operational during mandibular movement.

The *masseter* is made up of two main bundles of muscle fibres originating from the lower border of the zygomatic arch and running downwards and slightly backwards, to be inserted on the lateral side of the ramus of the mandible. Its major function is to close the jaws together with great force, although it may also protrude the mandible slightly during this movement.

The *temporal* muscle has a broad origin from the lateral surface of the parietal bone and its anterior fibres run more or less vertically, its middle fibres obliquely, and its posterior fibres almost horizontally, all to be inserted into the coronoid process. It is used to position the mandible during closing movements. Usually, the anterior fibres contract first, elevating the mandible, followed by the others to control fine positioning.

The activity of the temporal muscle is extremely complex and unilateral contraction is involved in lateral mandibular excursions. The muscle is extremely important in dysfunction (Chapter 26), since the pain arising from its spasm is reported by patients as headache.

The *medial pterygoid* muscle originates in the pterygoid fossa and its fibres run downwards, backwards and outwards to be inserted into the inner aspect of the ramus. It is able to elevate the mandible and position it laterally. During protrusive and lateral movements, the activity of this muscle is greater than that of the temporalis.

The *lateral pterygoid* muscle has two heads, one arising from the outer part of the lateral pterygoid plate and the other from the base of the sphenoid bone. The two heads come together and are inserted into the neck of the condyle and, through the anterior wall of the capsule, into the disc. The main function of this muscle is to draw both the head of the condyle and the disc forwards during opening movements. Unilateral contraction will produce lateral movement of the mandible in association with the other muscles.

There are *minor muscles of mastication* which include the *digastric* and the *buccinator*.

The digastric is an opening muscle running from the mastoid process to a bursa on the hyoid bone and up to the genial tubercles of the mandible. Contraction draws the chin downwards, but this is aided considerably by gravity so that the muscle is most prominent in the final opening movements.

The buccinator muscles are concerned with maintaining the muscular activity of the cheeks and retaining food on the occlusal surfaces of the teeth.

Temporomandibular joint function

The TMJ is capable of two movements:

● Rotation
● Sliding (translation)

Rotation occurs in the lower joint compartment and the axis for this is the mandibular *hinge axis*. When the condylar heads are in their most posterior superior (retruded) positions in the glenoid fossae, the axis of rotation is referred to as the *terminal hinge axis*. The path of rotation is then called the *retruded arc of closure* or *reflex arc of closure*.

Sliding or translation occurs in the upper joint compartment. The disc should locate on the head of the condyle throughout, though during sliding it lags behind the condyle somewhat so that the condyle comes to bear on the anterior fibrous thickening. The lateral pterygoid muscles are the principal protruders of the mandible, moving the discs anteriorly as well. The return movement of the mandible is caused by the elevator muscles of mastication but the disc is returned posteriorly only by elasticity of the bilaminar zone.

If the discs get out of phase with the condylar heads or the bilaminar zones lose their elasticity, then 'clicks' occur during movement. The disc may become trapped anteriorly to the condylar head on closure and the click occurs as the condylar head rides backwards on the posterior band. On the next opening movement the disc is released and moves sharply posteriorly as the condylar head moves forward.

When the mandible moves to open the mouth from its retruded position with the teeth touching, it will initially describe an arc about the terminal hinge axis. At about 15 mm open, further hinge movement is impossible and the condyles slide forwards, taking their discs with them, and continue the rotation on a wider arc until maximum opening is reached (*Fig. 8.2*). The pathway described forms the posterior boundary of the envelope of border movements (*Posselt's envelope*). The superior boundary of the envelope is determined by the teeth and the remainder to a large extent by the ligaments around the TMJ.

Lateral movement of the condyles within the fossae occurs as the mandible moves to the left or right and is called *side shift*.

Teeth

Centric occlusion

Centric occlusion (CO) is the position of maximum intercuspation of the teeth and is also referred to as the *intercuspal position* (ICP). Because it is usually the position where exact interdigitation occurs, it may be called the position of 'best fit'.

CO is used in function to stabilize the mandible for swallowing or as a position for resting during mastication. Most individuals swallow with their teeth together with the lips forming the anterior oral seal. Whilst individuals close their teeth into CO automatically, the position is learnt behaviour and appears to be in the short-term memory.

As a minority behaviour, tooth apart swallowing is recognized. This may be caused by discrepancies in arch form, tooth position or soft tissue morphology; the reader is referred to texts on orthodontics for further reading on this subject.

CO is a position that is used hundreds of times each day for swallowing saliva and is the major reference position for occlusal restoration. The vast majority of restorations are adjusted to CO with the patient being asked to 'close together on to your back teeth'.

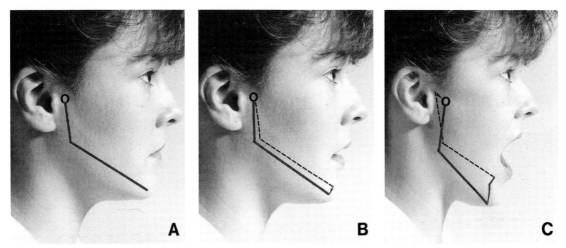

Fig. 8.2 Opening the mouth from the retruded contact position (**A**), the mandible first describes an arc on the terminal hinge axis (**B**), followed by protrusion and rotation to wide opening (**C**). This movement is the posterior border of Posselt's envelope. Opening from centric occlusion would trace an arc slightly anterior to this

The basic unit of centric occlusion is the *cusp/fossa relationship*, with a *supporting cusp* occluding with a *centric stop* (*Fig. 8.3A*). The centric stop may be a fossa or a pair of marginal ridges or a single sluiceway (*Fig. 8.3B*). Each cusp will rest in a fossa in a stable relationship, having reached this position by eruption. The position of the teeth in CO is maintained as *occlusal stability* with either inclined planes opposing each other (*Figs 8.3 and 8.4*) or by the tips of cusps occluding with flat areas – either as a result of wear or because of a natural shallow fossa anatomy. The palatal cusps of the upper teeth and the buccal cusps and incisal edges of the lower teeth are all supporting cusps occluding into central fossae, marginal ridge or cingulum contacts.

If three inclined planes interact to form the cusp/fossa relationship, this is called a *tripod* (*Fig. 8.4*). Some authorities believe this to be a fundamental occlusal relationship. It is, though, exceedingly difficult to reproduce in restorations and even if it is, the properties of the restorative material may not maintain it (see Chapter 14).

Loss of the cusp/fossa relationship contacts leads to loss of occlusal stability and tooth movement may follow, leading to overeruption, tilting or rotation.

The buccal cusps and incisal edges of the upper teeth and the lingual cusps of the lower teeth do not participate in the arrangement for occlusal stability and are termed *non-supporting cusps*. These cusps have no opposing contacts in centric occlusion but may contact teeth in the opposite arch in lateral excursions and protrusion (see later). An alternative terminology uses *stamp cusp* instead of supporting cusp and *shear cusp* instead of non-supporting cusp.

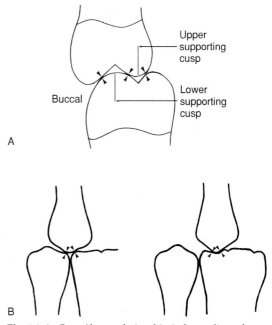

Fig. 8.3 A: Cusp/fossa relationship in bucco-lingual section. Stability is provided by the accurate meeting of the inclined planes. **B** Cusp/fossa relationships in mesio-distal section. The upper supporting cusp may occlude with two marginal ridges, or into a sluiceway

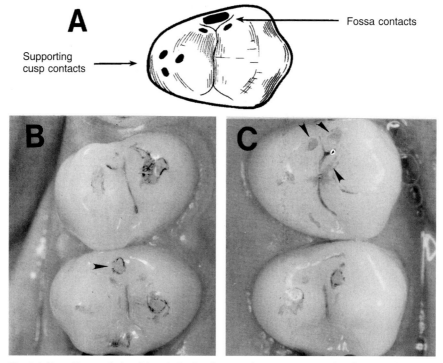

Fig. 8.4 Cusp/fossa relationships. **A** Occlusal view of an upper premolar showing classic tripod contacts, one set in the sluiceway fossa and the other on the tip of the supporting cusp. **B** and **C** Clinically this may be obscured by folding of the articulating paper in the fossae, or by natural variations in relationships. The fossa contact in **C** is almost a tripod, whilst that in **B** is a flat contact on the top of the marginal ridge

Centric relation

When centric occlusion has been lost, in full dentures for instance, or is unsatisfactory, another reference position must be used for restoring the occlusion. This is *centric relation* (CR). It is important to recognize that this position has been defined for the convenience of restorative dentists and is not a physiological position. This may explain the several definitions that exist for the position.

CR, sometimes referred to in prosthetic dentistry as centric jaw relation (CJR), is a position of the condyles within the glenoid fossae unrelated to tooth position. The most common definition used in the United Kingdom is 'the most retruded position of the condyles in the glenoid fossae from which unstrained lateral movements are possible'. However, this is a difficult concept to operate in practice and a rather better definition for practical, clinical use is 'the most superior, posterior position of the condyles in the glenoid fossae'. Some American authorities prefer two other closely related positions: 'the most superior position' and

'the most superior anterior position'. It is outside the scope of this book to consider the arguments proposed for these but the most important consideration is to obtain a *reproducible* and *symmetrical* mandibular position around which to reconstruct the dentition.

CR is usually found by manipulating the mandible and pushing the condyles upwards and backwards. The condyles will then be centred on the terminal hinge axis and the mandible can be 'rotated' by the operator on the retruded arc of closure.

As the operator moves the teeth together, there will usually be tooth contact before CO; this is the *retruded contact position* (RCP), and the teeth involved exhibit a *premature contact*. The movement of the mandible from RCP to CO has a superior or 'vertical' component, an anterior or 'horizontal' component and perhaps a lateral component (*Fig. 8.5*). The magnitude of this *mandibular slide* is often defined as the ratio between the vertical and horizontal movement. The shorthand for the ratio is either Vh (pronounced 'big V, little h') where the vertical component is greater than the horizontal or

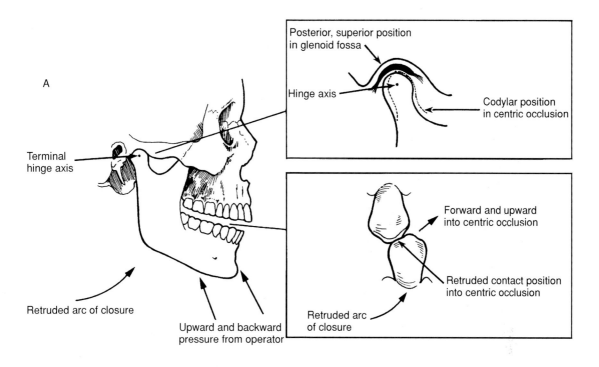

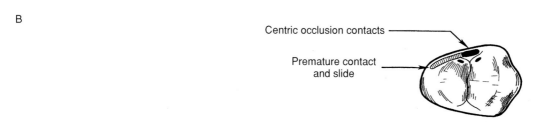

Fig. 8.5 A The retruded arc of closure and a precentric premature contact on two premolars. Following this contact, the mandible slides upwards and forwards into centric occlusion. **B** Plan view of articulating paper contacts made during the movement in **A**

Hv (pronounced 'big H, little v') where the horizontal component is greater.

In a minority of patients no mandibular displacement will be seen, such that centric relation is coincident with centric occlusion. However, this diagnosis can be suspect in view of the difficulty that can be experienced in the manipulation of the mandible (see Chapter 14).

The significance of mandibular slides is disputed. A posterior–anterior slide with Vh is very common and it would appear that a separation of CR and CO is natural. The condylar position in CO is between 0.5 and 2 mm anterior to centric relation in the majority of individuals. This discrepancy appears to be physiologically necessary, though the reason is unknown. When reconstructing the dentition, the new centric occlusion is made with the condyles in CR, though some limited evidence exists to suggest re-establishment of a more posterior CR within two years of reconstruction in dentate patients.

Lateral slides are less common as are those with Hv. It is possible that a slight asymmetry in mandibular position might lead to muscle fatigue, as might a long horizontal component in the mandibular displacement. This is discussed in more detail in Chapter 26.

When individuals close naturally into CO, the prematurities are not contacted; it is part of the learnt behaviour mentioned above to avoid them.

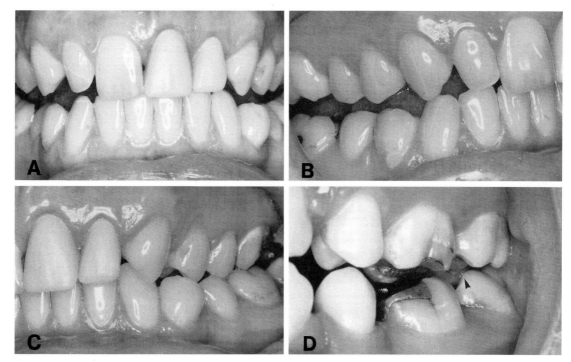

Fig. 8.6 Tooth guidance. **A** Incisal guidance. In sliding forwards with the upper and lower incisors together, the mandible also moves downwards, discluding the posterior teeth. This patient has a high incisal guidance. **B** Canine guidance. The movement of the mandible to the right and downwards is dictated by the contact of the upper and lower canines and the slope of the condylar guidance on the left, non-working side. **C** Group function. There are multiple contacts between the upper and lower teeth when the patient moves to the left. **D** Non-working interference between the upper and lower second molars (arrowed)

Closure occurs straight to CO on a favoured arc of closure. Intrusion by stress, anxiety, and so on into the central nervous system may interfere with the co-ordination of this behaviour; this may lead to temporomandibular dysfunction (Chapter 26).

Mandibular guidance

The hard tissue guidance of mandibular movements comes from the condyles and their relationship with the glenoid fossae – the *condylar guidance* and, if the teeth are in contact, the tooth to tooth contacts – *tooth guidance*. Tooth guidance is made up of *anterior* (incisal and canine) guidance and *posterior* guidance.

Because the condyles can turn and slide and thus adapt to tooth positions, in practical terms the condylar guidance is not as important as the tooth guidance.

Protrusion

Anterior movement of the mandible from CO results in contact of the lower incisors with the palatal surfaces of upper incisors and the mandible has to open. It moves forward and downwards to incisal edge contact. The posterior teeth are *discluded*, but the amount of disclusion depends upon the height of the incisal guidance, the steepness of the curve of Spee, the cusp height of posterior teeth and their slopes (*Fig. 8.6A*). The anatomy of these features must be in harmony so that the posterior teeth do not prevent incisal edge contact.

Lateral excursion

This is also referred to as *mandibular side-shift*. The lateral movement is usually accompanied by a downwards movement caused by the tooth guidance. The side towards which the mandible is moving is the *working side*. The opposite side is the *non-working side*. In complete denture prosthetics the non-working side is referred to as the *balancing* side because of its relationship to denture base stability (see Chapter 24).

During lateral excursions, the non-working or *orbiting* condyle moves smoothly down the articular slope and medially towards the working side. The angle of the medial movement is the *progressive side-shift*. The working side condyle merely turns without coming forward. In some individuals, there may be also a bodily movement of the mandible and both condyles as soon as the lateral movement commences – the *immediate side-shift*.

The tooth guidance for the lateral movement may be *canine guided/protected* or in *group function*. In canine guidance, the lateral movement is guided only by upper canine to lower canine contact, coupled with the condylar guidance from the non-working side condyle (*Fig. 8.6B*). All other teeth should be discluded. In group function, on the other hand, multiple contacts of the cheek teeth occur (*Fig. 8.6C*).

There have been arguments as to which of these guidance arrangements should be used in reconstruction of the dentition. The 'popularity' of group function as a restorative scheme arose from studies of primitive peoples who ate an abrasive diet, thus losing cusp tips and bringing several teeth into contact in lateral movement. Therefore this is argued as the 'correct' scheme for man. However, in western races, canine guidance predominates in people under 40 years of age, whilst group function occurs after this age due to tooth wear. To favour one scheme to the exclusion of the other would seem illogical. As described later, it is better to conform to the scheme already present unless there are positive contraindications.

In both canine guidance and group function there should be no tooth contact on the non-working side. If there is contact, this is referred to as a *non-working interference*. Classically, on lateral excursion, the second molars of the non-working side may be in contact (*Fig. 8.6D*). This is considered to be a departure from occlusal norms and might be a predisposing factor in temporomandibular dysfunction. The 'proper' relationship is that the mandible should have tooth guidance on the working side, but only condylar guidance on the non-working side.

Tooth contacts in function

The teeth do not usually meet during mastication since the food is between them. They attain tooth contact in centric occlusion for swallowing or for rest between a series of chewing strokes. During eating, the mandible describes some form of 'tear-drop' pathway, with a favoured chewing side.

Mouth empty movements, *parafunction*, may involve tooth contacts and these may be habitual. In terms of restorations, it is important to reproduce exact and accurate tooth morphology so that this type of subconscious movement is not impeded, with the possible result of occlusal dysfunction.

Physiology of mastication

When an individual is at rest, with maximum relaxation of the jaw muscles, the teeth are not in contact but are separated by the so-called *freeway space* of about 2 mm. This is the physiological rest position of the mandible. There appears to be electrical activity in the jaw muscles even when at maximum rest, suggesting that the freeway space is maintained by muscle tone monitored by muscle spindles (see below), rather than by the elastic properties of the muscles and surrounding tissues.

The control of mastication is an extremely complicated activity and only the main principles can be covered here (*Fig. 8.7*). In so far as brain mechanisms are concerned, it appears that there are centres in the cortex, in the hypothalamus and limbic systems, and in the brain stem itself, each of which has central pathways to the trigeminal nucleus and thus controlling the muscles of mastication. In addition, the jaw movements used during speech are controlled quite separately. Disturbances in the central mechanisms controlling mandibular movements may result in clinical conditions such as bruxism (Chapter 26).

The direct control of the muscles of mastication is via the trigeminal motor nucleus lying in the middle level of the pons. Each individual muscle is innervated by a motor neurone in a particular region of the motor nucleus. The activity of the muscles is monitored continuously via their proprioceptive reflexes, that are largely controlled via the muscle spindles that exist in all the masticatory muscles. They are found in large numbers in the jaw elevator muscles, but much less in the depressors. The muscle spindles consist of specialized intrafusal fibres enclosed in a thin capsule and lying parallel to the main extrafusal muscle fibres or ordinary contractile fibres. Each muscle spindle contains both nuclear bag and nuclear chain fibres, the stretch in which is monitored by primary myelinated group I afferent nerves and thinner myelinated group II nerves. Stretching of the main muscle results in stretching of the muscle spindles, resulting in information being sent to the central nervous system. These spindles therefore monitor the stretch reflex of the muscles.

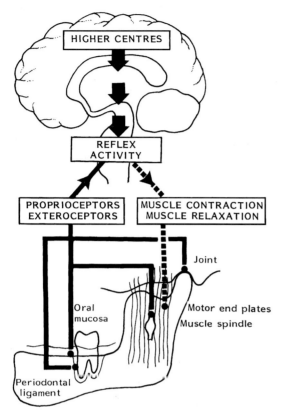

Fig. 8.7 Schematic diagram of the neural control of mastication. Proprioceptive and exteroceptive information from the muscles and oral tissues is processed in the brain stem. Under the influence of higher centres, motor impulses are relayed to the muscle end organs

Information from the central nervous system and alpha efferent nerves returns to the extrafusal or main muscle fibres, causing them to contract. The sensitivity of the muscle spindles is adjusted by motor enervation of the intrafusal fibres within the spindle. These consist of two types, called static and dynamic fusimotor fibres, and are supplied by gamma I or gamma II nerve endings. This system means that when normal muscle tone is maintained, the spindles are detecting stretching or shortening of the muscle.

However, if the muscle contracts considerably, the spindles no longer detect slight changes of length. At this point, the gamma motor neurones shorten the spindle, so that it is again able to monitor muscle tone. Information is also sent to the central nervous system from Golgi tendon organs that are much less sensitive than muscle spindles. Information from these appears to have an inhibitory effect on the motor neurones, so the muscle

spindles and Golgi tendon organs work together to maintain functional activity of the muscles.

These reflex arcs control various reflexes in the masticatory cycle. They are jaw opening reflexes, a variant of which is the horizontal jaw reflex occurring in lateral or horizontal movement.

There is also a jaw closing reflex, that 'operates' the reflex arc of closure. However, the normal path of closure is not the reflex one, but the habitual one that achieves centric occlusion efficiently.

In addition to the information from the muscle spindles and Golgi tendon organs, information is fed to the central nervous system from receptors in the joints, particularly in the capsule of the TMJ and in the peripheral parts of the articular disc. There are also receptors in the periodontium that range from non-specialized nerve endings to more complex structures. Pain is monitored via sensory nerve endings and directional sensitivity may be associated with mechanoreceptors. The presence of food in the mouth is monitored by exteroreceptors in the oral mucosa.

Masticatory cycle

It seems that when food is placed in the mouth its contact with the oral mucosa initiates, through sensory nerve endings, the commencement of the masticatory cycle. The size, hardness, taste and texture of the food is appreciated and this information is processed by an 'oscillator' system in the brain stem close to the trigeminal nucleus, so that rhythmic chewing movements begin. These movements are modified by reflex activity originating from nerve endings in the muscles of mastication, the periodontium, the oral mucosa and the TMJs, and are modified by the guidance planes provided by the joints, but more particularly by the teeth themselves.

When information reaching the central nervous system suggests that the food is well comminuted and formed into a bolus, *deglutition* begins. The relevant part of this is that the mandible goes into centric occlusion to be 'locked' in that position so that the pharyngeal constrictors and the tongue can operate from a firm base, and an anterior seal can be provided.

In such a complex system, instability of teeth, missing teeth, teeth in malocclusion or premature contact, pain in any tissues of the mouth, disturbances in the joint itself or influence from the central nervous system frequently result in facial pain arising from either the muscles themselves or referred to the masticatory apparatus, including the joint. Clinical dental procedures are aimed at restoring the harmony between all these components of the masticatory system.

Functional anatomy of the occlusion – Summary

Anatomy and physiology of the temporomandibular joints, ligaments and muscles of mastication and their relationship to the function of the teeth is the basis of occlusion.

Many terms used in describing the function of the teeth and the joints are a source of confusion and there are conflicting forms of terminology proposed by different authorities. The terms defined here are used throughout the book.

Success of much restorative dentistry depends upon the correct shaping of the functional surfaces of restorations to comply with the functional anatomy described here.

9

Properties of restorative materials

Understanding the formulation, basic properties and clinical behaviour of restorative materials is the key to their correct usage. All materials have limitations and must be used to their best advantage within a well considered treatment plan. Restoration design is to a large extent governed by the properties of the material chosen. This chapter considers the commonly determined physical and chemical properties of materials, how these compare with those of tooth substance, and the implications in general terms for clinical practice.

The mouth is a hostile environment for restorative materials. Within this environment they are subjected to physical and chemical stresses from the occlusion, the diet, plaque and the behaviour of the patient. The various effects are listed in *Table 9.1*. It is against their behaviour in this environment and their ability to be handled easily that materials must be judged.

The requirements of an ideal restorative material can be listed as follows:

- Physical properties equivalent to those of tooth
- Insoluble in oral fluids and diet
- Adhesive to tooth
- Dimensionally stable
- Chemically inert, non-toxic
- Cariostatic and bacteriostatic
- Tooth coloured
- Easy to handle
- Cheap

In relation to the first requirement, various physical properties of tooth tissues are shown in *Table 9.2*, but what these values do not reveal is the way in which a tooth, a very complex composite structure, functions. Also, as with many physical properties, the physical values vary not only with the site of the tissue, but also with the way in which it is tested.

Whilst enamel is a brittle crystalline solid, dentine is viscoelastic, being able to deform under load and recover subsequently. The combination of the

Table 9.1 Possible deleterious effects of intraoral function on restorations

Function	Agent	Possible effect on restorations
Mastication	Acids in diet or plaque	Surface degradation
	Abrasive food	Discoloration
		Dissolution
	Deformation by load	Fatigue and fracture
	Temperature change	Dimensional change and adhesion failure with tooth
	Saliva and dissolved or suspended compounds	Discoloration
Habits		
Tooth brushing	Abrasive	Surface loss
Pipe smoking	Pipe stem	Surface loss
Bruxism	Opposing teeth	Fatigue and fracture

Table 9.2 Some properties of restorative materials compared with tooth substance (indicative values)

Property	Enamel	Dentine	Amalgam	Composite	Glass ionomer cements	Cement base	Gold type III
Modulus of elasticity (GPa)	85	15	55	Hybrid 15 Microfine 10	Acid base 4 RMGIC 8	Polycarboxylate 3 Zinc oxide – eugenol 2	100
Compressive strength (MPa)	380	300	350	300	Acid base 250 RMGIC 300	Polycarboxylate 80 Zinc oxide – eugenol 40	N/A
Tensile strength diametral (MPa)	10	105	40	30–70	Acid base 10 RMGIC 20	Polycarboxylate 12 Zinc oxide – eugenol 3	450 (Uniaxial)
Vickers hardness kg/mm-2	300	60	100	60	40	40	150
Thermal coefficient of expansion $\times 10^{-6}/°C$	11.4 (Across crown)	8.3	25	30–50	Acid base 10 RMGIC 15	35	14.4

two make a very interesting engineering structure with the response to an applied load revealing it to be very durable, much better than if the two tissues acted alone. However, in analytical terms their combined constants are almost impossible to determine absolutely. Add to this the elasticity of the periodontal ligament that absorbs some occlusal loading, and the puzzle is complicated even further.

Table 9.3 Physical properties of restorative materials

Mechanical properties
  Modulus of elasticity
  Creep
  Compressive strength
  Tensile strength
  Flexural strength
  Fracture toughness
  Abrasion resistance

Physical constants
  Coefficient of thermal expansion
  Thermal conductivity and diffusivity
  Dimensional changes on setting

Degradation
  Sorption and solubility
  Corrosion
  Colour stability

Handling characteristics
  Mixing time
  Working time
  Setting time
  Surface finishing

Therefore, one can only sympathize with the biomaterials scientist who is called upon to design replacements for lost or excised tissues.

Physical properties of restorative materials

Various physical criteria may be used to describe materials and test their ability to restore teeth. *Table 9.3* lists some physical properties that are often quoted to justify clinical usage. Historically, the basis for acceptance of a new material was to select a group of clinically successful materials and characterize it by laboratory tests. The new material could then be judged against the values for the materials already in use for that particular application. Unfortunately, this approach is very restrictive of new developments, and the application and significance of some 'standard' tests is open to question.

Mechanical properties

Mechanical properties give an indication of material quality, but the testing method may not mimic the forces applied clinically; these vary in nature, magnitude and rate of application. Whilst considerable efforts have been made to develop clinically realistic tests, such as the 'artificial mouth', these are inevitably complicated and costly.

Mechanical properties tests also give an indication of possible handling problems, in that specimen preparation is often as crucial as the method of test. If a material causes problems, inconsistent specimens and a large scatter of results will be seen. This point is illustrated by the problems of adhesion testing, where clinical inconsistencies are also reflected in a very wide scatter of results in the laboratory.

Modulus of elasticity (Young's modulus)

This is a fundamental property that characterises the *rigidity* of a solid in tension or compression, when it is deformed elastically.

Stiff materials, such as ceramics and metals, have high elastic moduli and materials like impression rubbers have low moduli, with polymeric materials such as methyl methacrylates forming an intermediate group. The modulus reflects the amount of *deformation* or *strain* a material will undergo when a certain load or *stress* is applied.

When stress is plotted against strain, a characteristic curve is produced (*Fig. 9.1*). The slope of the linear portion where stress is proportional to strain, is the modulus.

The *proportional limit* shows where the plot ceases to be linear and the *elastic limit* indicates the onset of plastic deformation, where the removal of the load is followed by incomplete *recovery* to the original dimensions (*Fig. 9.2A*).

Before the elastic limit, removal of the load is followed by full recovery. If the recovery takes time to occur (*Fig. 9.2B*), the material is *viscoelastic* and this is a characteristic of the majority of restorative materials.

Full recovery is an important property of impression rubbers after they have been removed from undercut areas of the mouth, so that these may be reproduced accurately. However, because of their

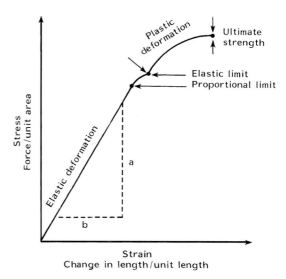

Fig. 9.1 Stress/strain curve. The ratio a/b is the modulus of elasticity

viscoelasticity, recovery is not instantaneous and they should not be cast for at least an hour, to allow recovery to take place first. If, though, the undercuts were severe, the material might be taken beyond its elastic limit and recovery would not take place – it would have a *permanent set*.

On the other hand, if *ductility* is required of a metal for swaging, then permanent deformation beyond the elastic limit, but before the *yield point*, is an essential property.

A complication of viscoelastic behaviour is that the rate at which loading takes place influences the strain, and results for modulus will vary accordingly.

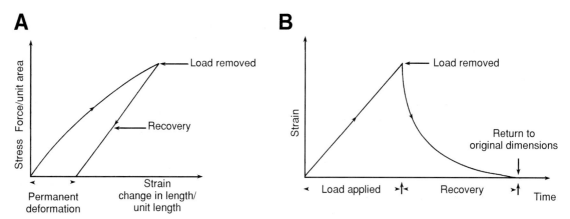

Fig. 9.2 A Stress/strain curve showing loading of a specimen past its elastic limit, resulting in a permanent deformation after the load has been removed. **B** Strain plotted against time for a viscoelastic material. After the load has been removed, some time is necessary for full recovery to take place

Brittle materials, such as ceramics, do not have an elastic limit, and exhibit rapid *brittle failure* when the stresses exceed the proportional limit. Visco-elastic materials subjected to low loads that are intermittent, may eventually *fatigue*, i.e. show reduced recovery and then deterioration by *ductile failure*.

As a concept it is important to decide which type of failure mode will occur in a given circumstance, and it is then possible to design a material for the application. However, as both types of failure may be seen intraorally, depending on the material in use, design decisions are difficult, if not impossible!

Progressive time-dependent permanent deformation under load is termed *creep*, which is a particular failing of dental amalgam. The loading by the occlusion causes the restoration to deform, and the margins, being thin, are the first areas to fatigue during the repeated loading. Corrosion of the metal hastens the fatigue cracking. The more successful amalgams have low creep values and lower corrosion rates. Interestingly though, the very lowest creep values do not seem advantageous, possibly because this is accompanied by brittle behaviour, with the material being too rigid to absorb stress.

Creep is measured by applying a *static* load for a given time and measuring the change in length of the specimen. However, intermittent loading is more realistic and *dynamic creep* is the measure of this.

Compressive strength

This is determined by applying a steadily increasing compressive stress to a cylindrical specimen until the specimen fractures (*Fig. 9.3*). It might represent the loading of a restoration by the occlusion, but takes no account of the support provided by the cavity walls or absorption of stress by the periodontal ligament. Further, the incidence of compressive loading depends upon the site of the restoration, with class III and V types receiving none.

The test gives some indication of the quality of a material but is not a definitive guide, since there is little point in having values above that of enamel, and this could be deleterious to opposing teeth. It is also not a very discriminatory test in terms of differentiating between materials of similar generic type.

The rate of loading of the specimen can significantly affect the results; strain rates during test of 1 mm/min are common, but apparently higher strengths can be recorded if higher rates are used. Attempts have been made to relate strain rates to those encountered during chewing, and 190 mm/min has been suggested.

Misleading results can also be obtained in composite materials whose filler particles will be compacted during testing, increasing the forces recorded prior to fracture.

Rapid attainment of an adequate compressive strength is an essential requirement for a cavity base that must resist the subsequent forces of restoration insertion. Compressive strengths of lining cements measured at 24 hours, rather than the realistic 10 minutes, are therefore not clinically relevant.

There is some correlation between the early (1 hour) compressive strength of amalgam and its clinical success.

Tensile strength

To determine this property, two opposing pulling forces are applied to the specimen in its long axis (*Fig. 9.3*). Tension is quite likely to be encountered in the mouth, for instance across the occlusal isthmus of a class II restoration under occlusal load.

It is a better test of material quality than compression, but the test specimens are more difficult to make and alignment during testing is critical to ensure the loading is uniaxial. The results are much lower than compressive strengths, partly due to sensitivity to the specimen defects mentioned above, as well as the difficulties of test. As with the compressive strength test, the results are strain rate dependent.

To overcome these difficulties, *diametral tensile strength* has become popular. Here, the load is applied to a cylindrical specimen on its side (*Fig. 9.3*). The application of a compressive load in one plane is converted to a tensile strain at right angles to it. It is, however, only suitable for brittle materials since it is assumed in the calculation that there is no distortion of the specimen prior to fracture. This is not the case with polymers and quite erroneous results can be obtained that flatter the material under test.

Flexural strength

The application of a bending force to a beam (*Fig. 9.4*) induces both compressive and tensile forces, and therefore the results should indicate a combined property. The test is useful for polymers and ceramics, and is simple to perform. Again, the results are strain rate dependent and can be affected by specimen defects as with other tests.

More recently *biaxial flexure* tests have become popular. Here the specimen is a disc supported on an annular knife edge and the load is applied to the centre of the disc. This removes the concerns about edge effects as these are outside the area of the specimen under test. In both uniaxial and biaxial

COMPRESSION

TENSION

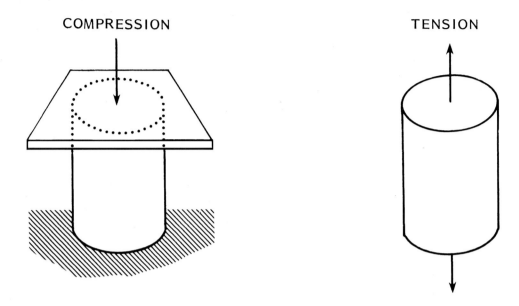

DIAMETRAL TENSION

Plane of
tensile
forces

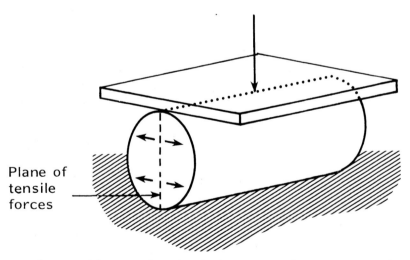

Fig. 9.3 Schematic diagrams of the test configurations for determination of compressive strength, tensile strength and diametral tensile strength

BENDING - FLEXURAL STRENGTH

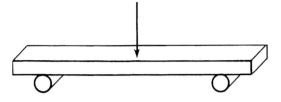

INDUCED COMPRESSIVE STRESS

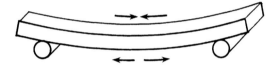

INDUCED TENSILE STRESS

Fig. 9.4 The fracture of a beam to determine flexure strength by three point loading. During bending, the upper surface is subjected to compression and the lower to tension

flexural strength tests, if the deflection of the specimens exceeds more than 10%, the theory for calculation is invalidated.

Fracture toughness

A series of complex tests under this heading endeavour to measure the energy required to propagate a crack within a material and create new surfaces. This is superficially attractive since crack formation is an integral part of intraoral failure. However, results are often modulus dependent and ranking of materials by some tests has been at variance with clinical findings.

Hardness and abrasion resistance

These properties give some guidance on the possible effects of surface degradation by physical as opposed to chemical agents. However, because of the very complex processes involved intraorally, their results can be very misleading.

Several types of wear tests have been devised that try to mimic oral conditions, but these have been disappointing as they tend to produce a ranking order that fits only one generic group of materials.

Physical constants

Coefficient of thermal expansion

A mismatch of the coefficients of thermal expansion of the restoration and tooth will result in differential expansion and contraction during intraoral temperature changes. This stresses the restoration/material interface and a space will form between the two, allowing ingress of fluids and bacteria, known as *microleakage* (see below).

These temperature changes can range from 5 to 65°C and the effects are made worse by capillary action as the expansion/contraction occurs. The worst material from this respect is unfilled acrylic resin, whilst the best are ceramic and glass ionomer cement.

Thermal conductivity and diffusivity

Thermal conductivity indicates the amount of heat passing through a standard volume of material when the specimen and its surroundings are at a steady temperature. This steady state is rarely reached in the mouth and it is better to consider the thermal diffusivity of any material which shows the rate of temperature change from one side of a specimen to the other during transient changes in temperature. This type of change is typical of intraoral conditions.

With metals, these properties are of considerable significance since the heat transference is so rapid that the underlying structure will be at the ambient temperature. With polymers the rate of heat transfer is considerably slower and composites show a surprising range of diffusivities that may relate to filler loading, size and type.

The ideal would be to match the material's diffusivity as closely as possible to that of dentine, as this acts as a very effective heat sink, both because of its bulk and its low diffusivity value.

Dimensional changes

Ideally, materials should undergo no change after placement in the cavity, but almost all setting materials shrink as new compounds are formed.

Polymerization of resins leads to contraction that may be quoted as volume or linear shrinkage. Whilst this gives some guide as to the amount of space that may form around restorations, its effects are moderated by the strength of mechanical or chemical bonds between the cavity wall and the material, and its configuration. The development of high molecular weight monomers of low shrinkage is very important.

Conversion of monomer to polymer during setting is usually inefficient in dental materials, about 40% for chemical initiation and 60% for light activation, and exposure to temperature changes intraorally induces further reaction leading to a *post-cure* shrinkage.

Water sorption causes expansion of dental polymers, but the effect is reduced by the containment of the material by the cavity and compensation for shrinkage does not occur.

The acid/base setting reactions of cements such as zinc cements and conventional glass ionomer cements are usually dimensionally stable if they are maintained at constant humidity. Loss of water leads not only to shrinkage but to weakening of the cement matrix, hence the need to coat glass ionomer cements with an impervious polymer layer during cement maturation.

The setting reaction of amalgam is complex, with an initial shrinkage caused by solution of the components, followed by expansion caused by crystallization of new phases. The net result in modern mechanically mixed materials is shrinkage.

Intraoral degradation

As was mentioned at the beginning of this chapter, the hostility of the mouth towards restorations causes many forms of degradation. All materials are affected in some way or other.

Sorption and solubility

Ideally these properties should have values of zero. The sorption of fluid by resins depends on their degree of cross-linking. Polymethyl methacrylate absorbs about 2% by weight of water and, in the long term, this reduces its physical properties. Other polymer-based materials, such as composites, exhibit less uptake, but the amount still has a significant effect on their properties.

Similarly, there is a loss of material from most polymers with time, as the lower molecular weight compounds slowly dissolve out. The solubility decreases as the molecular weight of the polymer increases and as more efficient conversion occurs during polymerization.

These properties are usually measured over a period of seven days for standard tests, but in the mouth they continue for a considerable time until equilibrium is reached; this is frequently many months.

Loss of material, which tends to include plasticizers, inevitably affects the mechanical properties adversely.

Whilst water is the recognized test medium, other solvents found intraorally, such as ethyl alcohol, and acetic and lactic acids, are likely to have deleterious effects. The solubility values for luting cements are important as an indicator of these materials' durability. Polycarboxylate and glass ionomer cements, when fully matured, have the lowest values.

Corrosion

This affects both metals and glasses, but by different mechanisms.

Amalgam   There may be some advantage in some corrosion of amalgam since the products are bactericidal and also block the cavity wall/material interspace. However, the corrosion occurs in the weakest phase of the set amalgam and causes the whole structure to weaken and particularly leads to 'ditching' of the margins.

The main product of the setting reaction of conventional alloys is a cored structure of unchanged alloy powder surrounded by the silver–mercury γ_1 and the tin–mercury γ_2 phases. Removal or reduction of the latter phase has been the prime objective, since it is by far the weakest of the phases. The presence of saliva and plaque sets up corrosion cells that results in the slow breakdown of the γ_2 phase with the formation of sulphides and chlorides, and also the liberation of mercury that continues to react with the unchanged alloy.

The high copper amalgams show a marked reduction or even elimination of the γ_2 phase. The copper has a greater affinity for the tin than the mercury, and copper–tin complexes are formed preferentially. These are themselves not entirely resistant to corrosion but the rate of corrosion is considerably reduced. The end products take some time to form and the elimination of the γ_2 phase is very dependent on mercury concentration during mixing.

Corrosion and creep are all increased by the presence of excess mercury and the mixing and handling of the materials must be carefully controlled. Certain high copper materials perform better than others and there is an overlap in performance with the poorer high coppers and the best conventional materials.

Glasses   The ceramics employed in composite materials as reinforcing fillers, and as inlays and crowns, are corroded by saliva.

In the composites, water is absorbed by the resin and comes into contact with the filler. Metallic ions pass from the glass and the accumulation of corrosion products causes stress cracking in the resin. Long-term immersion studies have shown dramatic decreases in strength of conventional composites. Glasses containing barium, strontium or zinc salts to confer radio-opacity are more vulnerable than alumino-silicate combinations.

However, the microfine materials are more resistant to corrosion because the filler particles are surrounded by heat-cured resin that exhibits a lower water uptake. The clinical durability of the microfines is greater than would be expected from simple mechanical properties tests and this illustrates another problem in predicting clinical performance. Their performance clinically is very similar to the more highly filled composite resins.

Colour stability and staining

This applies principally to the polymer-based materials. Loss of tooth matching colour may be due to setting reaction by-products, degradation of the base polymer, or accumulation of extrinsic stains on a degraded surface.

Amines are used as initiators in both chemically cured and light cured materials and they remain after the reaction as potential discolourants. If the amine concentration is too high, perhaps in order to accelerate setting, then colour instability will result in the long term. Accelerated ageing tests will reveal this.

The principal base monomer of many composites is bis-phenol A glycidal dimethacrylate (bis-GMA) and this yellows gradually when exposed to ultraviolet light. U-V absorbers are added to counteract this, but they are not wholly satisfactory. The polymer also changes colour due to sorption.

However, the most critical aspect of the composites is their tendency to accumulate stain on the surface. This is partly due to the degradation of the silane coupling agent that bonds the filler to the resin and partly to the abrasion of surface resin, leaving a rough surface. Porosity, that results from air inclusions during mixing and placement, also collects stain.

Microleakage

The interface between restoration and cavity wall is an area of weakness that is under the influence of the properties discussed above. In the absence of an adhesive, mechanical interlocking between tooth and restoration is all that maintains a seal. As shrinkage and subsequent temperature changes occur, the links are broken, and fluid and bacteria pass in. The space becomes an area of transit for all types of compounds that cause staining and pulpal sensitivity. Bacteria are the least welcome as they are able to colonize the dentine surface and are implicated in the pulpal reactions to restorative materials.

Various techniques and materials have been developed to overcome the problem, the first being the cavity varnishes used with amalgam. Even these were soluble and the success of the restoration depended upon corrosion products blocking the space. The development of dentine adhesives or restoratives that adhere to dentine offers the best hope for the elimination of the problem (see below).

Ion exchange across the interface is of considerable interest. For example, fluoride migrates from the glass ionomer cements and inhibits caries initiation at the restoration margins. The fluoride is incorporated in the glass as a flux to aid manufacture and intraorally it slowly diffuses into the surrounding matrix, from which it passes into the tooth tissue (*Fig. 9.5*). More recently fluoride releasing polymer-based restoratives have also become available.

Handling characteristics

Materials must be formulated so that they can be manipulated easily. Any material that is difficult to use or is oversensitive to handling techniques is likely to be a failure, no matter how good its final properties.

Mixing

The most efficient way of ensuring the correct proportions of components and a satisfactory mix is to use encapsulated materials. With amalgam, encapsulation has the added advantage of improving mercury hygiene.

The cements, particularly glass ionomers, are the most sensitive to errors in proportioning and mixing. Care must be taken to follow the manufacturer's instructions exactly.

Mixing also incorporates air into the material that may lead to surface problems. Single component materials, particularly those such as the light cured composites, that are vacuum packed as well as being delivered in single dose 'compules', help reduce the problem.

Working time

Adequate time must be available to mix and form the restoration before the setting reaction increases the viscosity of the material to a level at which it is not workable. The chemically cured composites are the most dramatic example of this problem. They tend to be overinitiated to please the clinician, with a short setting time. Unfortunately, this severely restricts the working time, leading to poor cavity wall adaptation and surface clefts if placement is not rapid.

This problem has been improved by the 'command setting' materials. These use external energy,

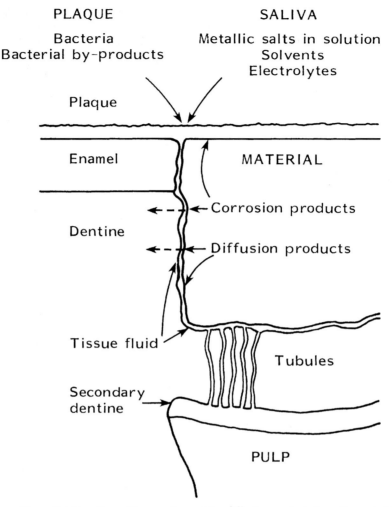

Fig. 9.5 Microleakage. Tissue fluid together with corrosion and/or diffusion products from the material passes out and bacteria, toxins and various salts in solution pass in

currently light of the wavelength 410–490 nm, to excite an initiator in the material. However, the working time is not unlimited as the operating light also emits light of the critical wavelength. Unless an appropriate filter is fitted to the operating light, the working time can be quite restricted.

Rapid setting amalgams, mainly spherical particle or microcut types, also have a restricted working time. If this is exceeded, increments may not amalgamate with each other, leading to 'layering' within the restoration.

Setting time

A rapid set seems to be clinically desirable to reduce chairside time. However, this brings with it the loss of working time discussed above, and also in polymeric materials the chain growth is restricted, leading to inferior physical properties. A long setting time can be equally deleterious, since great patience is required from the clinician. The early glass ionomer cements were very slow setting due to the low reactivity of the glass and early contamination with saliva led to rapid breakdown of the restoration.

Surface finishing

The final restoration should have very low surface energy so that it does not collect plaque and other intraoral deposits. Often, the 'as set' material will require a finishing stage to impart a smooth surface. This must be as simple as possible and ideally done at the placement stage. However, very few materials have achieved their optimum properties at this time and finishing must be delayed until maturation has occurred.

Adhesion

Many attempts have been made to achieve chemical attachment of the restoration to both the enamel and dentine. These may be divided into two distinct groups:

- Bonding directly to the substrate by the restorative (polyacid-based) cements
- Bonding to the substrate by the use of an intermediate bonding resin

Bonding directly

The oldest successful adhesive system is that using polyacrylic acid as found in the polycarboxylate and glass ionomer cements. Two reactions appear together. The first is a simple chelation reaction in which the calcium in the enamel and dentine reacts with the polyacrylate ion. The carboxylic acid groups of the cement polyacid displace phosphate and calcium from the hydroxyapatite surface, with the formation of an intermediate layer of fluoridated carbonoapatite. The second is a limited chemical reaction between the organic phase of the dentine and the polyacrylate ion. This mechanism of attachment has not been clearly defined but it is reported that the bond to *decalcified* dentine is very difficult to break.

The bond appears to be a dynamic phenomenon. The polymeric nature of these cements ensures a multiplicity of bonds between substrate and cement so that under clinical conditions the severance of a single bond does not lead to failure. Though the bond strength of glass ionomer cement to dentine is not high in comparison with other adhesives, the bond appears to be the most durable and reliable of the currently available materials.

The surface must be clean and free of pellicle. Various cleaners, or *conditioners*, have been used, starting with citric acid. This, however, produced pulpal irritation and more recently the use of tannic acid and, more commonly, polyacrylic acid has become more accepted. However, it is now thought that the bond strengths to freshly cut dentine are no different from those found with treated dentine.

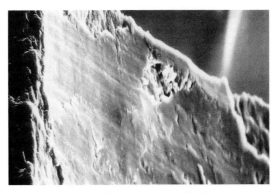

Fig. 9.6 A scanning electron micrograph of a smear layer at the cavity margin. It is an incomplete layer with some patches of underlying enamel showing through

Use of an intermediate bonding resin

Smear layer

The cutting of both enamel and dentine produces a layer of amorphous material, rich in calcium, that is smeared over the surface of the enamel and dentine – the *smear layer* (Fig. 9.6).

The amount of smear created depends on the type of bur used. The ranking order from most to least is white stone, metal blank, diamond and tungsten carbide burs. The tenacity of the smear layer has never been determined, but it appears to be rather variable. Its presence confers two advantages:

- Sealing of the dentinal tubules
- Provision of a calcium rich layer

The smear layer blocks the cut ends of the dentinal tubules and therefore may be a factor in pulp protection from microleakage.

Bonding mechanism

Bonding to dentine has passed though a number of development phases during the past decade and there is still some difficulty in determining the real mechanism that produces the bond. It appears to be established that the bonding is of a micromechanical nature and this is achieved by some form of alteration of the dentine/smear layer continuum with a primer. This is then coated with a low viscosity monomer that is inherently hydrophilic in nature. A final methacrylate polymer is then bonded on to the surface.

The increase in the surface calcium effected by the smear layer was originally thought to be of use with many of the early adhesive systems that claimed to bond to the inorganic component of the tooth. Currently there is a requirement that the smear layer be either modified or removed. The more recently developed systems bond by intimate micromechanical interlocking and entanglement of the polymer within the collagen matrix of the dentine or by 'total etch' to the dentine walls. There was originally some concern as to the effect of the adhesive primers on the underlying dentine structure and the odontoblast processes but this appears to be unfounded except where the floor of the cavity is close to the pulp

The current method of surface preparation of dentine requires use of an agent, usually an acid, to modify and partly remove the smear layer. The acids currently used include nitric, phosphoric, maleic and citric acids. These materials partly remove the smear layer and widen the lumen of the dentinal tubules. They also partly demineralize the intertubular dentine, leaving the collagen as a fibre web. This is then impregnated by the hydrophilic monomer, producing micromechanical entanglement within the fibre scaffolding. It is to this intermediate polymer/collagen layer that the methacrylate polymer is bonded.

The effect is confined to the outer 3–6 μm of the dentine. Care must be taken during the priming process since excessive demineralization of the dentine leads to a collapse of the collagen network and less penetration of the monomer, with a resulting reduction in bond strength. Currently the

bond strengths that are obtainable are in the region of 20 MPa (close to the bond strengths found to enamel). However, the results are somewhat variable and depend on the type of dentine used to conduct the test and the method of test itself (see below). Manufacturers have tried to reduce the conditioning and priming stages to avoid complex procedures and so-called 'single component' adhesives, that are in reality mixtures of primers, conditioners and monomers, have been marketed. The number of compounds in the mixture may reduce the activity of each, thus leading to lower efficiency.

Methods of adhesion testing

Bond strength

The demonstration of effective bonding and its absolute measurement is desirable to support the efficacy of a particular system. Mechanical bond strength measurement is unfortunately fraught with potential systematic and random errors.

Forces designed to rupture the bond can be applied in several ways. The most common are tensile and shear forces (*Fig. 9.7*) and many individually designed test apparati have been proposed to apply these.

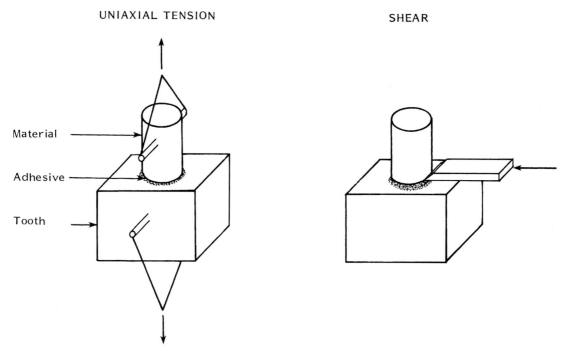

UNIAXIAL TENSION   SHEAR

Material

Adhesive

Tooth

Fig. 9.7 Adhesion testing. The arrangement for the determination of tensile and shear bond strengths

Sources of error in testing may be due to use of an incorrect substrate, surface preparation and standardization, specimen handling and peel and shear forces created as a result of the alignment of the specimen during testing.

In view of the shortage of human teeth, a number of substitutes have been used. These include animal teeth, particularly bovine, and synthetic hydroxyapatite. Both types of substitute are similar chemically to human teeth, but have structural differences. They are useful in screening potential adhesives, but finally there is no substitute for human teeth.

Variations in bond strength are also found in parallel with compositional differences of the teeth. For example, age or position of dentine in relation to the pulp will vary the mineral content of the specimen surface.

The surface area for bonding must be carefully and accurately defined and the method must not contaminate the surface. For ease of analysis, the surface must be flat and, to avoid mechanical interlocking contributing to the bond, as plane as possible. Handling the specimen after bonding will need extreme care if the bond is not to be stressed prematurely.

A universal joint system is usually incorporated into tensile testing assemblies to align the specimen and substrate with the direction of the applied force. However, during this alignment the bond can be stressed non-axially by peel and shear forces.

Measurement of microleakage

The measurement of the intrusion of an agent, such as a dye, into the space between the material and the tooth also is a common test for the demonstration of adhesion. This should reflect the effects of inclusion in a cavity rather more than the simple flat surface bond strength tests.

Many intrusion agents have been used such as radio-isotopes, bacteria, electrolytes and air. However, the hydrodynamics of the dentine cannot be reproduced, and results may not correlate with clinical observations.

Biological compatibility

Biological compatibility is of paramount importance for any material that is placed permanently in living tissues. By virtue of compounds leaching from the material, local or systemic effects are possible.

Dental materials are often placed at a time when they are chemically active, after which they set and become essentially inert. A series of *in vitro* and *in vivo* tests have been devised to screen the biological properties of restorative materials.

The *in vitro* tests begin with a simple screening of cell cytotoxicity, after which the material is tested in animals. The animal tests are implantation in the tissues and simulated in-use tests in the teeth.

For the in-use tests, the material is placed in standardized cavities and the pulpal response noted at various time intervals after placement. There are a number of problems with this test in terms of reproducibility and variability but, in the absence of any reliable alternative, it is the best guide to compatibility for restorative materials.

The laboratory tests at the cellular level tend to eliminate materials that are acceptable in other tests. For instance, cytotoxicity is reduced if fully set material is used instead of freshly mixed material.

The presence or absence of an intervening layer of dentine between material and pulp alters the response of pulp tissue to the material very considerably. Zinc oxide/eugenol cements are the classic example of this, in that if they are applied to exposed pulp, they induce inflammation, whilst they are obtundent to the closed pulp.

Clinical testing

Following laboratory testing, the materials are subjected to clinical trials. An initial *explanatory trial* using controlled conditions and a small number of clinicians is followed by a *field trial* where the material is used by many operators in general practice conditions.

The time scale for these assessments is inevitably long and the trials are costly. It might be as long as five years between invention of a material and its marketing, but there is no avoiding this. Realistic accelerated tests are difficult to devise in primates and are not representative of human intraoral conditions.

Conclusion

The combination of laboratory tests, animal studies and clinical trials ought to provide the clinician with considerable valuable information on the likely behaviour of a material when it is placed in the mouth.

Unfortunately this is not the case, since there are so many unquantifiable biological factors that influence clinical success. Not least of these is the skill of the clinician in handling materials. Proper attention to detail and understanding the quirks of each material is an essential component of the dentist's education.

CLINICAL MANAGEMENT AND TECHNIQUES

10

Intracoronal restorations

Evolution of materials, cutting instruments and techniques, together with a better understanding of the structure of the dental hard and soft tissues and of the carious disease process, has resulted in modifications to the principles of cavity design propounded by G. V. Black over a hundred years ago. The advent of adhesive materials coupled with the more precise diagnosis of caries by radiography has led to different concepts. The need for retention created by the cavity shape has been reduced and the lesion is treated at a much earlier stage. These factors have led to smaller cavities and greater conservation of sound tooth tissue. The range of materials available for restoration of an intracoronal cavity has increased dramatically in the last five years.

Indications for treatment

Primary carious lesions

There is considerable evidence to support the remineralization of the early carious lesion in enamel (Chapter 6). Only when the lesion shows positive evidence of having reached the dentine should operative treatment be commenced. *Figure 10.1A* shows a radiograph of an early lesion for which the application of topical fluoride coupled with regular radiographic review would be appropriate.

Figure 10.1B, on the other hand, shows clear evidence of caries in dentine, and this lesion should be excised and the tooth restored. The diagnosis of caries must be aided by high quality radiographs that have been taken and processed by standardized techniques.

Failed restorations

Restorations may fail because of recurrent caries, failure of restorative materials or fracture of the surrounding tooth. The diagnosis of these was discussed in Chapter 3, as was the difficulty associated with accurate diagnosis of when to replace a restoration or when to accept apparently minor faults.

Cavity design and preparation

The extent of excision of caries and the final shape of the cavity depend upon:

- The size of the lesion or cavity to be re-restored
- Its position with regard to aesthetics
- The need to conserve tooth substance
- The choice of restorative material
- Caries incidence and oral hygiene

These factors are interrelated considerably. The sequence for cavity preparation is:

1. Obtain access and explore the lesion
2. Choose the restorative material
3. Complete the cavity design and preparation

This is in total contrast with the old traditional teaching of cavity preparation, blamed on Black though perhaps aided by subsequent teachers, where particular 'standard' cavity shapes were defined and applied without thought being given to the lesion, the tooth and its environment.

Lesion

An initial assessment of extent of the lesion is based on clinical and radiographic appearance. However, both methods may underestimate the actual size

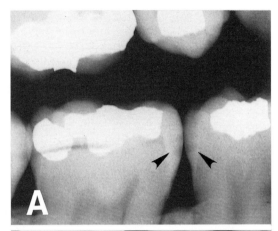

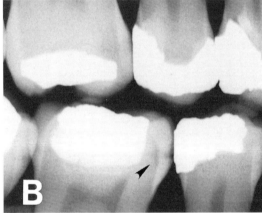

Fig. 10.1 Bitewing radiographs. **A** Early enamel caries (arrowed) which should receive topical fluoride application rather than restoration. **B** Approximal carious lesion (arrowed) that extends into dentine. This lesion should be excised and the tooth restored

and exploration is essential prior to making a decision on restoration type. Remember that enamel and dentine cannot be replaced once removed, so a cautious approach is necessary. Use small rotary instruments to gain direct access to the lesion, clear the enamel–dentine junction and the dentine floor and then consider the likely restoration type.

Choice of restorative material

The choice for intracoronal cavities is often a compromise between aesthetics and long-term durability. Principles of the material types and adhesion to tooth are discussed in Chapter 9. The range of materials and techniques available for intracoronal restorations is large. It includes:

- Amalgam
- Direct composite resin
- Glass ionomer cement
- Compomers
- Composite resin inlay
- Ceramic inlay
- Gold inlay

Amalgam

The material of choice in the posterior teeth where the cavity involves occlusal contacts remains *amalgam*. It is simple to use and durable. The major question is over its safety and a review is cited in the bibliography; to summarize:

- Mercury is a tissue poison and the prime risk is to the dentist and staff. Improvements in mercury hygiene with capsulated amalgam and the careful control of waste have reduced this risk to a minimum.
- Environmental concerns have led to legislation in some countries seeking to eliminate amalgam from use. Other legislation concerns the disposal of amalgam waste into the public sewers and amalgam separators may be installed on dental units to prevent this. However, it is possible that normal particle filtration systems found in suction and spittoon units are as effective as some separators.
- The most emotive area is the allegation of health risks to the patient. Reports on this are far from conclusive and, to date, no clear unequivocal scientific evidence exists to support the elimination of amalgam from dental practice; notwithstanding this, advice has been given that removal or placement of amalgam restorations should be avoided in pregnant women when clinically reasonable.

Clearly, reduction in the use of amalgam is possible. Where restorations will be lost in a short period, as in deciduous teeth, then other materials may be used. However, the current amalgam replacements are all relatively new materials that introduce technical difficulties in placement and their long-term performance in equivalent cavities is not as cost effective and durable as amalgam.

Direct tooth-coloured materials

Composite resin
Thirty years of relatively successful usage has seen this group of materials become well established for anterior use. In spite of developments, their use in occlusal load-bearing restorations must be viewed with caution since they are technically much more demanding to use than amalgam and may not maintain occlusal contacts as well. They have acceptable wear characteristics in small cavities but

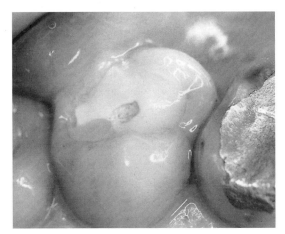

Fig. 10.2 Occlusal wear of a direct composite resin restoration

in larger cavities surface loss may be seen within five or so years (*Fig. 10.2*). Marginal breakdown may be associated with the occlusion and late effects of polymerization shrinkage.

Current materials are almost exclusively of the blue light/camphoroquinone initiated type with two component self-initiating materials being reserved for practice locations with poor electricity supply. The by-products of the amine–peroxide self-curing system lead to colour instability, and in light activated materials there is no peroxide, and the amine concentration is reduced. However these materials will change colour slightly during the polymerization process and will still darken with age.

Light activated materials are dispensed in a single component format and this permits the manufacturer more flexibility in the production of the material, and multifunctional monomers are common. These have enhanced physical properties. Further, the single component can be packed at the factory under vacuum, mixing is eliminated, and the risk of air inclusions is reduced.

The other principal development has been in filler technology with denser, fine particle hybrid materials now being the commonest formulation. The microfine materials have provided good clinical service but the vagaries of the market place have reduced their usage.

The restriction of the light cured materials is their *depth of cure*. Only those parts of the material reached by the light are initiated, and therefore if the light source is too far away or the unpolymerized layer is too thick, there will be incomplete polymerization. Restorations that are deeper than 1.5 mm must be built in separately polymerized layers. This makes the restoration tedious and costly to construct.

Glass ionomer cement

Glass ionomer cement (GIC) has undergone the greatest developments in the past 10 years. The original acid–base reaction setting materials are still regarded as being effective but the incorporation of polymers in the composition has led to several different material types – the *resin modified glass ionomer cements* (RMGIC). These materials were produced to counter the limitations of the conventional GIC, namely slow build-up of mechanical properties and sensitivity to moisture.

All RMGIC have, to a greater or lesser extent, an acid–base setting reaction that accompanies a polymerization reaction. The accompanying water soluble monomer system, usually *2-hydroxyethylmethacrylate* (HEMA), may be polymerized by:

- Blue light via a photosensitive initiator, usually camphoroquinone – *light cure*
- A redox amine–peroxide self-initiating system – *dark cure*
- A combination of the two – *dual cure*

Monomer substitution of the water using HEMA has produced a range of materials that have early mechanical properties similar to those of a mature (3–4 months old) conventional GIC. The initiation of the polymerization reaction by light provides a form of command set, although the acid–base reaction continues for some time afterwards. The materials leach fluoride in a similar manner to the GICs but they are less susceptible to changes in moisture content.

Addition of HEMA has led to a setting exotherm that is markedly greater than the composites and there is substantial polymerization shrinkage. It has been suggested that this can be compensated for by the high water sorption, but saturation of the restoration takes several weeks.

Marked polymerization shrinkage subjects the bond to tooth tissue to substantial stress during the setting stage and the durability of the bond is uncertain. On the evidence currently available the RMGIC are more appropriate for the restoration of anterior teeth.

Attempts to achieve radio-opacity in acid–base GICs have been made with varying degrees of success. The majority have been associated with the modification of the glass to include a radio-opaque element, frequently strontium.

Silver particles may be sintered with the glass during its production to form a *cermet*. Another method is the addition of amalgam alloy particles at the chairside. Both these methods provide radio-opacity and also enhance the mechanical properties if added in appropriate proportions.

The cariostatic properties are advantageous. Fluoride ions released from the glass during the

Table 10.1 Comparison of glass-ionomer cements, composite resins and their derivatives

Property	Composite resin	Glass ionomer cement (Acid–base reaction)	Resin modified glass ionomer cements (Blue light activated/dual cure)
Adhesion	Intermediate agent(s) required	Inherently adhesive	Intermediate agent(s) usually required
Fluoride	Mostly none	Good diffusion	Good diffusion
Setting reaction	Blue light–rapid	Slow	Blue light–rapid Self-cure component of dual cure–slow
Setting shrinkage (average)	Significant (1–2%)	Minimal	Significant (3%)
Abrasion resistance	Good except under occlusal load	Poor	Moderate
Flexural strength (average)	High (120–150 MPa)	Low (60 MPa)	Moderate (80 MPa)
Finishing	Immediate	Delay until mature	Immediate
Aesthetics	Good	Variable	Good

setting reaction leach out from the filling matrix to the surrounding tissue. There is also evidence that there is a reverse flow when fluoride ion concentration in the surrounding medium is raised. It is now inferred from this that the GICs may act as reservoirs for various ions. This is of considerable significance as it has been demonstrated in a number of studies that there is caries inhibition around these restorations.

Compomers
These materials, also called 'acid modified composites', combine some aspects of GICs with those of composites. Their monomer contains a number of carboxylate groups and sets in the same way as the blue light initiated composites. However, once the restoration is exposed to saliva, water is absorbed and an acid–base reaction is started. The carboxylate groups react with the alumino–silicate filler to form a salt matrix, and fluoride is released. Their mechanical properties are similar to the microfine composites and an intermediate dentine bonding agent is needed to achieve adhesion.

Direct tooth-coloured materials – summary
This bewildering array of materials can be regarded as a spectrum ranging from pure acid–base reaction 'salt matrix' materials at one end to purely polymer-based materials, the composites, at the other. How many of these will survive in a very competitive market place remains to be seen. Clinical choice is to a large extent personal and empirical and in *Table 10.1* the basic properties are compared. There is no doubt that the average

general dental practitioner is attracted to a rapid setting material that can be finished immediately, is not sensitive to water content and has good aesthetics. These criteria reduce the popularity of the original acid–base reaction GICs in favour of RMGIC and composites. This implies that dentists are willing to accept the use of additional bonding agents and the deleterious effects of polymerization shrinkage.

Indirect restorative materials

Composite inlays
To overcome the direct composite's restricted depth of cure, difficulty in achieving an approximal contact and lack of durability in the occlusion, these materials have been developed for processing outside the mouth either at the chairside or in the laboratory. Curing ovens using heat, light or pressure alone or in combination polymerize the materials more effectively. The occlusion and approximal contacts can be adjusted more easily and there is better control of placement.

The cavity must be prepared to be non-undercut to allow insertion of the inlay. A low viscosity composite luting agent is used in association with the acid etch technique and, perhaps, dentine bonding agents.

The disadvantages of the systems are the cost of the additional processing and inherent weakness of the luting composite. The inlay still appears to be vulnerable in occlusal contacts, and marginal staining where the lute has broken down is common.

Ceramic inlays

Ceramic is the most durable of the tooth coloured materials and has been in use for many years as a very successful crown material (see Chapter 15). Refinements in formulation and firing technique have now made the construction of accurate inlays possible. They have the advantages of maintaining the occlusion more reliably than polymers and they have far superior colour stability.

Disadvantages are the inherent brittleness of ceramic that leads to marginal fracture and the problem that besets all indirect restorations, the lack of durability of the cementing material.

Gold inlays

Gold inlays are very much out of favour even though when well constructed they are arguably an excellent restoration. They are the restoration of choice for maintaining occlusal stability and have no adverse effects on the opposing enamel surface. However, the skills required, coupled with the weakness of the cement lute, make them inferior in the majority of operator's hands to the average amalgam restoration. This is not to say that the placement of amalgam does not require a high level of skill – it does – but the technique is more forgiving.

Treatment of the minimal dentine lesion

Occlusal caries – the preventive resin restoration

A minimal lesion in an occlusal fissure should be treated by local excision of the carious dentine through the overlying enamel. The access should be of sufficient size to allow good vision of the affected dentine. The other fissures on the occlusal aspect should be inspected for evidence of caries, rather than just staining, and should not be removed unless carious dentine can be seen under them. Occlusal stops will be unlikely to be removed by such a preparation, and therefore glass ionomer cement can be used because of its adhesion to dentine, low pulp irritation and fluoride diffusion.

The remainder of the fissure pattern should be acid etched prior to the insertion of the GIC, and fissure sealed after insertion. The fissure sealant should be extended over the GIC to protect it from water (*Fig. 10.3*).

If the fissure is very steep, so that the sealant will not enter it fully, or there is suspicious staining, then fissure widening may be used. A fine tapered diamond is run along the fissure at the depth of the enamel–dentine junction. Any caries revealed by this can be removed locally by a small round bur, run at slow speed. The whole cavity can now be restored with GIC, or acid etch retained composite resin.

If, after exploration of the lesion, the cavity is found to be larger than expected with occlusal function then amalgam will be the material of choice (*Fig. 10.4*).

Approximal caries

Several minimal designs have been suggested. All of these rely on very precise control of fine cutting instruments, and the unique properties of glass ionomer cement. It is essential to use magnification for accurate vision whilst cutting this type of preparation.

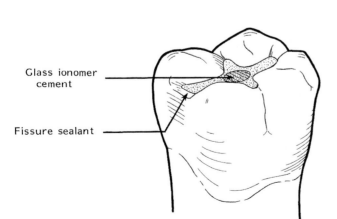
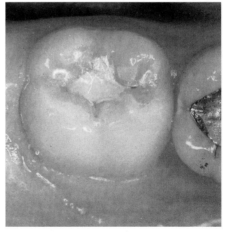

Glass ionomer cement

Fissure sealant

Fig. 10.3 Preventive resin restoration. The deeper part of the cavity is filled with glass ionomer cement and this, plus the fissure system, has acid etch resin applied to it

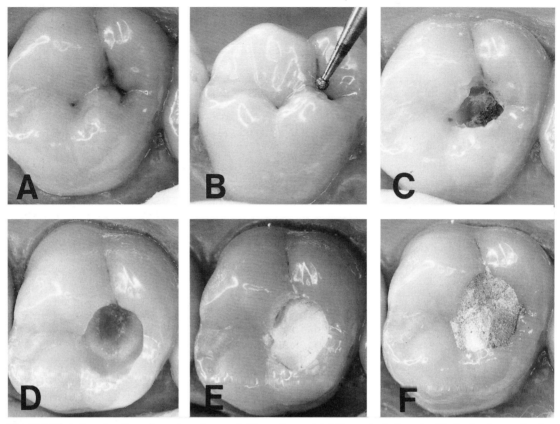

Fig. 10.4 Clinical exploration of a carious fissure. **A** The occlusopalatal fissure is darkened with shadowing under the enamel. **B** A small round bur is used to obtain access to explore the lesion. **C** The lesion turns out to be large. **D** The periphery is cleared and then the pulpal floor is excavated. Some residual staining is left. **E** A calcium hydroxide liner is placed on the stained area and a zinc oxide–eugenol base restores the cavity to minimal depth. **F** Completed amalgam restoration.

The commonest of these is the *tunnel preparation* (*Fig. 10.5*) that maintains the marginal ridge, but care must be taken not to touch the adjacent tooth as the tunnelling emerges approximally. Sight of the approximal lesion is obtained by widening the occlusal access bucco-lingually. GIC is suitable for small lesions; in a larger cavity it can be used for the approximal part, but it may be surfaced with composite resin occlusally. Modern condensable GICs may be an alternative material for the whole restoration.

Moderate lesions

Conservative class II cavity

Preparation is begun by obtaining access to the approximal lesion to inspect its extent and make a provisional decision on the likely restorative material. The occlusal section is prepared in accordance with any carious attack in the fissures and the need to provide mechanical stability for the restoration. The overriding considerations are to:

● Conserve as much tooth substance as possible
● Maintain occlusal contacts on enamel

Approximal section One of the main problems associated with the approximal box preparation is a failure to determine the site of the carious lesion in all three planes prior to the commencement of the preparation. The tendency is to cut standard shaped cavities without locating the lesion properly, which results in extension either too far lingually or buccally. Slightly rotated teeth are a particular problem. The initial penetration of the marginal ridge should be made directly towards the lesion, and not simply to remove the entire proximal surface in one go.

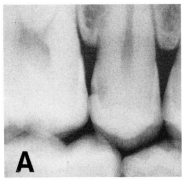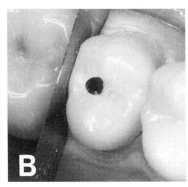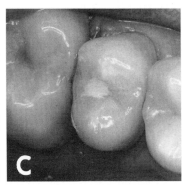

Fig. 10.5 Tunnel preparation. **A** Bitewing radiograph of ⌐5 showing minimal approximal caries in dentine. **B** The approximal lesion is approached via an occlusal access having placed a section of matrix band to protect the adjacent tooth. **C** Glass ionomer cement is placed to restore the 'tunnel'. This must be chemically cured since the marginal ridge will obscure the approximal section from the curing light. The glass ionomer cement and the fissures are covered with fissure sealant

The margins of the preparation should just clear the contact with the adjacent tooth buccally, lingually and cervically, meaning that the outline follows the embrasure shape, though with straight edges. The box profile is therefore naturally undercut (*Fig. 10.6*).

Clearing the contact means that the restoration margins are accessible for finishing and for oral hygiene. It also allows a matrix to be placed (see below).

Occlusal section
The *occlusal key* is cut to one-quarter to one-fifth the intercuspal distance (*Fig. 10.7*); this reduces to a minimum risk of weakening the remaining tooth structure.

Any further reduction in cavity width here is determined by the restorative material that has been chosen. Adequate space must be provided for the entry of the amalgam condenser, though less is required for composite resins, since they flow under pressure.

The cavity design should avoid cutting enamel centric stops, since none of the direct materials is capable of maintaining occlusal stability over long periods. In particular, evidence to date indicates that successful use of composites and glass ionomers in the posterior region requires that they are placed in non-stress-bearing areas. Also, freehand carving, by either carvers or rotary instruments, of accurate occlusal morphology is unreliable (Chapter 14). Proper occlusal stability is unlikely to be produced.

The extent of the caries may prevent such minimal outlines, but as a general rule and where possible, adoption of this principle would extend the life expectancy of any restoration.

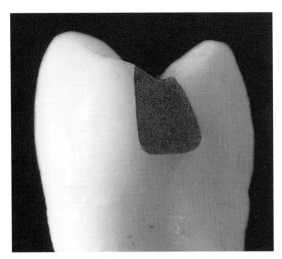

Fig. 10.6 Approximal box outline for a conservative cavity

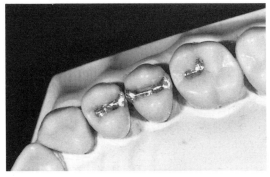

Fig. 10.7 Conservative cavities for amalgam

The cavity should extend just below the enamel–dentine junction occlusally, so that this may be inspected for caries and the restoration can be based on dentine, which has more resilience. Localized areas of caries should be removed either with excavators or slow running large round burs. The irregularities in the floor of the cavity may be filled later with some form of structural base.

The extension of the cavity into the fissures and embrasures should be determined by the patient's predisposition to caries and, with a large number of carious lesions in fissures, fissure extension would be advisable. Tooth morphology also affects the decision. Deep convoluted fissures will predispose towards recurrence of caries and should be excised.

Stability   In spite of the advances in adhesives, it is unwise to rely on any of the current types to provide stability for class II restorations. Conventional retention is still required to prevent displacement by having the base of the cavity fractionally wider than the outline, which provides a mechanical key, and having a flat floor for stability.

The approximal box requires resistance to prevent displacement towards the adjacent tooth, and this should be provided by the occlusal portion of the cavity.

When using composite resins, microleakage is reduced by the bond to acid etched enamel. To achieve this bond, prisms must be etched in their long axis and bevelled margins are necessary to expose prism ends in certain areas. The proximal box margins should be bevelled, but not the occlusal section. Here the enamel is cut transversely by the normal preparation because of its slope towards the fissure.

Instrumentation

Limits on the extent of cavity preparation are imposed by bur dimensions, the precision and state of handpiece bearing, and the visual acuity of the operator.

Burs   Burs used may be divided into those that *abrade* away the surface and those that *cut* the surface. The first category includes the diamond instruments that have a fine grit of diamond embedded in the matrix of the bur. Their method of production limits their effective diameter to not less than 0.8 mm, and the wear on a bur of such a size is very rapid. These abrade away the surface of the dentine, producing a surface of uniform roughness.

Tungsten carbide burs have blades with cutting edges that may be serrated to increase the cutting

rate. Even these burs tend to grind the tooth rather than truly cut the surface. Here again there is a limit to how narrow these burs can be before the risk of fracture of the metal becomes unacceptable; their diameters must be greater than 0.8 mm. At any thickness, though, they are very prone to fracture if any lateral stress is placed upon them. The fracture occurs either at the shank or within the structure of the bur itself, depending on the design. This limitation plus the eccentricity of the handpiece means that the minimum possible width of cavity that can be obtained realistically is about 1 mm.

Burs with a sharp terminal profile, such as the inverted cone or flat fissure, introduce stress concentrations in the line angles of a cavity, and round profile burs, such as the dome fissure, are preferred.

Anterior restorations

Here all that is required is excision of the lesion with the minimum removal of tooth substance. The old kidney-shaped class V cavity is aesthetically unsatisfactory and quite unnecessary.

Cervical lesions may be restored with composite resin, compomers, GIC or RMGIC if they have enamel margins by GIC if they are sited in dentine alone. In this region, the composite currently provides the best aesthetics and bonds well to acid-etched enamel. GIC has durable bonding to dentine and the important advantages of fluoride exchange and better stain resistance. The compomers, the fluoride-releasing acid modified composites, may also be used but there is currently inadequate evidence to determine their long-term performance and they show polymerization shrinkages that are similar to those of composites. RMGIC show even greater polymerization shrinkage and are therefore less suitable. Where cervical root caries has appeared in areas of gingival recession, or in sensitive abrasion cavities, GIC is the material of choice.

Because adhesion of both composite resin and GIC is variable, it is unwise to rely on it totally for retention, and mechanical undercuts must be provided. However, as discussed in Chapter 9, marginal leakage is considerably reduced.

For class III lesions it is desirable to adopt a palatal approach for the approximal lesion wherever possible for aesthetic reasons, and to angle the bur into the lesion under the marginal ridge to maintain enamel in the occlusion (*Fig. 10.8*). The labial extension should be just through the contact, and whilst this may result in a very thin layer of enamel and dentine or enamel alone, the modern aesthetic materials offer the advantage of

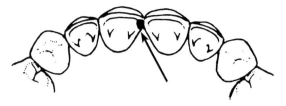

Fig. 10.8 Direction of access to a mesial lesion on an incisor. The marginal ridge is preserved by this line of approach

supporting this layer through bonding; this produces a better aesthetic result. The necessity for the palatal extensions or dovetails frequently included in the older class III cavities has been obviated by the advent of the acid etch technique and the newer dentine adhesives. As with the class V, though, it is still preferable to include some mechanical retention as well; this would take the form of gingival and incisal pits and grooves, providing these do not weaken the remaining tooth.

The choice of restorative material is between GIC and composite resin and their hybrid relatives, with the GIC having a positive advantage in individuals with high caries rates. Composites and compomers have a slight advantage in respect of early colour match.

Where teeth are to be restored with composite resin, a bevel applied to all enamel margins will improve the etching characteristics, but will result in a thin wedge of composite resin at the periphery of the restoration. If the bond fails, chipping and staining will occur and so it might be better to avoid bevelling, provide mechanical retention and use the acid etch technique to improve marginal adaptation only.

Cavity finishing

Differing opinions exist as to whether cavity walls should be left as they are cut or smoothed with some form of blank or multi-bladed finishing bur. The surface differences produced by different burs is striking, but did not seem to be critical for clinical results until the arrival of adhesives.

The quality of the adhesive bond is dependent to a large extent on the morphology of the substrate to which it is applied; this will vary according to the instruments used. The rougher the surface, the more difficult will be the wetting of this by the adhesive. The result is air pockets under the restoration that provide a route for microleakage, in spite of the adhesive. Theoretically the smoother the surface, the more efficient will be the adhesive process.

Several cavity cleansers have been proposed for use with amalgam. Some of these have proved harmful, such as the dehydrating alcohol varieties. The blander ones are designed to remove bacteria that have been implicated in pulpal reactions under restorations. This may be desirable, but they also remove the smear layer that is better left alone. The best and most biologically acceptable cleanser for use prior to placing amalgam seems to be the air and water from the triple syringe.

Pulp protection – linings

On completion of the cavity a decision should be made regarding the need for further pulpal protection. In the majority of minimal cavities, the protection afforded by the dentine from both chemical and mechanical irritation is adequate. But once the cavity extends beyond minimal size, additional pulpal protection is required.

Lining materials may be divided into three groups:

● Bases
● Liners
● Varnishes

Bases

The primary purpose of these materials is to protect pulpal tissue from mechanical and chemical irritation. Their properties also allow their use as a dentine replacement. They are usually used in thick section to act as thermal insulators. For clinical use, it is important that they reach a substantial strength quickly, otherwise the restoration placement, particularly the condensation of amalgam, will be compromised.

Zinc phosphate cement

This material is still used routinely by some operators as it is easy to manipulate. The main constituents are buffered phosphoric acid and a mixture of zinc oxide and magnesium oxide, and it sets by the formation of a hydrated zinc phosphate.

Biologically, there are reservations about the cement since a considerable amount of free acid is available for some time after mixing. This may be responsible for pulpal irritation and pulpal necrosis, but bacterial ingress might be more important in the aetiology of pulpal problems. Its other main drawback is its susceptibility to fluid contamination, especially during the early stages of setting.

The cement is stronger than any of the other bases in compression and therefore provides stability in thick section when the restoration is placed.

Polycarboxylate cement

The powder consists of a mixture of zinc oxide and magnesium oxide with vacuum dried polyacrylic acid; this is simply mixed with water.

The resulting material, that has a zinc poly-acrylate matrix, has similar properties to those of phosphate cement, but its main advantage is that it possesses adhesive properties to tooth structure. Pulpal irritation is reported to be significantly below that of phosphate cement, which may be due to the high molecular weight of the polyacrylic acid. The material is therefore rather better than phosphate cement, but it has more difficult handling characteristics. Addition of fluoride salts permits a limited short-term release of fluoride ions.

Zinc oxide–eugenol cements

These are derived from the original simple zinc oxide–eugenol (ZOE) cement that was used as a sedative dressing. In its crudest form the material was not strong enough to be used as a base or as a long-term temporary dressing. It did, however, have an obtundent effect on pulp symptoms as long as dentine remained over the pulp. On exposed soft tissue, the material is an irritant.

The basic ZOE cements have been modified by the addition of a variety of materials. *Zinc stearate* and *zinc acetate* were first included as a means of increasing the strength and shortening the setting time, and either *polystyrene* or *ethoxybenzoic acid* have been added to reinforce the materials further.

Whilst still the weakest of the bases, mixed correctly it provides good service. However, incorrect proportioning is common, which means that the material is used at powder: liquid ratios well below those which would achieve the optimum properties.

The importance of having a strong base has been demonstrated by work that shows that there is a displacement of the restoration under load, and the displacement is directly related to the type of cement used as a base.

The other disadvantage of the eugenol-based materials is that they are not compatible with all restorative materials. Polymer-based materials are plasticized by the eugenol and their polymerization is retarded.

Glass ionomer cements and resin-modified glass ionomer cements

This family of materials has, in addition to the restorative materials described earlier, derivatives for use as linings. The conventional GICs provide a material with similar compressive strength to phosphate cement and having a tenacious bond to tooth. The RMGICs offer greater mechanical strength initially but at the expense of a considerable polymerization shrinkage and a marked exotherm during this setting phase. This may well affect the adhesive properties of the cement. Some concern has been expressed about the monomer addition to these materials, 2-hydroxyethyl methacrylate (HEMA). This has been reported to have adverse effects on skin, and allergic reactions have been reported.

Liners

These materials form a thin layer over the pulpal floor of deep cavities and the commonest form is the calcium hydroxide cements whose therapeutic action is discussed in Chapter 11. The calcium hydroxide is combined with a polymer base that may be self curing or light activated.

Self-curing liners have poor mechanical properties in comparison with the bases discussed earlier, but they are valuable as chemical insulators in shallow cavities and as sublinings in deep ones. In deep cavities, it is desirable that they should be covered by a structural base because of their weakness.

The development of light activated resin-based liners has changed the materials considerably. Their advantage is the increase in mechanical properties, but there is a reduction in the pH of the cement from pH 11 to 7, and this reduces secondary dentine deposition. It is possible that these materials will not be as effective as pulp-capping agents. They also set by an exothermic reaction, and this can lead to substantial temperature rises.

Cavity varnishes

These materials are usually based on resins such as copal varnish and polystyrenes in a volatile solvent. Their main purpose is to prevent the ingress of bacteria and microleakage into the dentine tubules. They are not thermal insulators, and have high solubility. They have been replaced in anterior restorations by the adhesives and their long-term durability with amalgam is questionable.

Conclusion

Use of bases is reduced in current clinical practice because of the use of dentine bonding agents and the total etch techniques referred to in Chapter 9. The ease of use of the calcium hydroxide liners has resulted in these being the most popular lining for amalgam restorations.

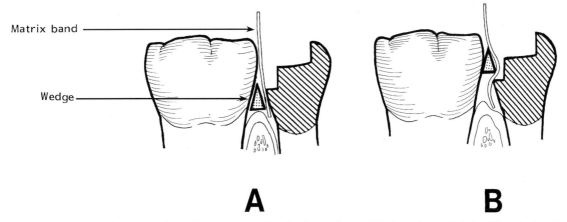

Fig. 10.9 Wedging technique. **A** shows the correct position for the wedge, and **B** shows it too high, buckling the band

Matrices

A plethora of matrix retainers and bands is available and it is difficult to single out any one particular type as being the ideal. However, there are a number of desirable features for any system:

- The approximal contour should be reproduced accurately
- The band should be thin enough to provide an adequate contact and yet be rigid enough not to buckle or crease
- The bands must be of sufficient variety to match various tooth shapes
- The retainer should be stable and allow correct tightening of the band at the cervical margin
- For light-cured materials, the bands must allow transmission of light

The difficulties of all the current systems are that none of them produce the concavo–convex outline of the natural tooth and most produce a flat surface, with the contact usually at the marginal ridge rather than one-third of the way down the approximal surface.

The Siqveland type is usually the easiest to use but will produce a poorly-contoured approximal surface unless it is burnished to shape. It should also be cut after packing, so that it can be removed laterally through the contact. If this is not done, there is a danger that removal will take the marginal ridge with it.

It is essential to wedge all bands, and failure to do this will result in overhangs that are difficult to remove in amalgam but almost impossible to detect or remove with composite resins without damaging the tooth.

The choice and use of wedges is also important. The wedge must hold the band against the cervical margin of the cavity. Frequently this is not achieved and the wedge rests on the margin, interfering with the contour (*Fig. 10.9*).

Matrices for the anterior region are ill developed, and improper use can ruin the restoration. The most difficult restoration is the class V, since the acute convexity of the buccal aspect together with the complex shape in the longitudinal plane of the teeth will frequently result in poor contour. The contoured soft metal matrices are the most satisfactory but are unusable with light-cured materials.

Restorative materials – handling

Amalgam

The variables that can seriously alter the properties of the material and the durability of the restoration are:

- Proportioning
- Mixing
- Condensation
- Carving
- Polishing

Proportioning

For hand mixing it was necessary to use an excess of mercury, with mercury/alloy ratios of 8:5 or 7:5 and even after condensation excess mercury remains, with consequent reduction in physical properties. This problem has been reduced considerably by mechanical mixing and encapsulation which, because it is more efficient, requires a ratio of about 1:1.

Mixing

The correct ratio must be mixed for the correct time. An under-mixed amalgam will be dry and crumbly. The ideally mixed material should be a cohesive ball that can be pushed to thin film without breaking up, with the over-mixed material being soupy, difficult to remove from the capsule and frequently hot to touch. Over-mixing reduces the working time and increases creep values, whilst under-mixing leads to an unusable mix.

Condensation

Undercondensation by using inadequate pressure or a large surface area condenser will result in inadequate expression of excess mercury and also lead to microporosity. Here the admixed and spherical particle alloys show some advantage, since they may be condensed with less pressure, and puddling of the alloy produces a satisfactory restoration. In fact, the use of a small condenser is contra-indicated with these alloys as the tip will push through the amalgam and leave subsurface porosities. Mechanical condensation is also disadvantageous.

Carving

Correct reproduction of the occlusal contacts, together with removal of the mercury-rich excess layer, is essential. In Chapter 8, the difficulty of reproducing exact anatomical cusp/fossa relationships was described. Occlusal stability can be achieved, together with axial loading of the tooth, by carving flat centric stops to receive the opposing supporting cusps, rather than attempting tripods (see *Fig. 14.8b*). If the tripods have one or more contacts missing, the tooth will move to find a stable position. This may create occlusal interferences.

The amalgam restoration should hold shimstock, and if it does then a shiny mark(s) will be seen on its surface; this is not necessarily a 'high spot', and an amalgam with no shiny marks will be out of occlusion. Unfortunately, the majority are taken out of occlusion for this reason and occlusal instability ensues.

Polishing

Polishing should correct any carving errors, such as excess at the margins or occlusal problems, but must not eliminate the occlusal stops already produced. When using finishing burs or polishing pastes, it is undesirable to produce local hot spots on the surface, since this will probably cause changes in the phases of the amalgam. It also causes excess mercury to come to the surface and this, in turn, weakens the material.

Composite resins

Clinical usage of light activated composites is complicated by:

- Restricted depth of cure
- Activation by the operating light
- Occlusal shaping
- Deterioration in the activating light unit

The activating light intensity is reduced if it is obstructed by tooth or is some distance away from the material, as with the floor of the approximal box in a class II restoration, and therefore the restoration must be built in individually-cured increments that are no more than about 1.5 mm thick. The depth of cure is also reduced by a darker shade.

The light output from each commercially available light unit varies and this can seriously affect the curing potential of the system. It may also be affected by variations in the power supply voltage that reduce the energy emitted at the 470 nm wavelength. A reduction in the voltage shifts the energy distribution toward the higher wavelengths. The bulb should also be changed at least every six months to maintain efficiency, and the continuity of fibres in the fibre optic type should also be checked regularly as these are prone to breakage. Devices are now available for testing the light output and this should be done regularly.

Class II restorations

The placement of composite resin in a class II cavity requires meticulous execution of each stage in turn, and consequently much time.

The sequence of placement, which should be done under rubber dam, is:

1. Pre-wedge to open contact area
2. Prepare cavity with rounded line angles and bevelled approximal box
3. Line with eugenol-free base
4. Acid etch enamel, apply thin layer of 'enamel bonding agent'
5. Place dentine bonding agent
6. Place transparent matrix, re-wedge
7. Apply and cure 0.5 mm of composite at the cervical margin to avoid shrinkage and marginal failure (*Fig. 10.10*)
8. Build and cure the remainder in 1.5 mm increments
9. Complete occlusal surface

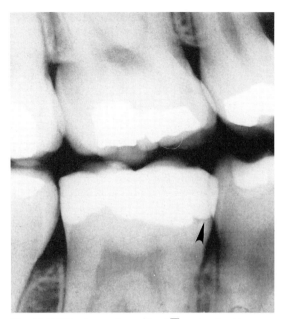

Fig. 10.10 Bitewing radiograph of $\overline{6}$ restored with posterior composite. There is a failure of adaptation at the mesial cervical margin (arrowed)

placement. However a certain amount of water is essential for the setting reaction, and they must not be allowed to dry out, otherwise they will crumble.

Mechanically mixed encapsulated materials provide a much more reliable and consistent material since the method of mixing is the greatest problem with GICs at present. Poor results are usually due to incorrect proportioning and mixing, and the materials are often blamed rather than the operator's or nurse's inability to follow the instructions.

Inlay techniques for gold, composite resin and ceramic

The basis for all indirect restorative techniques is the cutting of a non-undercut preparation, the reproduction of this through an impression and laboratory model, laboratory construction of the restoration and finally its fitting and cementation in the mouth.

Variations around these basic principles are brought about by the physical properties of the inlay material and the cementing medium.

The occlusion is difficult to restore, as free hand carving leaves an oxygen-inhibited surface that should be cut back. This may be avoided by overfilling and cutting back after curing. This is tedious and produces a relatively inaccurate occlusal morphology with the inherent risk of removal of tooth tissue, since differentiation between tooth and restorative is frequently difficult. An occlusal index can be prepared preoperatively to mould the composite, or, rubber dam permitting, the patient can close into centric occlusion with the composite covered with a piece of cling film. This latter technique gives a quick and simple guide to the occlusal stops.

There is a higher incidence of postoperative pain following composite placement. The polymerization shrinkage causes cuspal flexure and marginal leakage, and the light is a potent source of heat. Some materials stick to instruments and are thus pulled away from cavity floors, leading to leakage (*Fig. 10.10*).

Glass ionomer cements

All the materials are sensitive to water contamination in the early stages of setting and should be protected from early exposure to saliva after

Gold inlays

Here the technique has been developed over many years to compensate for the lack of adhesion and the solubility of the cement, originally zinc phosphate. Gold inlays have to be mechanically retentive without the cement being present. This is achieved by near-parallelism of cavity walls and by having a single and long path of insertion. A cavity taper of 5–10° is necessary.

The cement is protected from oral fluids by a bevelled margin on the inlay that can be swaged on to the tooth surface, covering the cement lute. The excellent strength of gold alloys allows this thin layer to be manufactured and manipulated.

The cement provides the final stability for the inlay by mechanical interlocks with the cavity wall.

Composite resin and ceramic inlays

A bevel cannot be constructed in these materials because they are not strong enough in thin section. There will therefore be no protection for the cementing medium that is exposed to both oral fluids and the occlusion. Processing problems have led to the requirement that the cavity taper is of the order of 25–30° and therefore there is no inherent mechanical stability to the restoration. Retention of these inlays is totally dependent on the adhesion of the cementing material.

The cements are fluid polymer composites of low filler concentration whose physical properties are considerably lower than those of restorative composites. These are literally the weak link. Their degradation leads to marginal staining and lack of support for the inlay margin, that is then prone to fracture.

Clinical studies suggest that these problems are seen at about five years service.

Intracoronal restorations – Summary

Techniques for small restorations have changed dramatically in the last few years. Advances in the diagnosis of caries, materials and cavity design have eclipsed Black's original concepts. Understanding the pathology of caries, the anatomy of the tooth and the properties of restorative materials is essential for the design of modern cavities. These designs are based on individual circumstances and not learnt by rote.

Tooth tissue should be regarded as a precious resource, only to be removed if essential. Small cavities cause less trauma and do less harm to the natural occlusal relationships.

A large range of restorative materials is available. All have limitations and some have not been in general clinical service for long enough for their longevity to be established.

11

Management of the deep cavity

Management of the deep cavity requires accurate assessment of the pulpal condition, the restorability of the tooth and the method of restoration.

This chapter discusses pulp testing, pulp capping, the use of auxiliary retention and the choice of restorative material.

In distinction from the treatment of the small to moderate carious lesion, the deep cavity requires not only a decision on the restorative technique to be used, but also, and most importantly, an assessment of the state of the pulp.

Clinical assessment of pulp conditions can be unreliable, and for this reason it is far preferable to institute regular and routine 6-monthly examinations to avoid, amongst other things, the problems of managing deep caries. This is particularly important in the young patient, where there is less mineralization of the dentine, and the response to carious attack by the pulp cannot keep pace with the advancing lesion.

In the older patient the rate of spread is slower, and the pulpal response of laying down secondary dentine and increasing the mineral content of the dentine is able to provide some chance of pulp defence (see Chapter 6).

Pulp assessment

The clinician has very poor information to guide him – there is no opportunity to biopsy the diseased tissue! The clinician needs to make the fullest use of:

- Symptoms
- Clinical appearance
- Vitality tests
- Radiographic appearance

The correlation of symptoms with pulpal pathology is poor. However, the following sequence may act as a guide:

1. Transient low grade pain on eating sweet foods – *early lesion in dentine, pulp normal*
2. Transient mild pain on hot and cold foods – *deeper lesion in dentine, pulp normal*
3. More severe pain lasting after the stimulus has gone – *pulp pathology*

Provided the symptoms are transient, it is fairly certain that the pulp tissue is not involved in the pathology, and the response can be regarded as essentially physiological. It is only if the pain continues after the stimulus is removed that there is a strong possibility that the pulp has started to respond at a cellular level. The more severe the pain, the less chance there is of pulp recovery after removal of the caries.

Of course, this nicely ordered picture may not be seen, since the chronic nature of the lesion may not give rise to symptoms at all. Alternatively, there may be odd diffuse pain which is poorly localized. Unfortunately, the absence of pain is no guarantee of pulpal health and the possible maintenance of vitality.

The visual appearance of the lesion – extent of breakdown, colour of tooth and so on – provides a valuable indication of the likely depth of the lesion. This, coupled with the radiographic appearance and the results of vitality tests (Chapter 2), will put the clinician on the right track on the flow chart (*Fig. 11.1*)

Operative treatment

This is best done under rubber dam to reduce the risk of salivary contamination of any exposure to a minimum.

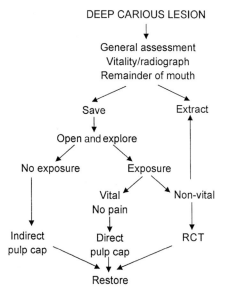

DEEP CARIOUS LESION

↓

General assessment
Vitality/radiograph
Remainder of mouth

Save   Extract

Open and explore

No exposure   Exposure

Vital   Non-vital
No pain

Indirect   Direct   RCT
pulp cap   pulp cap

Restore

Fig. 11.1 Management of the deep carious lesion. RCT, root canal treatment

The objective is to remove all the peripheral caries, thus obtaining good access to the body of the lesion, and then to remove carefully the caries that lies directly over the pulp.

The ideal is to excise the whole lesion, leaving sound dentine as the base of the cavity. However, when a pulpal exposure might result, it is permissible to leave a zone of altered dentine at the base.

It is the identification of the proximity of the pulp and the dentine that may be left that presents the problems. It is very difficult to be sure of the three-dimensional relationship of the lesion with the pulp, though, with experience, an educated guess is possible.

In all circumstances, soft mushy dentine must be removed. However where there is slight softening but the dentine appears structurally intact, it is possible to leave this if the risk of exposure is high. The means of determining the extent of the penetration of the caries are very limited and use of the conventional dental probe to detect softening could easily lead to penetration of a very thin layer overlying the pulp.

Two layers within the dentinal caries are important clinically:

1. *Superficial* – extensively demineralized, containing a large volume of bacteria
2. *Deep* – slightly demineralized, containing no bacteria

The structure of the first layer is totally disorganized, whilst the second retains the basic ordered structure of dentine. It is the deeper layer that can be remineralized in favourable conditions (*Fig. 11.2*).

Dyes that are able to differentiate between these layers in the dentine may be used instead of clinical experience. The dye acid red (1% in propylene glycol solution) has been shown to stain the superficial layer only, leaving the deeper layer unstained. The dye is applied, washed off and the stained area removed with an excavator. This operation is repeated until the base of the cavity remains unstained. This is a possible method of detecting caries but it must be used with caution as there is some doubt as to the precision of the dye

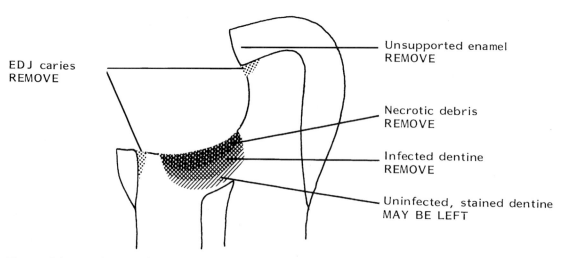

EDJ caries
REMOVE

Unsupported enamel
REMOVE

Necrotic debris
REMOVE

Infected dentine
REMOVE

Uninfected, stained dentine
MAY BE LEFT

Fig. 11.2 Schematic diagram of the zones of a deep carious lesion. EDJ, enamel–dentine junction

penetration. Injudicious or heavy-handed removal of the infected tissue may result in a pulpal exposure.

Once the removal of the infected material has been completed, and no exposure has resulted, and if the tooth is restorable, an *indirect pulp cap* is placed.

The most reliable material is calcium hydroxide, usually in a resin base, which has two effects. Its high pH of 9–11 reduces the activity of any bacteria still remaining as the environment changes from acid to alkaline, and it provokes remineralization of the softened dentine and the deposition of secondary dentine beneath the lesion by the pulp. Since this effect appears to relate to pH, there is some concern about the therapeutic efficacy of recently produced materials that have a pH of 7. However, these new materials do have the advantage of being stronger mechanically and can more readily withstand the occlusal load transmitted via the restoration. The older materials required an extra structural base to absorb this load.

If removal of the softened dentine results in an exposure, then the whole lesion should be excised immediately. Contamination of the pulp will have occurred and infected dentine should not remain in the area. It is now necessary to consider *direct pulp capping*.

Again, success depends upon the absence of cellular changes in the pulp, as may be indicated by symptoms. A number of physical criteria also determine the success of the procedure:

- *Size of the exposure.* The larger the exposure, the less likely is a successful outcome since contamination of the pulp with infected dentine debris will have occurred. Also haemorrhage will be increased. Ideally the exposure should be less than 0.5 mm in diameter, and any over 1 mm in diameter have a very poor prognosis
- *Contamination with saliva.* This reduces the success rate greatly since there will be bacterial contamination
- *Marginal leakage.* Any leakage can result in bacterial ingress and direct access to the pulp

Once the exposure has been located, all the dentine debris should be removed. Any haemorrhage must be arrested, preferably without massive blood clot formation. Evidence suggests that the presence of a large clot reduces the success rate.

The exposure is then treated with calcium hydroxide materials that are free from zinc oxide/eugenol. Again, use of a structural base to prevent displacement of the calcium hydroxide liner is necessary.

Success rate is variable for carious exposures, whilst that for traumatic exposures is considerably better.

It is, of course, very important to see that there is pulp tissue present. Calcium hydroxide applied to an empty pulp chamber has little value.

Pulpotomy may be attempted for large exposures. This involves opening the pulp chamber and amputating the coronal pulp, leaving what is hoped to be healthy pulp in the roots. The root canal pulps are covered with calcium hydroxide.

The success of the procedure depends on the infection being limited to the coronal pulp, and this will be far from certain. However, if the root canals cannot be negotiated by conventional instruments, pulpotomy gives some hope of retaining the tooth.

Postoperative assessment

The patient should be warned of possible pulp symptoms and told to return immediately if there is pain. Regular review using vitality tests and radiographs is essential to ensure that any changes in pathology of the apical tissues may be detected. Calcium hydroxide may cause excessive deposition of secondary dentine that may occlude the root canal. Should this occur, intervention and endodontic therapy may be indicated before the canal is obliterated.

Restoration

In many cases where indirect or direct pulp capping has been necessary, the tooth will have lost a considerable amount of tissue. The plan for restoration should consider, in particular, retention and stability of the proposed restoration, and the occlusion. Interim temporary dressing should be avoided if possible, since subsequent removal of this and more preparation can insult the pulp further.

Anterior teeth may be restored by pinned or acid-etch retained composite resin but, as discussed in Chapter 15, this may have some limitations aesthetically and functionally. Once large amounts of what are small teeth are lost, then elective devitalization, root filling and a post crown are almost inevitable.

In posterior teeth, where all cusps remain intact, or only a single cusp has been lost, restoration with amalgam is the most reliable solution. Here retention is usually obtained from the remaining tooth substance and free-hand carving reproduces occlusal stability adequately.

Where more tooth has been lost, then the accurate reproduction of the occlusion will almost certainly require a cast gold crown or inlay. In order to provide a proper foundation for the casting, a core is necessary.

Choice of core material

Three materials may be used for core construction:

- Amalgam
- Composite resin
- Glass ionomer cement

Amalgam

Amalgam has several advantages. It can be well condensed around pins and may be contoured to anatomical form easily. It has good long-term durability if crown construction is to be delayed, perhaps whilst oral hygiene is being improved. If there is any dissolution of the cement lute during the life of the crown, corrosion of the amalgam provides a barrier to leakage.

Composite resins

These materials are more operator sensitive and appear to have a higher failure rate. They are difficult to adapt around pins and cases of crown failure have been reported due to separation of the core from the pins. Unless a specific core building material is used, there is no colour contrast between it and the tooth. This could make seeing the finishing line difficult during crown preparation.

Glass ionomer cements

Currently it is desirable that GICs are supported by a considerable volume of tooth structure for their successful use as core materials. Cermets and condensable glass ionomers have increased the applications of GIC derivatives for cores, but clinical results are few. Whilst the presence of fluoride, adhesive properties and their dimensional stability are advantages, manipulation is more difficult, and amalgam has the proven durability. It would be unwise to rely on the adhesion of GICs to support a crown and not use pins.

Amalgam core placement

Amalgam will always require auxiliary retention, though when it is not to be reduced by subsequent crown preparation, careful use of the remaining tooth tissue to provide undercuts can be successful. It is important to remember that any additional aid to retention will weaken the tooth and the dangers of excessive use of pins must be recognized.

The principal means of adding retention are:

- Pits and grooves
- Pins

Pits and grooves

The objective is to place the grooves or pits in opposing walls to resist the displacement of the restoration either vertically or laterally. However, their effectiveness can be limited, and they certainly weaken remaining walls. To be of use, any groove must be opposed by another groove or other retentive feature. The two features will then act in concert.

Unless they are of adequate depth and undercut to allow for the setting contraction of the amalgam, they will serve little purpose. It is also imperative that the amalgam is adequately condensed into them.

Pins

Pins, whilst aiding retention of the restoration, also introduce planes of weakness in the material and stress concentrations in the tooth. A balance must be established between adequate retention and a restoration that fractures under occlusal stress.

Three types of pin are available:

- Self threading
- Friction grip
- Cemented

Self threading   The pin hole is prepared by a twist drill, the diameter of which is slightly smaller than the pin. The pin, usually integral with a bur shank, can then be tapped into place using slow speed. The pin shears off the bur shank as it meets the resistance at the base of the pin hole. These are the most convenient and safest of the types available, but a number of difficulties can occur during placement:

1. *Oversized pin hole*. This is either the result of the handpiece chuck running eccentrically due to a worn bearing, or lack of positive control of the handpiece as the hole is cut.
2. *Dentine failure*. The speed of rotation or weakness of the dentine can lead to the thread that has been tapped shearing as the pin reaches the bottom of the hole. The pin then comes back with its shank.
3. *Incomplete seating*. This is a particular problem with the self-shearing varieties and can be caused by running the handpiece too fast, or by variations in elasticity of the dentine resulting in the pin shearing early.

The first two may be corrected by either cutting the next larger hole and trying again with the larger pin, or cementing the pin in place. The latter is difficult, but may be the only solution.

Failure to seat properly may lead to excess pin intruding into the occlusion and also weakness in the support for the pin. If the pin is secure, then it

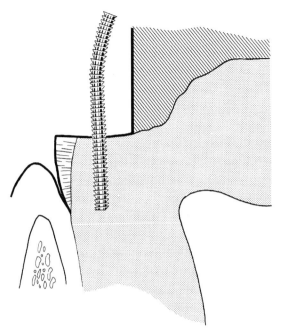

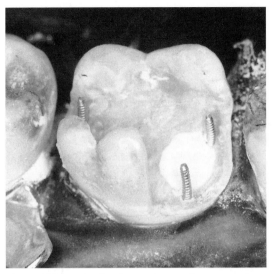

Fig. 11.4 Three pins in place and correctly contoured

Fig. 11.3 The position of a pin. It should be surrounded by dentine, 1 mm inside the enamel–dentine junction, 2–3 mm deep and bent to fall within the contour of the restoration

will need bending or cutting. It is better, though, to try to remove it and start again.

Even successful placement of this type of pin is potentially damaging to the dentine, causing crazing and stress concentrations.

Friction grip   Here again the pin hole is prepared to a slightly smaller size but the pin is pushed home using a holder. This type of pin relies on the elasticity of the dentine to accommodate and retain it, and again there is a risk of stresses and fracture of the dentine under load.

Cemented   These pins are cemented into place in slightly oversize holes using low viscosity polycarboxylate or cyanoacrylate cements. Increased retention may be obtained by sandblasting the pin to produce a mechanical interlock between the dentine, cement and pin. Introduction of the cement into the pin hole may be aided by the use of a spiral root filler.

Pin placement

This is particularly important since the pin must be placed in an area that provides support for the restoration and does not weaken the tooth. It must also not perforate the pulp or periodontal tissues.

There are, therefore, a limited number of sites where pins may be positioned.

Pins should be placed in dentine and to ensure an adequate bulk of dentine surrounding them (*Fig. 11.3*), they should be about 1 mm inside the enamel–dentine junction. Any closer to the junction, and there will be a high risk of fracture of a plate of enamel and dentine away from the side of the tooth. Repair of this, so far below gingival margin level, can be impossible.

The anatomy of the pulp chamber and the interface between the root and the periodontal ligament dictate the angulation of the pin. The pin hole should be parallel to the external root surface and a good guide to this is to place the tip of the bur, or the blade of a flat plastic, in the gingival crevice against the root. The bur may then be placed at the same angle on the dentine.

Commencement of the pin hole may be assisted by cutting a small depression with a small round bur. The pin hole itself should be cut to a depth of about 2–3 mm, with some brands having a collar fitted to the burs to limit the depth of the hole. The pin should extend the same length above the surface.

After placement, pins should be bent to fall within the contour of the final restoration and sufficient amalgam must overlie the pin so that it does not crack away either during carving or subsequent crown preparation (*Fig. 11.4*).

Considerable care is necessary during bending since injudicious bending will stress the dentine and cause crazing. A number of devices are available to do this and they work on the principle of gripping the pin just above the point of entry

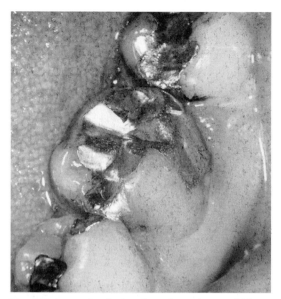

Fig. 11.5 A completed pinned amalgam that would be suitable as a medium-term restoration

into the dentine. The cemented pins offer the advantage of pre-bending prior to cementation.

Adequate clearance must be obtained between the top of the pin and the surface of the restoration. Failure to do this will result in the exposure of the pin either during carving or subsequently during crown preparation. Reduction of the length of the pin is dangerous, and the most effective way is to use a diamond in an airturbine. Under no circumstances should a tungsten carbide bur be used, as it is likely to fracture. Care should be taken with both self-threading and friction grip pins that they do not start to work loose during this procedure, and the patient's pharynx must be protected against swallowing or inhaling the pin.

A rough guide to the number of pins that should be placed is one per cusp lost, with a minimum of two. There should be at least one at each end of a core so that when the occlusal reduction for the crown preparation is done, one section of the core does not drop away (*Fig. 11.4*).

Matrices

Placement of matrices on the badly broken-down tooth presents a particularly difficult problem. The Siqveland can be very difficult to use, since as the band is tightened, it may ride up the tooth and slip over the cavity margin, resulting in a negative margin or a space through which amalgam will be exuded. Careful stabilization of the retainer by one hand during packing can help.

The Tofflemire holder, with its larger selection of bands, may be better and is usually easier to adapt to irregular margins.

Wedging is essential for any matrix so that the band is firmly adapted to the margins of the tooth. Care is necessary to avoid the wedge riding up over the preparation margin (see *Fig. 10.9B*). Failure to establish a stable, adequately contoured matrix for a core will lead to failure.

Packing and carving

Several successive mixes of amalgam should be used, rather than one large one, since the later ones will be workable at the end of packing. Carving of a core should aim to maintain the contacts with adjacent teeth and stabilize the occlusion. Elaborate anatomical detail is not necessary, provided the crown is to be prepared within a short time.

However, if the aim is to produce a medium-term restoration, then tooth anatomy should be reproduced to maintain periodontal health (*Fig. 11.5*).

Management of the deep cavity – Summary

Assess the pulpal condition as accurately as possible

Remove all peripheral caries

Remove pulpal caries with caution and attempt to prevent an exposure

Can the tooth be restored?

Indirect pulp cap/direct pulp cap with calcium hydroxide

Provide auxiliary retention, usually by pins

Restore with amalgam posteriorly, composite anteriorly

Review pulpal and apical condition regularly

12

Root canal treatment

> The field of endodontics, and root canal therapy in particular, has seen a large number of changes in techniques, equipment and materials in the last few years.
>
> There are now more methods of preparing and filling a root canal than any other small restorative procedure – the subject is 'technique intensive'!
>
> Fortunately, the basic principles underlying all methods remain the same and this chapter considers these to the exclusion of detailed descriptions of all the various twists and turns of new techniques.

The maintenance of pulp vitality should be one of the primary objectives of restorative dentistry. However, as more teeth are retained by a population of increasing average age, so the incidence of pulp pathology increases. Whilst prevention of the need for root canal treatment is very desirable, knowledge of its techniques is essential for modern day practice.

The *object* of root canal treatment is to maintain a functional tooth with a healthy periodontal ligament in the dentition following pulp pathology and its sequelae (Chapter 6).

Diagnosis and treatment planning

The choices in formulating the treatment plan depend very much on the general factors discussed in Section I, and the local need to keep a particular tooth within the context of the mouth as a whole.

Investigation of the deep cavity and the principles of pulp management were discussed in Chapter 11 and the present chapter deals with the extremely local problems of dealing with the restorable, non-vital tooth or a tooth chosen for elective devitalization.

Diagnostic procedures for root canal treatment follow the same basic guidelines presented in Section I, but particular note should be made of:

- Symptoms
- Problems of pulp testing
- Radiographic appearance
- Restorability of the crown

The first two relate to the achievement of a precise diagnosis of pulp condition, the third to the mechanical problems of preparing a root canal, and the fourth to the subsequent and final stage of restoration.

Following the decisions that the pulp is non-vital and the tooth should be conserved if possible, the crucial factors are that the root(s) must be amenable to root filling and that the tooth should be restorable afterwards. The treatment plan should include a provisional decision on the restoration type.

The *technical objectives* of root canal treatment are to:

- Remove all infected and contaminated tissue
- Shape the canal to an appropriate form to receive the chosen filling material
- Obturate the whole canal to block and seal the dead space

To remove all infected tissue, which includes both pulp and dentine, the full length of the root canal must be prepared to the apical constriction.

The root filling material must be chosen before the preparation is started, so that the preparation is shaped accordingly. For example, an apical master cone system will require precise preparation of the apical region of the root, whilst a fluid injectable system might be able to penetrate areas that simply have had infected tissue removed.

Root canal morphology

As a basis for successful root canal therapy the dentist must have a comprehensive knowledge of the anatomy of the pulp chambers and root canals of all teeth. Variations in anatomy are common and canals cannot be regarded as simple tubes running from crown to apex. Single roots often contain more than one canal and there will be other features such as transverse anastomoses, fins, lateral canals and apical deltas. Accessory canals are important also; these may pass from the pulp chamber into the furcation areas of molars or occur in the main root area.

The most common variations in root canal anatomy are:

- A single canal running to the apical foramen
- A root containing two separate small canals that unite in the apical region and exit through a single foramen
- A root containing two completely separate canals that exit through separate foramina
- A root containing a single canal that divides in two in the apical region and exits through two foramina

The most likely teeth to have more than one canal in a single root are, in descending order of incidence:

- Lower molars: mesial roots
- Single rooted upper premolars
- Upper first molar: mesio-buccal root
- Lower incisors
- Lower premolars

The canal anatomy for an individual patient, though, must be assessed by radiography and the radiographs must be of high quality and free from distortion.

When looking at the radiographs, each root to be treated should:

- Have evidence of a patent, unobstructed root canal reaching the apex
- Be negotiable by conventional instruments, i.e. not excessively curved

The actual canal, though, is usually nothing like the rather reassuring image seen on a conventional radiograph. *Figure 12.1* shows a lower incisor X-rayed in the usual labio-lingual view, together with a mesio-distal view. Far from being a conical tube, the canal is irregular, probably has two main branches for part of its length, and exhibits sharp curves. In addition, the microscope would reveal connecting branches of pulp, blind and patent lateral canals, and various fin-like projections.

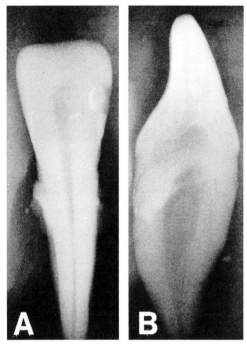

Fig. 12.1 Radiographs of a lower incisor, showing **A** the conventional labio-lingual view, **B** the 'unknown' shape of the canal when seen from the side

Difficulties in interpretation can be produced by overlying anatomical structures – such as the zygomatic arch in the upper molar region, sclerosis of root canals, hypercementosis and overlap of individual roots. The last problem must be overcome by re-angulating the X-ray tube to throw the roots clear of each other (*Fig. 12.2*).

In some cases, sclerosis may not be complete but the radiograph may not show a canal. Here it is worth trying to find canals operatively.

Very thin roots may not have sufficient radio-density to be visible within the denser bone. An instrument in such a root can sometimes appear to be leaving the crown through a perforation. The X-ray tube angle should be changed to concentrate on the problem root.

Apical anatomy

The apical foramen is not usually at the anatomical apex of the root and is likely to be on the side of the end of the root. The foramen may be single or multiple and can lie at the confluence of two (or more) root canals. The mature root shows an apical constriction where the canal narrows dramatically at its apex, caused by dentine and cementum

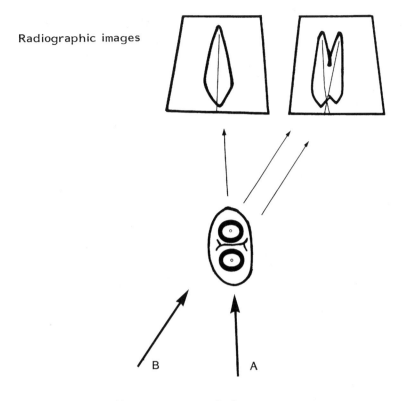

Radiographic images

X-ray tube angulation

Fig. 12.2 Angulation of the X-ray tube to separate the images of two roots on a single tooth. **A** Conventional periapical view. **B** The tube is moved mesially to give separate root images

deposition (*Fig. 12.3*). The apical constriction is the upper limit of the ideal canal preparation and is located 0.5–1 mm from the anatomical apex.

The radiographic apex can be distorted by the angulation of the X-ray beam in relation to the film, and precise detail of the apical foramen is not usually clear on radiographs. Occasionally, though, an apical delta can be seen, as can lateral canals.

Pre-endodontic preparation

Before root treatment is commenced:

● The tooth must be caries free
● The crown should be provisionally restored

The latter stage should aim to maintain tooth position, seal the entrance to the canal(s), provide support for the rubber dam, and restore aesthetics.

The removal of caries might well have been done at the provisional planning stage to assess restorability, but all stained dentine and unsupported enamel must be removed prior to root canal preparation so that disease progression is stopped.

Posterior teeth will often need pinned amalgam cores or well-retained temporary crowns. Some thought must be given to the final restoration, because when the root treatment is completed, a new core will be required and the old pins could well be lost. Some 'free' dentine should be left to receive the permanent pins later.

When constructing the pre-endodontic restoration, it is important not to obstruct access to the root canal(s). If, for example, the whole crown was filled with amalgam, it would be exceedingly tedious and dangerous to find the root canals through this. The roof of the pulp chamber should be overlaid with a weak cement that is easy to remove later.

Anteriorly, if enough coronal dentine is present, a composite resin provisional restoration is satisfactory. Problems arise if a crown is necessary. A technique that was commonly used was that of a hollow tube temporary post crown, e.g.

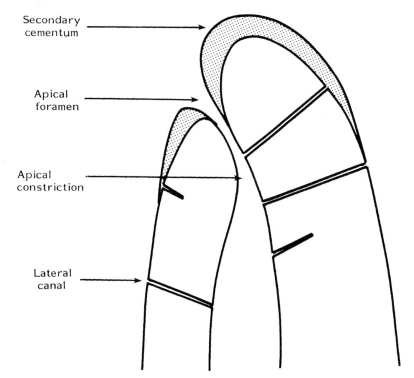

Secondary
cementum

Apical
foramen

Apical
constriction

Lateral
canal

Fig. 12.3 Diagram of the anatomy of the root apex. The apical constriction is between 0.5 and 1 mm below the apical foramen

McGibbon's tube. Whilst superficially attractive, the internal diameter can restrict canal preparation. It is now common practice to make a conventional provisional post crown that is removed at each preparation and filling stage. Of course, this brings complications for rubber dam placement (see below).

Canal preparation

Isolation

Rubber dam is essential to:

- Protect the oro-pharynx
- Minimize contamination of the open root canal
- Retract soft tissues

In some areas, it is possible to avoid the use of clamps; this has the advantage that the radiographic appearance is not obscured by metal.

The problem of isolating the crownless root has to be dealt with using the adjacent teeth for stability, and joining the holes in the dam (*Fig. 12.4*).

Access

Pulp chamber

Access must be obtained through the coronal tissues to reach the apical constriction. The preparation of the access cavity must remove the 'roof'

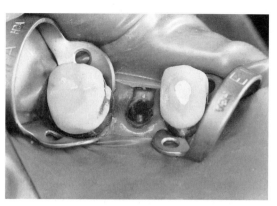

Fig. 12.4 Rubber dam applied to ⌊5 which has had its temporary post crown removed to allow root canal treatment

of the pulp chamber so that the floor of the chamber and the opening(s) of the root canal(s) can be seen clearly. The access cavity must be placed so that it lies in as near a straight line with the apex as possible; this allows efficient instrumentation with little bending of the instruments.

The final breakthrough into the pulp chamber must be done with slow speed, and not the air turbine, to prevent air or water under pressure entering the root canal and passing into the apical tissues. Also, and perhaps more importantly, when obtaining access to molars, the roof of the pulp chamber is often very close to the floor, and rapid cutting may perforate the roof, the floor and the furcation! In some circumstances the use of an excavator to remove the roof is a distinct advantage.

There is a compromise between excellent endodontic access, where removal of the crown to gingival level would expose the root canals very obviously (!), and the restorative requirement where as much tooth substance as possible should be conserved.

The access cavity must be extended to enable removal of all coronal pulp, particularly in anterior teeth where residual necrotic tissue may cause discoloration.

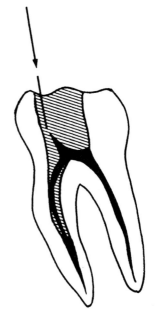

Fig. 12.5 The preparation of a curved root requires removal of the shaded areas, so that it is effectively straightened

Root canal orifice enlargement

Access into the root canal system and preparation of the coronal one-third of the root canal is performed at this stage. Fine canal orifices will be located with ISO 08 or 10 files and a knowledge of where to look is essential to avoid excessive removal of dentine.

Orifice enlargement should create a smooth entry route for files later and also begin the straightening of curved canals (*Fig. 12.5*). Once the orifices have been positively identified and slightly enlarged by filing, Gates–Glidden burs, size 1 or 2 initially, are used to remove dentine rapidly. Care must be taken to remove dentine appropriate to the canal straightening objective, and not to enlarge the orifice symmetrically around the original canal into areas of little dentine. The pulp chamber must contain irrigant during this procedure (see below).

Pulp extirpation

The timing of pulp extirpation, if necessary, is difficult. It is facilitated by orifice enlargement but it needs to be done at the peak of local analgesia. Pragmatically, many dentists choose to remove the pulp as soon as pulp chamber access has been done to avoid causing pain.

A barbed broach should be inserted carefully along the canal wall and kept short of the apex to avoid *apical perforation*. To engage the broach in the pulp tissue, it should be twisted and withdrawn in a smooth, gentle action. Sharp movements should be avoided to prevent tearing and incomplete removal. In fine canals, a Hedstroem file of small diameter may be better, since the barbed broach could bind and lodge in the canal.

If the tooth is non-vital, then necrotic tissue should be removed with a file and by irrigation with a 1% sodium hypochlorite solution. The apical portion of the canal must not be prepared in any way before the working distance has been determined.

The problems of obtaining local analgaesia for pulp extirpation were discussed in Chapter 3.

Working distance determination

The position of the apical constriction in relation to a fixed reference point on the crown of the tooth should be determined as accurately as possible, (± 0.5 mm). This is essential to ensure correct mechanical preparation that, if *short*, will leave:

- Necrotic material at the apex
- Untreated pulp space apically

If the working distance is *long*, the preparation will:

● Destroy the apical constriction
● Damage the apical tissues
● Make filling difficult

The sequence for working distance determination is:

1. Select the largest file that will pass easily into the canal for good radiographic definition
2. Measure the preoperative radiograph and compare the root length with average values. Decide on the likely working length and set a stop on the file to this length
3. Note the reference point on the crown (if no crown, use adjacent tooth)
4. Insert file slowly; stop and X-ray if obstructed
5. When at provisional working distance, X-ray (watch for bending of the film and tube angle, Fig. 12.6A)
6. Measure the image of the file on the film – it should be ± 1 mm of reality to indicate minimal distortion; retake if wrong

7. Measure the distance from the tip of the file to the radiographic apex
8. If this is greater than 5 mm, increase the insertion of the file, and re-X-ray
9. From an undistorted radiograph, and when the tip of the file is close to the apex, measure the distance from the tip to the apex and add this to the known file length, in millimetres
10. Subtract 1 mm from the measurement – this is the average position of the apical constriction and is the working distance (*Fig. 12.6B*)
11. Record the distance in the patient's notes

Mathematical formulae should be avoided since they take no account of unseen curvatures, make no adjustment for hidden radiographic distortions, and errors in measurement are multiplied.

Electrical conductivity methods for determining working distance are available, but these may give false values where there is contamination of the canal or in the presence of apical pathology. If such equipment is used, the working distance must be confirmed by radiography for the patient's record.

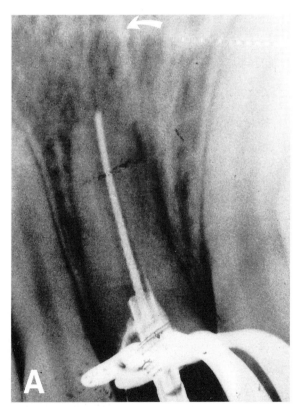

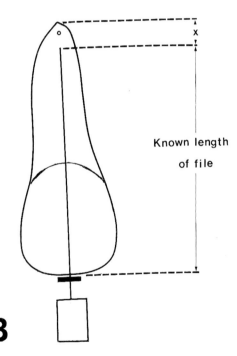

Fig. 12.6 A Periapical diagnostic radiograph with elongation of the apex due to bending of the film in the palate. The apex can just be seen (arrowed) as a faint white line. **B** Determination of the working distance. (x – 1) mm is added to the known length of the file, as long as the radiograph is not distorted and x is small

Canal preparation

The preparation must:

- Remove infected or degraded dentine
- Modify the shape of the pulp space so that it can be filled efficiently

The properties of the root filling material will influence preparation shape and this principle is the same as that applying to cavity preparation (Chapter 10). For example, a retentive cavity is required if amalgam has been chosen as the restorative material, and a non-undercut cavity is required if a gold inlay has been chosen.

Table 12.1 lists the types of root filling materials that are available. The ideal material would be:

- Easy to use within the canal confines
- Controllable during application to avoid over or underfilling
- Condensable into canal wall irregularities
- Biocompatible
- Unaffected by tissue fluid
- Non-resorbable

Table 12.1 Root canal filling materials

Material type	Principal components	Technique	Advantages	Disadvantages
Semi-solid	Gutta percha (GP)	Cones/lateral condensation with sealer	Compressible Controlled insertion	Difficult to use in fine, curved canals
		Thermomechanical compaction GP melted by friction of compacting instrument; minimal sealer	Good condensation	Excessive heat generated Shrinkage on cooling
		Warm vertical condensation with heated spreaders; no sealer	Good condensation	Time consuming Soft GP may pass through apex
		Thermoplasticized injection with vertical compaction	Time saving due to extraoral softening	Variation between systems Shrinkage on cooling Soft GP may pass through apex
Solid	Silver Titanium	Single cone with sealer	Ease of use in curved canals due to rigidity	Poor adaptation Canal space blocked with metal – difficult to remove Corrosion of silver
Hybrid	Gutta percha coated plastic	Cone heated to soften GP; then warm vertical condensation	Good condensation	Canal space blocked with plastic core – difficult to remove
Pastes	Zinc oxide–eugenol (ZOE)-based plus various additives: iodoform, paraform, steroids, antibacterials	Spiral paste filler in conventional handpiece spins material into canal	Simple to use	Difficult to control Extrusion/voids easily done Vital structure damage reported from paraform extrusion Resorbable
Root canal sealers	Zinc oxide–eugenol Calcium hydroxide/ ZOE	All used with master cones	Biocompatible Biocompatible	Solubility Solubility
	Epoxy resin		Slow setting	Apical irritation reported
	Glass ionomer cement		Biocompatible	Vulnerable to water contamination; rapid set

- Adhesive to dentine
- Dimensionally stable
- Radio-opaque
- Easy to remove in the event of problems

Currently the preferred technique is to use *gutta percha* (GP) in the form of a master cone and accessory cones together with a root canal sealer. Whilst tedious to use, the control provided in the positioning of the root filling exactly at the apical constriction and the density of the filling achieved is not provided reliably by any other material.

The optimum shape to receive laterally condensed and sealed gutta percha is a smooth walled tube with a continuous taper from the apical constriction to the access cavity. The last 1 mm of the apical region should be of round cross section to receive the *master cone.*

Perhaps the most important thing to remember during canal preparation is that canal morphology is extremely variable, some of which cannot be prepared mechanically. Therefore, all that is prepared are the main, accessible areas, with the hope that the other areas will be sealed and rendered harmless at the filling stage.

Instrumentation

There are several instrumentation systems for canal preparation; they all require the use of files, and these may be specially developed for the particular system. The principal method is the use of *hand files* but files may also be 'driven' by handpieces in *rotary* or *reciprocating* motion, by *vibrating* handpieces and by *sonic* or *ultrasonic* energy.

Hand files are necessary for the control and definition required in the preparation of the apical region but the mechanical systems may make bulk preparation of the remaining canal easier.

Of the mechanical systems, the sonic instruments have been shown to be the most effective. They also have the advantage that they combine irrigation with preparation.

The files themselves are also being developed rapidly. Whilst some files are sharp tipped and only cut on the withdrawal stroke, there are newer designs that have safe, blunt tips that can cut when moved in either direction. This latter design of file reduces the canal irregularities, such as zipping and ledges, that may be produced by sharp-ended files.

The precise manipulation of the file required to achieve the desired canal shape and remove debris has been the subject of considerable research. There are at least eight methods that have been advocated by endodontists in recent years – there will be more!

The most efficient way to prepare the apical stop and remove debris is to insert the file towards the apex until it binds, either at the working distance or short of it, and make a quarter to half a turn clockwise to engage the cutting blades into the canal wall.

Then, if using single direction cutting files, withdraw the file completely, bringing the debris out with the file.

If using two-directional cutting files with blunt tips, maintain the apical position of the file and turn it anticlockwise one turn. Provided the file being used can cut on the upstroke, this action will remove the dentine that had been engaged by the clockwise turn. This is the *balanced force technique.*

The preparation should be done with copious irrigation and with care to clean debris from both the canal and the files. The two preferred irrigants are normal saline and 1% sodium hypochlorite. Both act to lubricate the files and collect and displace debris, whilst the hypochlorite also dissolves organic matter and is mildly bactericidal. The advantage of saline is that it is non-irritant if passed through the apex.

When the file reaches the working distance and does not bind on turning, change to the next file up and continue with the chosen action.

Do not enlarge the apical stop any more when both:

- The diameter has reached the minimum size for the material (No. 25 for GP), and
- Clean dentine dust has been seen on the last file

The remainder of the canal (that excluding the apical 1 mm) should now be prepared by *circumferential filing* to flare it outwards towards the crown. It is now unnecessary to twist the file to engage the blades, since pressure can be applied via the handle. Also, the canal profile is oval and the simple turning and cutting action used for the apical stop will simply cut a round shape in the oval, leaving the periphery unprepared. The majority of radiographically straight canals have some degree of curve in the apical third and the *step back technique* provides a controlled method of negotiating and enlarging this curve.

The canal is prepared progressively short of the working distance with progressively larger instruments. Care must be taken not to create ledges or elbows by trying to take stiff instruments around the bend. Files larger than no. 35 will not negotiate a curve at the apex, even when pre-curved before insertion in the canal.

The danger of the progressively shortening preparation is the tendency for debris to remain ahead of the files. The working distance must be re-established at each progression by the original apical stop size file, with slight turning to engage and displace the debris. The shape will be determined basically by the original canal morphology,

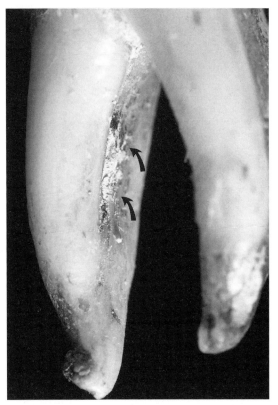

Fig. 12.7 Strip perforation on the inner aspect of the mesial root of a lower molar (the root canal has been fitted with gutta percha)

and it is necessary to remove an even amount of dentine from its periphery. Preparation should continue until the even tapered shape is achieved and clean dentine dust is brought out with the canal walls offering firm resistance to cutting.

Stiff files, used around a curve, may create a separate channel away from the main canal. A new apical foramen may be created and, whilst this is essentially a lateral perforation, the term *apical transportation* is used to describe the outcome. As with many of the canal preparation faults, it is very difficult to correct. Precurving a fine file and trying to re-establish access to the real apical constriction is the only solution.

Canals that are curved in their middle third should be prepared by filing the inner aspect of the curve, to 'straighten' the canal within the curved root – *anticurvature filing*. The danger here is of filing too much and perforating the inner aspect of the root – a *strip perforation* (Fig. 12.7).

Haemorrhage should not be seen during canal preparation. If it is, this may indicate:

- Pulp remnants still present at the apex
- Apical perforation

- Lateral perforation
- Furcation perforation

A radiograph should be taken with the apical stop file in place and the working distance checked. *Pulp remnants* may be removed by filing since they will often be inaccessible to a barbed broach; local analgesia is necessary. *Apical perforation* may allow extrusion of material at the root filling stage. The correct working distance should be re-established and an apical stop created. Small *lateral perforations* and *furcation perforations* can be sealed at the root filling stage after the correct line of the canal has been re-established. Large lateral and furcation perforations are difficult to seal and therefore have a poor prognosis.

After preparation, the canal should be dried first with a cotton wool pledget and then by careful use of paper points. To dry the apical stop, the paper point should be capable of passing into it, i.e. do not use no. 60 points in a no. 25 stop!

Medication

After preparation, canals may be filled by some type of dressing material that could have an antimicrobial effect. Many substances ranging from antibiotic mixtures to very irritant disinfectants have been used. No conclusive evidence exists regarding the efficacy of canal medication.

Waiting a week or so between preparation and filling does allow any acute apical reaction to pulp extirpation or debris being pushed through the apex to subside without pain. The inflammatory exudate can pass into the partly empty canal.

A mild antimicrobial with very low irritation is calcium hydroxide in a propylene glycol vehicle. This material is sometimes successful in resolving a persistently oozing canal if left for 4–6 weeks, though replacement is necessary every 10 days or so to maintain activity.

Single visit root canal therapy is possible, provided there is no infection present. This has the advantage that the canal is open for a relatively short period, there being no temporary dressing that may leak and contaminate the canal.

Root filling

After preparation, and before root filling, the tooth should:

- Be symptomless
- Not be tender to percussion
- Have no exudate in the root canal(s)

If any of the above are present, it indicates continuing pathology. Wash the canal to remove the dressing, dry it, re-establish the working distance with the apical stop file and re-dress. Review in a week to 10 days.

When obturating the canal, the master cone must match the file size as closely as possible, but some variation in the GP cones is inevitable because of difficulties in manufacture. After placement of the master cone, lateral or accessory cones are condensed into place together with the sealer. This means that the working time of the sealer should be sufficiently long to allow this.

The sequence for root filling is:

1. Remove the dressing from the canal, re-establish the apical stop with the appropriate file. Wash and dry
2. Select the GP point of the apical stop size and mark the working distance on it; insert it into the canal slowly
3. Make sure the point reaches the working distance and is a good fit ('tug back')
4. X-ray to check that the GP fits to the working distance

If the point does not fit to the working distance when tried in, or is short when X-rayed, repeat the preparation of the apical stop to either clear debris or extend the preparation if it is short. Re-check the diameter of the GP point on a gauge and, if necessary, try another one of the same nominal size. The GP try-in also checks the preparation in addition to checking the master cone fit.

Then:

5. Mix sealer and place a range of accessory cones with their tips in the sealer
6. Select a file size smaller than the apical stop and coat this with sealer and, with an anticlockwise rotation, coat the canal walls with sealer, up to the stop
7. Coat the master cone with sealer, insert it carefully (beware hydraulic effects of pain or extrusion) to the marked working distance
8. Using lateral spreaders, beginning with the smallest, make room for accessory cones alongside the master cone and build up the full filling sequentially
9. Take a postoperative radiograph and seal the access cavity

If the canal is overfilled, tell the patient and keep it under review. If the canal is underfilled because of technical error, remove the root filling and start again.

If this underfill goes to the working distance which is short because of some obstruction, then again tell the patient and keep it under review.

Problems encountered during root canal therapy

The almost blind instrumentation of a series of natural channels of variable anatomy is inevitably accompanied by risk. *Table 12.2* sets out the major problems that might be encountered during root canal therapy. Some of these have been or will be discussed in more detail within the text.

It is important that the patient understands the technical difficulties that may be encountered during root canal therapy. This will be the basis for their informed consent. In the event of a complication, such as a lateral perforation or a fractured instrument, the patient must be informed about what has happened and its likely outcome.

Fractured instrument

The current techniques of filing rather than reaming and the construction of modern files means that broken instruments are less common. Forcing instruments around canal bends or jamming them in the apical constriction are recipes for disaster.

The most likely instruments to fracture will be fine files in a curved apical region or the tips of Gates–Glidden burs in the canal orifice. The former are usually impossible to remove. The canal preparation should be completed, perhaps with by-passing of the fragment, and gutta percha condensed around it.

Overflexing is the usual reason for Gates–Glidden fracture and the main shank of the bur is supposed to be the fracture zone of the instrument. However, tips may break in the canal and because these are usually superficial, they can be retrieved using a file or excavator. Failing this, the Masserann kit (see Chapter 27) may be used.

Open apex

This may occur as a result of incomplete root formation (Chapter 3) or because of instrumentation beyond the apical constriction (apical perforation). It makes root filling difficult because there is no restriction to the escape of sealer into the apical tissues. In the immature root, the canal is funnel shaped, becoming wider towards the apex. Conventional condensation is then almost impossible.

Preparation of the immature canal should be done by careful circumferential filing, since the apical diameter is usually larger than the largest file. The root filling should be made up, by trial and error, from warming and coalescing several GP points into a large single cone of the right diameter. This can be tried-in in the usual way and then sealed carefully, avoiding extrusion into the tissues.

Table 12.2 Root canal therapy problems

Stage	Problem	Action	Comments
Access	Incomplete analgesia	1. Repeat LA with 3% prilocaine or 5% xylocaine 2. Steroid dressing for 48 hours; retry LA 3. If all fails, general anaesthesia for pulp extirpation	1. Second agent potentiates the first 2. Pulpal inflammation is reduced, neural pain pathway recovers, LA then becomes effective 3. Ensure that GA is justified on likely success rate of root canal treatment
	Perforation – furcation or lateral	Re-establish correct canal line If small, pack perforation with calcium hydroxide; this will be supported by the RCF later	Prevention is better than cure Note root angle before cutting, especially if there is an artificial crown present that may obscure the true angle
Canal preparation	Incorrect working distance from radiographic distortion	Retake radiograph	Avoid calculating working distance if: • the image of the file is not 1:1 with reality • the file does reach to within 5 mm of the apex
	Obstructions Secondary dentine, pulp stones	Dentine softening agent, e.g. EDTA, slow reaction – seal and leave	
	Canal anatomy Curves, fins, apical delta, lateral canals, accessory canals, internal resorption	Prepare only those major channels that allow file access	Use step back and anticurvature techniques
	Preparation faults Ledges, zips, elbows	Attempt to re-establish correct preparation path Pre-curve instrument, attempt to reach correct apex	
	Apical transportation	As open apex; see text	
	Apical perforation	Attempt sealing at RCF stage	
	Strip perforation, lateral perforation	If at the apex and tooth symptomless, root fill around fragment If in main body of canal, remove (see Chapter 27) or bypass using canal anatomy If irremovable consider apical surgery	Prognosis for large perforations is low. If accessible, consider surgery (see Chapter 27)
	Fractured instrument	See Chapter 3 See text	The round instrument will not obstruct all of an oval canal Always inform the patient
	Fractured root Open apex Post crown present	If crown sound, consider apical surgery. If inadequate, remove, re-root fill and re-restore	
Medication	Persistent exudate and/or symptoms	Check working distance and preparation; re-dress with calcium hydroxide Consider apical surgery	
Canal obturation	Overfilling	Radiographic review if symptomless If symptoms, remove or consider apical surgery	If found at review: leave if no pathology Re-root fill if to have new restoration even if no pathology
	Underfilling/undercondensation	Remove RCF and re-fill	

LA, local analgesic; RCF, root canal filling; EDTA, ethylenediaminetetra – acetic acid

Filling a canal with an apical perforation is also difficult. The length of insertion of the master cone must be controlled carefully, and it should be held against the crown whilst inserting lateral cones, so that the spreaders do not push it past the apex. Lateral condensation must be gentle, to avoid extrusion of sealer.

Review

Apical tissues take time to heal, and progress should be monitored radiographically at six months after filling, one year after that, and then every two or three years. There is an incidence of recurrent infection around apparently successful root fillings that may relate to lateral canals, or to short zones of unfilled apical canal.

Healing of the root end is by the laying down of cementum across the apical foramen and possibly the presence of clean dentine dust will help this. There may be a very small zone of clean compacted dentine chippings at the final extent of successful root fillings.

The final coronal restoration should be completed as soon as possible after the root filling. There is evidence to suggest that leakage from the crown will contaminate the root filling and promote bacterial growth.

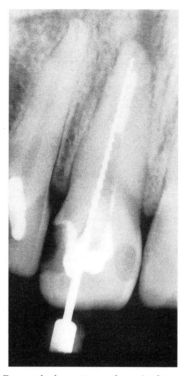

Fig. 12.8 Removal of a gutta percha point by a Hedstroem file. This file is ideal because of its rearward facing barbs

Recurrent infection

Symptoms, or radiographic appearance of an increasing area of radiolucency at the apex indicate pathology and failure of the root filling. Consider either:

- Removing and repreparing the root filling (*Fig. 12.8*)
- Apical surgery

Do not intervene in cases of long standing, symptomless over- or under-filled canals (*Fig. 12.9A*), though there could be an exception to this if the tooth were to receive a crown or be a bridge abutment. Residual static apical radiolucency may be accepted in the absence of symptoms provided that the apical area is less than 5 mm in diameter.

Apical surgery

The surgical approach to the root apex is required to place an apical seal when the conventional approach through the root is impossible, or when an apparently well-executed root filling has failed. Surgery should be reserved for these cases and should not be used to correct symptomless and signless filling errors.

The circumstances in which to consider surgery are, *in the presence of infection*, canals that are non-negotiable or difficult to fill because of:

- Secondary dentine, curves, pulp stones
- Fractured instruments
- Post crowns (*Fig. 12.9B*)
- Unremovable root fillings
- Lateral canals
- An open apex

Surgery may also be used to provide root canal treatment rapidly or to deal with infection that persists in spite of repeated dressing.

If the irremovable root filling is an apical silver point or a retrograde amalgam, and the remainder of the canal is empty, then the cause of the infection may be leakage past the filling into the canal. Bacteria can obtain their nutrient from the leakage and toxins pass out into the tissues. In these cases it is worth trying to prepare the empty canal and fill it up to the existing root filling (*Fig. 12.10*).

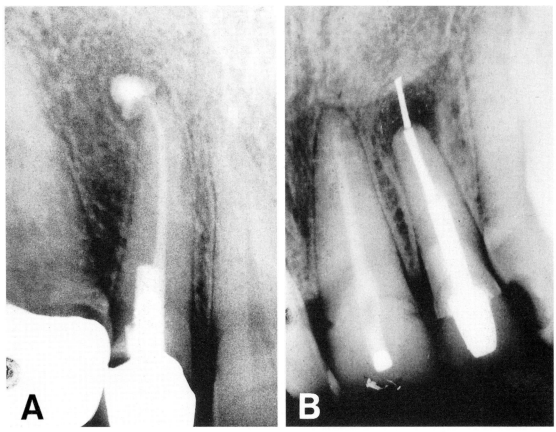

Fig. 12.9 A Extruded sealer associated with a long-standing and static apical area at 2|. No treatment is required. **B** Extruded gutta percha in |2 associated with symptoms and a sinus. There is a very good post crown present, and the extruded filling probably could not be retrieved anyway. The tooth was apicected. The postoperative radiographs are shown in *Figure 3.5*

Apicectomy technique

Local analgesia is usually acceptable for most single teeth. Intravenous sedation or general anaesthesia may be indicated for several teeth or apprehensive individuals.

The analgesia must be effective, with palatal and incisive canal blocks being necessary for upper anterior teeth.

The sequence is:

1. Analgesia
2. Raise full gingival flap with bevelled incision at the papillae (*Fig. 12.11*); this gives good access and little scarring
3. Identify the apical region by pressure with an excavator to try perforating the cortical plate over the infected area. Otherwise measure the root length from the preoperative radiograph
4. Remove cortical bone with slow speed burs with copious irrigation
5. Avoid scarring the root by working higher than the apical level initially
6. Obtain clear access to the root apex and identify any anatomical structures of relevance, e.g. antrum, mental nerve
7. Clear any soft tissue around the apex – *excision biopsy*
8. Reduce the apex by a bevelled cut, so that the root face is angled towards the operator
9. Cut a 2–3 mm deep undercut cavity in the root canal end
10. Wash, dry, and pack the bone with ribbon gauze to isolate the apex.
11. Place retrograde amalgam
12. Remove gauze and excess amalgam, irrigate, close and suture

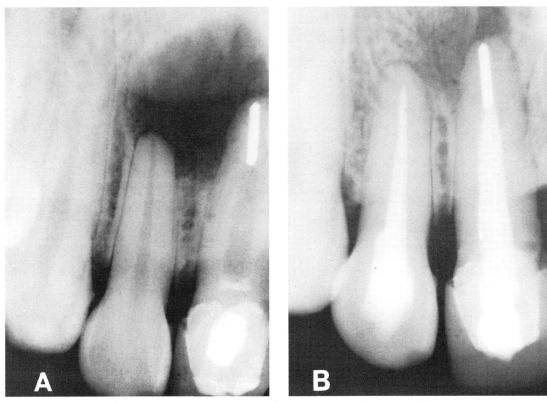

Fig. 12.10 A Apical infection associated with a non-vital 2| and an apical silver point in 1|. **B** This was treated by conventional root canal therapy of 2| and root filling the 1| up to the silver. The result was complete resolution of the infection without surgery

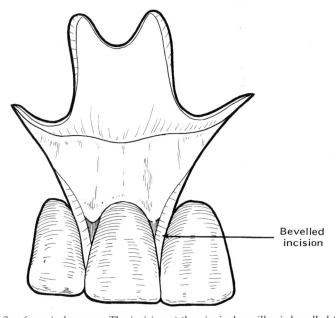

Bevelled incision

Fig. 12.11 Full gingival flap for apical surgery. The incision at the gingival papillae is bevelled to provide a broad area for replacement, which reduces recession

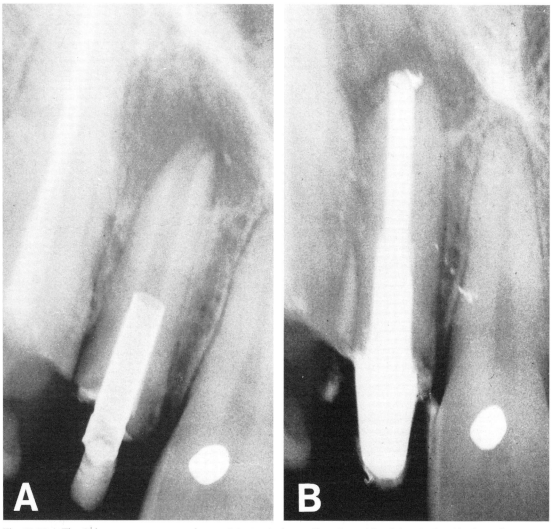

Fig. 12.12 A The 2⌋ has an open apex and a persistent apical area. Dressing with calcium hydroxide through a McGibbon's tube has been unsuccessful. **B** A long post has been inserted in 2⌋ at the time of apical surgery prior to the placement of the retrograde amalgam. A provisional crown is placed at the same time to wait for gingival healing

Systemic antibiotics should be prescribed pre-operatively for medical problems, or postoperatively for the prevention of infection in a large bony cavity.

The more posterior the tooth, the more difficult will be the surgery and the more likely there will be anatomical complications.

The palatal roots of upper premolars are difficult to reach and see. Palatal roots of upper molars would require a separate palatal flap, but these are straight and can usually be root filled conventionally. The buccal roots are easily accessible by surgery.

The maxillary antrum lies close to the upper premolars and molars. Antral perforation does not usually give rise to problems because the flap closes it. The patient should be given systemic antibiotics and told not to blow his or her nose.

The mental nerve is a complication with lower premolars, and the hazard of mental anaesthesia must be mentioned when consent to apicectomy in the region is sought. Many now consider that apical surgery of lower premolars is contraindicated because of the possibility of this complication.

The inferior dental nerve is close to the lower molars – do not apicect these.

Finally, always place a retrograde amalgam; do not rely on the sealing ability of the existing root filling, which may be disturbed when cut.

In view of the concerns about the toxicity of amalgam discussed in Chapter 10, alternatives for retrograde root filling have been suggested. The GICs and EBA reinforced zinc oxide eugenol (ZOE) cements have been used but limited data in support of these are available. The sensitivity to moisture of both materials and the solubility of the ZOE cements could be disadvantages when in contact with tissue fluids.

Where a post crown is to placed, the post should be made first before the surgery, in case the post preparation displaces the apical seal later. The surgery is performed by a *through and through* technique where the canal is open to both the mouth and the apical tissues. The canal is dried and the post cemented with the apical tissues protected from excess cement (*Fig. 12.12*). The through and through technique may also be used where there is an open apex and an empty canal. The canal is root filled with the flap raised and a retrograde seal placed afterwards.

Apical bone may take several months, sometimes over a year, to fill in. This should be monitored radiographically at regular review (see *Fig. 3.5*).

Success rate of root canal therapy

Outcome analysis in restorative dentistry is generally insufficient. Whilst success rate studies have been reported, these are often retrospective and therefore preoperative criteria are not established and various techniques may be employed. The studies often include a large number of operators. Clinical trials of restorative materials are an exception, probably because they are easier to conduct with clear trial entry criteria, proper control groups and pre-trial training of operators. Assessment criteria are well established and short-term analysis means that most of the original cohort of patients can be reviewed. On the other hand, the design factors for fixed prosthodontics are very difficult to study.

In root canal therapy, success rate studies rely to a large extent on radiographic interpretation and the reproducibility of some of these is notoriously poor. The acceptance of new instrumentation techniques is based on laboratory studies rather than clinical outcome.

The highest success is found with single rooted teeth with little or no infection (>90%) whilst the lowest is with multi-rooted teeth with established and long-standing apical areas particularly in the mandible (<60%). Bacteria can remain undisturbed in such tooth sites as lateral canals and non-obturated areas of main canals and within well established apical areas. The problems described in *Table 12.2* all reduce the success rate. Under-preparation and under-filling are associated with lower success than over-filling.

The clinical studies show that the principal factors influencing success are:

- Root canal morphology
- Quality of canal preparation and filling
- Presence of apical infection

The over-riding requirements of root canal therapy are to remove bacteria from the canal system and to prevent their re-establishing themselves there again.

Root canal therapy – Summary

Base treatment planning on accurate radiographs and a realistic assessment of outcome.

Thoroughly debride as much of the canal system as possible.

Shape the canals in accordance with the choice of root filling material.

Obturate all the prepared space.

Ensure proper sealing of the access cavity by the coronal restoration.

Review apical condition regularly.

13

Diagnosis, treatment planning and management of the periodontally involved dentition

This chapter considers aspects of diagnosis, treatment planning, treatment and follow-up for a patient having periodontal disease, together with comments on the broader restorative implications of the management of the disease.

Introduction

The planning and execution of treatment for any disease or condition is dependent on careful diagnosis. Having defined periodontitis in Chapter 7, the disease should be easily diagnosed by noting gingivitis accompanied by loss of attachment. Unfortunately, this alone is of little value to treatment planning for an individual patient and the diagnosis of periodontitis needs to be qualified. Such qualification requires:

- Identification of aetiological and predisposing factors
- Qualification of disease severity
- Appreciation of patient factors relevant to management

The disease itself arises from the interaction of a pathogenic subgingival flora on a susceptible host. Therapy aims to eradicate the former but can do little to alter the latter, so for this reason recurrence of the disease is always a possibility. Long-term successful treatment of the patient with periodontal disease depends on a considered management programme where pre- and post-treatment care is as important as the actual treatment itself.

Management of periodontitis is based upon initiatives for:

- Removal of subgingival plaque (*therapeutic phase*)

- Prevention of recurrence through the control of supragingival plaque (*preventive phase*)

The therapeutic phase is highly operator dependent whereas the preventive phase is highly patient dependent. Both are based on mechanical debridement of supra and subgingival plaques and clearly the efficiency of the procedures used, whether in the surgery or at home, will have a direct bearing on success.

Chemical agents, largely against microorganisms and antimicrobial, may be employed both locally and systemically. Modification of the host response to plaque is an alternative possibility.

Diagnosis – qualifying factors

Once loss of attachment in the presence of inflammation, based on clinical and radiographic examinations, has been established, the diagnosis of periodontitis is made. The diagnosis must then be qualified in order to prepare a treatment plan.

Plaque scores

Subgingival plaque is the major aetiological factor in gingivitis and gives rise to the subgingival plaque associated with periodontitis. Levels of plaque on all or selected teeth should be recorded using a suitable index or scoring method.

Plaque scoring at various time intervals forms the basis for diagnosis, oral hygiene instruction, assessing response to instruction and for patient information and encouragement. Clinical probing and radiographic examination provide information about the presence of subgingival deposits, notably subgingival calculus, and usefully directs treatment (See Chapter 2 for BPE or CPITN).

Local predisposing factors

Certain factors encourage plaque accumulation and some make plaque removal difficult by normal tooth cleaning methods. These include:

- Supra and subgingival calculus
- Carious cavities
- Subgingival restorations
- Overhanging restorations
- Poor approximal contact areas
- Fixed and removable appliances or prostheses

Perhaps surprisingly, mucogingival anomalies and tooth malpositions have little bearing on plaque accumulation and removal.

Modifying factors of the gingival or periodontal response to plaque

Local or systemic conditions referred to in Chapter 7 should be identified from the history and examination of the patient. Special tests to determine predisposition or susceptibility to periodontal disease are rarely needed and the important factors usually arise from the medical history. However, where unusual symptoms or signs are apparent, particularly in gingival inflammation, that appear outwith the known medical history or local factors, consideration to haematological investigation and urinalysis must be considered.

It is worth noting that at present the use of microbiological methods to qualify the bacterial aetiology of periodontitis are of no value in the treatment planning of individual patients with chronic adult periodontitis and of little, if any, value to rapid onset types of disease.

Severity

It is essential to qualify the diagnosis of periodontitis for severity, particularly in respect of the patient's age. The following aspects should be examined to determine the severity of periodontitis:

- Gingival inflammation and associated recession or enlargement

- Loss of attachment
- Mobility
- Bone loss
- Tooth position
- Tooth vitality

A determination of severity is usually based on standard clinical and radiographic assessments particularly using a graduated periodontal probe to record pocket depth and loss of attachment. The same instrument provides information on distribution and severity of gingival pocket inflammation assessed as bleeding in response to probing. Loss of attachment, or more usually pocket depths, are recorded in millimetres. Multisite probing (6 per tooth) is often recommended but a considerable amount of information can be derived from mesial and distal probing and probing to the furcation areas of molar teeth.

Examination of the gingiva may reveal inflammation demonstrated by bleeding on probing and gingival enlargement that may be local or general. Local inflammation is most likely to be due to local predisposing factors such as poorly adapted crowns. There may be exudation of pus from periodontal pockets.

Gingival recession may be local or general, where again a differential diagnosis based on aetiology may be required. Gingival recession may lead to sensitivity of dentine and poor aesthetics. These may need to be considered in the general treatment plan.

Mobility is assessed using the handle of the probe alone or together with the handle of the dental mirror and typically graded on a 0 = none through to 3 = severe basis. Sophisticated instruments are available to measure mobility but their value to the assessment and follow-up of the individual patient is perhaps questionable. Vertical mobility is usually a poor prognostic sign and care must be taken in distinguishing pathological mobility resulting from bone loss and physiological mobility due to increased tooth loading, particularly as they may coexist.

Radiographs should be taken to show the teeth and supporting structures at appropriate areas of the mouth, using the lowest dose of radiation possible. Recent guidelines support the use of radiographs based on clinical need. Full mouth periapical radiographs for diagnosis and follow-up of the periodontal patient are for this reason now rarely required. One cannot be dogmatic concerning which radiographic views are required, but long cone periapical films usually provide the best definition.

Tooth position may indicate that drifting and/or overeruption has occurred. Particularly at anterior sites, aesthetic considerations may have major treatment planning implications, and decisions concerning orthodontic and restorative treatments have to be made.

Bone loss both in extent and type (horizontal or vertical) should be noted with particular reference to furcation defects, the latter being poor prognostic indicators to treatment success. The type of bony lesion will influence decisions concerning non-surgical and surgical periodontal treatment and the use of guided tissue regeneration.

Tooth vitality should be assessed by conventional thermal and/or electrical methods where clinical or radiographic evidence dictates. Periodontal lesions may compromise tooth vitality and, conversely, endodontic lesions may create apparent periodontal or furcation lesions. Distinguishing an endodontic–periodontal lesion from a periodontal–endodontic lesion is important because of the poor treatment prognosis of the latter compared to the relatively good treatment prognosis of the former. Again, both can co-exist, making definitive diagnosis difficult. Sinus formation may be important in the differential diagnosis of apical from periodontal infections.

Most assessments of disease severity must be correlated to *age* since this provides information concerning disease susceptibility and rate of disease progression, prognosis and therefore treatment planning.

A number of methods using chairside test kits have become available to evaluate disease activity and outcome of treatment. Whilst these are of interest, particularly in respect of the pathogenesis of periodontitis, the test kits appear to provide no more information concerning disease activity or lack of it than bleeding on probing. The consensus of opinion at present is that test kits are of no value in determining the need for treatment, or to the success of treatment that cannot be obtained by conventional clinical methods.

Patient factors

Patient factors are of considerable importance to treatment planning since they can influence the disease itself and the ability and willingness of the individual patient to participate in the treatment plan. Firstly, there is a need to assess whether an individual can fulfil the long-term commitment to the prevention phase of management alone or with assistance from third parties. Secondly, it is important to determine whether an individual can receive the ideal treatment for the disease. Some of the answers to these complex questions can be determined easily from direct discussions with an individual and a consideration of their psychosocial and medical backgrounds. Other aspects of assessing their ability to participate in the management programme are difficult, sometimes

impossible, to evaluate, particularly during initial appointments.

Patient factors that may be relevant to the preventive phase of management are probably numerous but at present many are ill understood. At the extremes, why some individuals appear able to practise good plaque control, and others not, often cannot be explained. It may be simply related to their apparent compliance and dexterity with oral hygiene practices that has been determined in retrospect, rather than predicted prospectively at the initial diagnostic and treatment planning visits.

Nevertheless, some factors that may contribute to difficulties with oral hygiene can be identified:

- Physical and/or mental handicap
- Chronic medical conditions, particularly of painful nature, may influence co-operation
- Social or occupational commitments may limit time available
- Social problems can affect ability and willingness

Patient factors that can influence the receipt of treatment are usually more obvious but potentially large in number and variable in their impact.

The age and general medical and psychological health of an individual are most important. As an example, in the aged it is possible to judge retrospectively the susceptibility to periodontal disease and plan treatment accordingly. In such circumstances treatment is likely to be conservative, even palliative. Conversely, in the young healthy adult, particularly with advanced periodontitis, treatment planning may have to be aggressive.

Specific aspects of the *medical history* can place individuals at risk from periodontal procedures, both non-surgical and surgical. These include:

- Congenital and acquired heart valve defects and artificial heart valves
- Bleeding diatheses and other acute haematological disorders
- Anticoagulant therapy
- Long-term steroid therapy

Medical disorders or conditions may influence the timing of periodontal procedures, for example:

- Pregnancy
- Coincident medical or surgical procedures

Concurrent pharmacotherapy may influence the periodontal state and therefore treatment decisions, notably those associated with gingival hyperplasia.

Medical conditions or present pharmacotherapies can influence the decision to employ chemotherapy within the periodontal treatment plan. These include where the periodontal chemo-therapy could induce:

- An adverse patient reaction due to allergy, for example penicillin or aspirin
- An adverse interaction with current medica-tion, for example aspirin and coumarin anti-coagulants
- An antagonism of an existing medical condition, for example aspirin and peptic ulceration
- Potential deleterious effects to the foetus during pregnancy, for example metronidazole

Medical and social problems can affect the patient's ability to attend for treatment, particularly since periodontal treatment is often protracted and recalls are regular and continuous. These could include occupation, travel distance, availability of transport and finances.

Treatment planning

Accepting that periodontal disease arises when suitable pathogens act on a susceptible host sug-gests three possible approaches to treatment:

- Remove the pathogens
- Alter the host response
- Reduce or change susceptibility

The mainstream approach to management of peri-odontal diseases has been and remains the removal of the subgingival pathogens and the prevention of recurrence through supragingival plaque control.

The host response can be altered to advantage by drugs such as non-steroidal anti-inflammatory drugs (NSAIDs). The role of NSAIDs in therapy is not established at present with clear concerns over benefit to risk ratio due to potential serious side-effects. At present NSAIDs are of interest in researching pathogenesis of periodontal diseases. Low dosage tetracyclines and non-antibiotic tetra-cyclines appear of interest for potential effects on host collagenase; further data are awaited.

Susceptibility is poorly understood and therefore nothing can be done at present to change the susceptibility of most individuals with period-ontitis. Specific aspects of the medical history that increase susceptibility, notably those influencing polymorph function, usually cannot be altered but have to be taken into account in treatment plan-ning. Present knowledge indicates that patients with periodontitis should stop cigarette smoking. Logically improving diabetic control in type I and type II diabetics should decrease susceptibility, but data are lacking.

Based on the antipathogen approach to manage-ment the following phases form the basic treatment plan for periodontitis:

1. Hygiene phase
   - Advice and instruction in supragingival plaque control
2. Therapeutic phase
   - Thorough debridement of the root surface
   - The use of surgery to improve access
   - Adjunctive use of antimicrobials
   - Recall and maintenance.

Interestingly, this 'modern' treatment plan can be found almost in its entirety in periodontal text books from the beginning of the century. Before considering the specifics of the treatment plan applied to the average case of periodontitis, impor-tant factors concerning individual patients have to be considered, since these may modify treatment planning to a lesser or greater degree. These include:

- Susceptibility factors needing to be removed
- Predisposing factors that affect plaque accumu-lation and retention
- Severity factors as they affect prognosis

Susceptibility factors include the modification of a smoking habit, diabetic control and the use of antimicrobials where polymorph function is compromised.

Predisposing factors that are outside patient con-trol need to be removed or modified. These have been discussed earlier and frequently involve restorative procedures.

Extractions may have to be considered when:

- Periodontal therapy cannot or is unlikely to resolve the disease
- Aesthetics can only be improved by prostheses
- Comfort and security problems can be improved only by prostheses
- Coincident restoration problems exist, making the tooth unsavable

Decisions concerning the above may have to be taken in consideration of the patient's wishes, attitude, age and medical history.

Patient factors are of considerable relevance to treatment planning since they can influence needs and demands for treatment and affect the type and delivery of treatment. Some of the important patient factors that are identifiable from personal details, occupational, social and medical histories have already been mentioned. Most cannot be changed and therefore, when possible, the treat-ment plan has to be modified to accommodate them.

It is not unusual, particularly where aesthetic considerations are important to the patient, that collaboration with restorative and/or orthodontic colleagues is necessary. Based on these consulta-tions, restorative and/or orthodontic procedures may be planned to improve aesthetics and function. It is essential to appreciate that such procedures should only go forward consequent upon a successful outcome to periodontal treatment. There is evidence to suggest that restorative and, more particularly, orthodontic treatments which place increased loading upon individual teeth can act as aggravating factors in the progress of active periodontal disease. In the presence of treated periodontal disease, such effects appear irrelevant. Therefore, a sound basis for other treatments to the dentition must be a healthy periodontium.

Hygiene phase

Advice and instruction in oral hygiene methods must be tailored to individual needs. There is no scientific basis for providing any particular type of advice and instruction and there is little evidence that any method or device is superior to others. It would seem reasonable that patients or, where indicated, a caring third party understands the problem. Information on plaque, gingivitis and periodontitis should be provided and can include verbal and written instruction. The main aim is to achieve a level of supragingival plaque control compatible with gingival health. To achieve this the professional must identify individual factors which can affect compliance and dexterity with tooth cleaning habits.

Many individuals appear not to find interdental cleaning easy and do not follow advice on interdental cleaning. Some may have dexterity problems of varying magnitude and may require assistance. Certain sites appear difficult to clean, with most people spending little or no time cleaning such sites; most notable are lingual and palatal areas.

Oral hygiene procedures

There is no evidence for the superiority of any one method and recommendations should be based on individual needs and ability. Interdental cleaning is important in long-term management. Oral hygiene involves:

- Toothbrushes
- Toothpastes
- Mouth rinses

Toothbrushes Toothbrushing with a toothpaste remains the primary method of oral hygiene in the developed world and the individual is the major variable in influencing the outcome of tooth cleaning. Twice daily brushing appears optimal and for brushing times of 1–2 minutes.

There is little evidence that variations in manual toothbrush design influence oral hygiene and gingival health significantly. However, it would seem reasonable to suggest that head sizes are not too large for the specific individual and filaments are soft to medium and end rounded.

Electric toothbrushes can be of benefit to handicapped individuals. Also, there are some recent data to show that electric brushes, other than reciprocal types, provide some benefit compared with manual toothbrushes. The cost implications of electric toothbrushes have to be considered for each individual.

Toothpastes Toothpastes contain ingredients such as detergents, that provide some plaque inhibitory effects but these are probably insufficient to benefit gingival health. Recent evidence is available that toothpastes containing chlorhexidine, stannous fluoride or triclosan (with either zinc citrate or polyvinyl methyl ether maleic acid) provide modest benefits to gingival health. (NB, chlorhexidine and stannous fluoride toothpastes have the potential to cause tooth staining due to interactions with dietary chromogens on the tooth surface.)

Mouthrinses Mouthrinses containing a small number of agents, of which chlorhexidine is still considered the 'gold standard', have been shown effective adjuncts to toothbrushing with a toothpaste. However, as part of the long-term commitment to plaque control, the use of such rinses may be questioned on the basis of cost, benefit and local side-effects. For example, mouthrinsing twice daily with a proprietary product requires an approximate expenditure of four times that spent on toothbrushes and toothpaste.

Use of antiplaque agents, notably chlorhexidine, in the hygiene phase may be questioned. Chlorhexidine in the short term provides little if any therapeutic action against established gingivitis and certainly established periodontitis, since subgingival deposits are relatively inaccessible to supragingivally delivered fluids. The considerable inhibitory properties of chlorhexidine against supragingival plaque make an assessment of the response to oral hygiene instruction almost impossible and therefore may be misleading.

The professional responsibilities in the hygiene phase are to provide oral hygiene advice and instruction and to monitor response using plaque and/or gingivitis scoring. In addition, it may be necessary to remove or modify factors predisposing to plaque accumulation and retention. This includes scaling and polishing of teeth to remove supragingival plaque and calculus and easily accessible subgingival deposits, and the correction of faulty fixed or removable restorations.

Therapy phase – mechanical

The therapy of chronic adult periodontitis is almost totally based on non-surgical and surgical mechanical debridement of the root surface. Indeed, the treatment of rapid onset periodontal diseases with few exceptions always includes these mechanical methods.

Non-surgical and, more particularly, surgical procedures result in variable, often unpredictable, gingival recession. The choice of procedure must be made on the full understanding by the patient of the possible outcomes, including the possibility of dentine hypersensitivity (see gingivectomy below).

Non-surgical subgingival scaling and root planing techniques are the first line of treatment for all forms of periodontitis with the expectation of reductions in inflammation and probing depth, gains in attachment level and beneficial shifts in the subgingival bacteria. Procedures can be performed with hand instruments or ultrasonic scaling devices. Ultrasonic devices appear particularly efficient but lack tactile feedback and may be usefully combined with manual instrumentation. Local analgesia may be used as necessary, based on patient wishes and comfort.

Surgical techniques are used primarily to improve, assess and facilitate removal of subgingival deposits. In the uncomplicated treatment of periodontitis, flap procedures aimed at minimizing loss of tissue should be first choice. Gingivectomy eliminates pockets at the expense of gingival tissue and this can create aesthetic problems.

Flap and gingivectomy procedures may be used as part of the restorative therapy, for example crown lengthening.

Guided tissue regeneration

The ultimate goal of periodontal treatment is to restore lost connective tissue attachment. The healing process following either surgical or non-surgical treatment involves the formation of a long junctional epithelial attachment along the root surface without regeneration of the periodontal tissues. *Guided tissue regeneration* at present is the most promising method for restoring periodontal structures. The aims of this treatment are firstly, to prevent apical migration of the epithelial attachment during the initial stages of healing and secondly, to create a potential space under the surgical flap so as to facilitate regeneration of periodontal ligament along the root surface.

The space can be created by inserting an exclusionary barrier membrane under the flap and covering the root surface and adjacent bone. Various materials have been developed which may be resorbable or non-resorbable. To date, most of the clinical evaluation has been concerned with a non-resorbable expanded polytetrafluoroethylene (e-PTFE) material. Clinically impressive results, in terms of pocket depth reduction, gain in attachment and bone fill have been noted in grade II furcation lesions and various infrabony defects, with less impressive results in grade III furcations in maxillary molars.

Recently developed resorbable membranes have the advantage of not requiring a second operation for removal. These materials are based on lactide/glycolide copolymers or collagen. Studies have found the copolymers as effective as e-PTFE membranes in terms of gain of attachment and reduction in pocket depth. Bovine and human type I collagen membrane sponges have been used in guided tissue regeneration with good results, but there have been no direct comparisons with other materials.

Other approaches to regeneration of lost periodontal ligament have included the use of growth factors and an enamel matrix derivative, which do not involve the use of a barrier membrane. These materials are simply coated on to the exposed root surface prior to suturing of the replaced surgical flap. At present it is too early to ascertain the long-term benefits of these biologically active materials, although initial studies appear promising.

Therapy phase – chemoprevention and chemotherapy

Since periodontitis is a bacteria-associated disease, antimicrobial agents may be used as part of treatment. These may have a primarily preventive role or a primarily therapeutic role and can be delivered locally or systemically.

Chemoprevention is usually directed against the potential adverse effects of plaque organisms locally or systemically. Chlorhexidine mouthrinses, irrigation and sprays are the usual forms of local treatment. Indications for their use include:

- Reduction of contamination of the operatory with oral organisms
- Reduction of bacteraemia in the at-risk individual as an adjunct to systemic antimicrobial prophylaxis (see Chapter 4)
- Control of supragingival plaque when mechanical cleaning may be compromised.

Chemotherapy, either local or systemic, is usually used as an adjunct to mechanical surgical or non-surgical techniques.

Local delivery of antimicrobials subgingivally has been by:

- Irrigation
- Slow release devices

This area of local delivery has been extensively reviewed and currently it is considered that local chemotherapy should not be used routinely. It is indicated where sites have not responded to mechanical debridement techniques. Irrigation with either a single agent or a variety has not been a convincingly proven adjunctive to root planing.

The potential side-effects of the development of bacterial resistance and overgrowth of opportunist organisms must also be considered.

A number of antimicrobials in slow release devices have been shown adjunctive to scaling and root planing as measured by a reduction in pocketing and/or gains in probing attachment levels. These antimicrobials include tetracycline, minocycline and metronidazole. The value of chlorhexidine in slow release vehicles is still debated.

Systemic delivery is usually by the oral route and currently systemic antimicrobials have little or no place in the management of adult periodontitis. They may be considered in the management of juvenile, rapidly progressive and refractory periodontitis. The use of systemic antimicrobials in individuals whose periodontal state is compromised by a medical condition, e.g. diabetes, while logical, is unproven. It would seem reasonable to delay the decision to determine if such an individual is refractory to conventional therapy.

Systemic antimicrobials that have attracted most research interest are metronidazole, tetracyclines and the combination of metronidazole and amoxycillin. The decision to use systemic antimicrobials must be balanced against possible side-effects, namely:

- Hypersensitivity (allergic) reaction
- Development of bacterial resistance
- Superinfection by opportunist organisms
- Toxic side-effects of the particular antimicrobial
- Drug interaction with concomitant chemotherapy

Mucogingival surgical techniques

A variety of mucogingival surgical techniques have evolved over a number of years These have been designed to:

- Remove fraenal attachments
- Deepen sulci

- Widen or replace the width of attached gingivae
- Recontour gingiva and/or replace missing papillae

It is now appreciated that neither the mucogingival problem nor the treatment outcome to rectify the anomaly have any bearing on the prevention of recurrence or treatment of periodontitis. Mucogingival techniques, therefore, rarely feature in the treatment plan for the disease. Clearly, these procedures may provide aesthetic and/or functional benefits and are usually reserved for such indications. For example, the gingivoplasty procedure may be required for control of gingival enlargement consequent upon a number of drugs that were listed earlier (see Chapter 7).

Maintenance phase

It has been established that whatever the outcome of treatment, long-term success is dependent on supragingival plaque control that is improved by the combination of professional and personal hygiene programmes. Periodontitis is a chronic condition in which susceptibility does not change and therefore recurrence is always a possibility. There is, therefore, a need for recall, reassessment and remotivation of patients. When necessary, professional prophylaxis should be given. The timing of recall appears arbitrary and should be based on patient needs rather than applying the same regimen to each patient.

Patients who are unable to maintain a satisfactory level of oral hygiene, or who are not followed up, tend to show relapse over time. Conversely, patients practising over-zealous toothbrushing may cause gingival recession and those who are subjected to frequent and repeated scaling of teeth, particularly at shallow sites, show iatrogenic loss of attachment.

To summarize, care and maintenance are essential but should not be overprescribed. The value of long-term chemical plaque control for the susceptible periodontal patient who has been treated is not established.

Periodontal therapy – Summary

The main aspect of pre- and post-treatment management or preparation for the periodontal patient is the achievement and maintenance of satisfactory supragingival plaque control. This is dependent on professional and personal involvement in a disease for which susceptibility cannot be altered by means available at present. For the foreseeable future, 'once a periodontal patient always a periodontal patient'.

14

Principles of occlusal management

> The functional anatomy of the occlusion was described in Chapter 8. This chapter discusses the clinical techniques associated with the occlusion, particularly the use of articulators.

Occlusal analysis

Whilst the examination of the occlusion is part of the examination of every patient, the term 'occlusal analysis' implies a more detailed examination and this will be aided by articulated models.

An occlusal analysis is necessary for:

- Planning fixed prosthodontics
- Diagnosing cases of occlusal dysfunction

Clinical examination of the occlusion

The following intra-oral aspects are of particular interest:

- Missing or malposed teeth
- Cuspal height and cuspal inclines
- Centric occlusion, crossbite
- Tooth surfaces – wear facets, irregular surface loss, attrition, erosion and abrasion
- Curves of Spee and Monson, overbite, overjet, incisal inclination
- Restorations/prostheses – accuracy of fit, occlusal form and function
- Centric relation and the retruded arc of closure, precentric prematurities
- Extent and direction of centric relation (CR) to centric occlusion (CO) displacement (Vh/Hv)
- Tooth guidance in lateral and protrusive excursions and interferences

The examination will be completed by the examination of the:

- Temporomandibular joints
- Muscles of mastication

Detailed examination

This may be done alongside an articulation to confirm it, or as a clinical procedure only. The exercise requires 8 μm metal foil (*shimstock*) and artery forceps, 40 μm smudgeproof articulating paper, red and blue, with reverse action tweezers.

Centric occlusion The shimstock is used to check the existence of stable, contacting cusp/fossa relationships. The patient should be asked to close until the teeth are just touching, since variable compression of the periodontal ligaments can bring uneven or open sites into contact. This point is of considerable importance when fitting restorations, since clenching can create apparent evenness of contacts.

Shimstock is placed between each area of likely contact, the patient closes, and the foil will either be held or pull out (*Fig. 14.1A*). This can be noted and checked against the articulation later (*Fig. 14.1B*).

Next, blue paper is used to mark CO contacts. The teeth should be dried and the patient asked to close the teeth together. A variety of markings are possible, from the classic tripod to single fossa contacts (see *Fig. 8.4*).

Centric relation Red paper is now used to mark the retruded contact position (RCP) and mandibular slide from CR to CO. The patient is manipulated onto the terminal hinge axis and closed into the retruded contact position (*Fig. 14.2*). Then the patient closes of his or her own volition into CO.

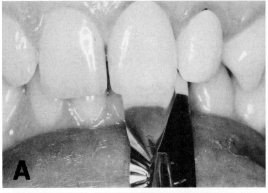

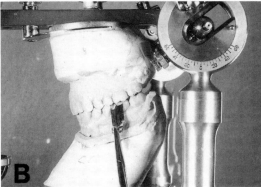

Fig. 14.1 A Shimstock being used to check the centric contact between the upper and lower central incisors. **B** Centric occlusion contacts on an articulator being checked with shimstock

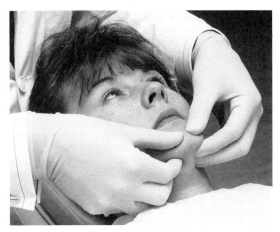

Fig. 14.2 Manipulation onto the retruded arc of closure. The operator's fingers and thumbs exert upward and backward pressure to locate the condyles into their most superior, posterior position and 'rotate' the mandible

This procedure leads to:

- Double marking of centric stops, i.e. red superimposed on blue
- Red alone marking the RCP and slide(s) (see *Fig. 8.5B*)

Lateral and protrusive excursions Examination of lateral and protrusive excursions should demonstrate either canine guidance or group function, and the length and height of the anterior guidance. This last characteristic is shown by the amount of posterior disclusion.

The most important aspect of eccentric excursions is to look for interferences, i.e. tooth contacts that are interrupting smooth and even sliding contacts. These contacts may cause deviations in side-shift or protrusion. In group function, all buccal cusps on the working side should be in contact. If, during the excursion, a pair of upper and lower cusps 'lift' the other cusps out of contact, this pair of cusps constitutes a *working side interference*.

Tooth contacts on the non-working side may interfere with condylar guidance and side-shift; these are *non-working interferences* (see *Fig. 8.6D*).

Temporomandibular joints These may be examined for movement and clicks by palpation with the fingers overlying the joints or in the external auditory meatus. In addition, a stethoscope may be used to listen to joint sounds.

Clicking in the joint may not be revealed by simple movement of the mandible, since the disc position may change when food is between the teeth. It can be useful to ask the patient to chew on some hard wax and listen during the series of functional movements.

Muscles of mastication Extraoral palpation of the temporalis origins overlying the parietal bones and the whole lateral aspect of the masseters is straightforward. Bimanual palpation of the masseter is more reliable with one digit within the mouth and one external. This same method can be used for the mylohyoid and digastric.

Intraoral palpation of the medial pterygoid requires a finger to be placed in the fauces area and this can be unpleasant. The most difficult muscle to palpate is the lateral pterygoid. The first finger is placed around the posterior aspect of the tuberosity and upwards to the lateral aspect of the lateral pterygoid plate of the sphenoid bone. This is uncomfortable also.

The discomfort induced by palpation may persuade the patient to report tenderness which, of course, is misleading. The muscles that can be palpated with reliable results are the temporalis and masseters.

Articulation of study models

Equipment

The equipment available for reproducing the occlusion in the laboratory, for either detailed the examination of the occlusion or for the construction of restorations ranges from the primitive to the esoteric, from bare hands to microcomputers!

The over-riding considerations, in the choice of equipment are to use that which is appropriate to the job in hand, and that both the dentist and his technician really know and understand the principles of the instruments they use. A badly used articulator is often much, much worse than using no articulator at all.

Incorrect articulation will lead to restorations that will require considerable chairside time for fitting whilst the occlusal surfaces are modified to suit the actual occlusion.

The very simple articulators, the average path and simple plane line, are too small to reproduce the relationship between the temporomandibular joint and the occlusal plane. For this reason they do not locate any hinge axis from the patient and may introduce errors if tooth apart occlusal records are used. These instruments are little more than a convenient way of locating two models in a fixed position

At the other end of the scale, the computerized *fully adjustable articulator* will provide the nearest equivalent to the patient, with curved condylar guides, immediate and progressive side-shifts, exact intercondylar width and an exact reproduction of the hinge axis.

The most practical type of instrument is the *semi-adjustable articulator* and its associated *face-bow*. There are several excellent types available and the choice depends to a large extent on personal preference. This book shows cases mounted on the Dentatus ARH and the Denar MkIIA (see Manufacturers' List, p. 281). The first is a good instrument for teaching the basic principles of occlusion and the latter is a light, simple instrument that is more suitable for fixed prosthodontics.

In order to illustrate the design of face-bows and articulators, the Denar MkIIA and its associated Slidematic face-bow will be described in detail.

Face-bow

The purpose of the face-bow is to locate the maxillary teeth in three planes (superior–inferior, anterior–posterior and lateral) to the temporomandibular joint (TMJ). Ideally, the articulator's hinge should be the terminal or *true hinge axis* of the joint. However, two pieces of equipment, a *hinge axis locator*, together with a *hinge axis transfer face-bow* are required to do this accurately.

For simplicity of use, most face-bows work in connection with an *arbitrary hinge axis*. A number of workers have determined the position of the true hinge axis for a group of subjects and correlated it with a surface anatomical landmark. Each worker has then derived an average position in order to dispense with true hinge axis location. These positions are usually claimed to be within 5 mm of the true hinge axis on all patients.

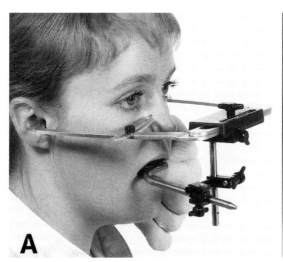
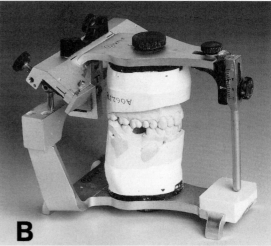

Fig. 14.3. A The Denar Slidematic ear-bow in place. The bow is self-centering and locates to the side of the nose for its vertical reference point. The bite fork is stabilized by the operator. **B** The Denar MkIIA articulator. This is a light arcon instrument, with adjustable condylar angles, progressive side-shift and immediate side-shift. The intercondylar distance is fixed

The most commonly used arbitrary hinge axis is a point 12 mm anterior to the posterior border of the tragus along a line drawn from the superior border of the tragus to the outer canthus of the eye. This position would be transferred by a face-bow to the condylar axis of the articulator.

However, it is easier to use an ear-bow that locates into the external auditory meatus, with the articulator having an ear-bow mounting site that is posterior to the articulator hinge (remember that the ear is posterior to the TMJ!). Alternatively, the design of the articulator and its mounting system takes account of this anatomy.

The Denar Slidematic face bow (*Fig. 14.3A*) is a self-centering ear-bow that can also measure the intercondylar distance. The bow is located in the vertical plane by an arbitrary point on the side of the nose, 43 mm from the upper lateral incisor edge.

The bite fork should locate the upper model accurately, but without engaging tooth undercut to avoid distortion of the wax. Three layers of base plate wax, softened and firmly sealed to the metal are sufficient, and a zinc oxide–eugenol wash can be added for extra accuracy if required.

In taking the record, ensure that:

1. The ear lugs are firmly engaged on bone
2. The reference plane locator points to the nose point
3. The bite fork is accurately and evenly located on all the teeth and stabilized by the clinician during recording
4. All screws, etc. are tightened firmly to avoid slippage during mounting

The record is assembled on the articulator by means of an index system that avoids the need to send the whole ear-bow to the laboratory. It is useful to have the articulator at the chairside to check the ear-bow settings and discover spurious recordings whilst the patient is still available.

Articulator

The Denar MkIIA (*Fig. 14.3B*) is a simple, light 'Arcon'-type semi-adjustable articulator. The 'Arcon' classification (short for ARticulator–CONdyle) describes the fact that the condyles are attached to the lower member, in comparison with the Dentatus ARH that is 'non-Arcon', having the condyles on the upper member (*Fig. 14.4*).

The arcon design is more realistic anatomically, since in protrusion the condyles move forward with the mandible. In the non-arcon, the condyles move backward in protrusion. Some minor technical advantages are also claimed for the arcon type.

The Denar can be set to vary the condylar angles, the progressive side-shift and the immediate side-shift. The antero-posterior position of the condyles

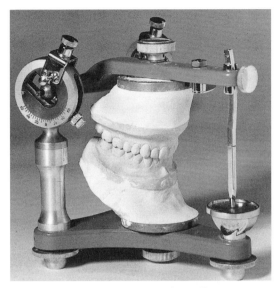

Fig. 14.4 The Dentatus ARH articulator. This is a non-arcon instrument, with adjustable condylar angles and progressive side-shift. It has no provision for immediate side-shift

can be adjusted to provide separate identifiable positions for centric relation and centric occlusion. It has a fixed intercondylar distance. The incisal guide can be 'customised' to the anterior guidance (see below).

Occlusal records

There are three types of static occlusal records, each for a different purpose. In addition, dynamic records can be used for certain articulators.

Centric relation record   This is a tooth-apart record, taken with the patient on the retruded arc of closure. It is used to carry out a preoperative occlusal analysis where problems have been diagnosed with the existing centric occlusion. Alternatively, it may be used for construction of restorations when centric occlusion is lost, as in complete dentures.

Centric occlusion record   This is a tooth-together record of the position of maximum intercuspation. This position is used for mounting preoperative and master models when no change to the existing centric occlusion is proposed. However, the best way of orientating the models is to avoid the use of an inter-dental record altogether, and place them into the position of 'best fit'. This position can be checked against the patient and marked on the models.

Lateral and protrusive check records   These are used to set the articulator condylar angles and the instruction manual of the articulator will specify those required for a particular instrument.

Dynamic records   A detailed description of these is outside the scope of this book. Basically, these are usually tracings or microcomputer signals from specialized kinematic face-bow systems.

They can be used to:

* Assess the amount of immediate and progressive side-shift
* Assess the condylar inclination
* Trace the condylar path shape
* Trace the incisal guide
* Trace the chewing cycle
* Assess muscle activity and functional disturbances

Recording media   The essential requirements are that the recording medium should:

* Not interfere with the path of closure of the mandible
* Record sufficient detail to permit accurate orientation of the models
* Be sufficiently rigid to stabilize the models during mounting on the articulator

The commonly used wax squash bite has the major disadvantage of interfering with the path of closure and also obscures the tooth position that is being recorded. Softer materials, such as alginate and impression rubbers, have been used to overcome this problem, but they give imprecise mounting positions for the models during articulation.

The technique to be described for a centric relation record offers rigidity and the minimum interference with closure.

The starting point is accurate study models, taken in an elastomer and cast with die stone occlusal surfaces.

The record consists of two thicknesses of very hard baseplate wax supporting a metal mesh. The mesh is cut to fit exactly to the palatal surfaces of the upper teeth and the wax is trimmed to the buccal surfaces (*Fig. 14.5*). This ensures good vision of the tooth relationships.

Bimanual manipulation of the mandible onto the terminal hinge axis or retruded arc of closure is now performed. The patient is asked to half open the mouth and relax. The operator's fingers and thumbs exert upwards and backwards pressure on the mandible to locate the condyles into the posterior, superior position in glenoid fossae (*Fig. 14.2*).

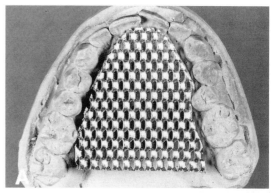
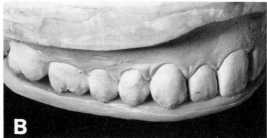
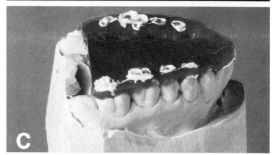

Fig. 14.5 A Occlusal record. Expanded metal mesh cut to fit to the palatal aspect of the upper arch. The mesh supports the recording wax and prevents distortion. **B** Two thicknesses of hard wax have been added to sandwich the mesh. The wax is trimmed to the buccal surfaces so that the occlusal relationship can be seen during registration. **C** The completed record has the cusp tips reproduced in zinc oxide–eugenol and should fit each model accurately

The wax wafer is softened in hot water and placed on the upper arch and the mandible manipulated on the hinge axis so that the lower teeth indent the wax by about 0.25 mm. The wafer is removed and chilled in cold water. This first stage creates a matrix to support the actual recording medium.

The detail of the tooth relationships can now be recorded using a zinc oxide–eugenol wash. The wash is 'dotted' into the tooth indents on both surfaces of the wax with just enough used to record the cusp tips only. Any more may record occlusal

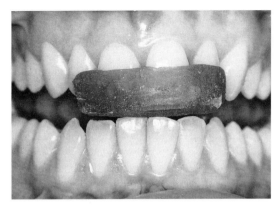

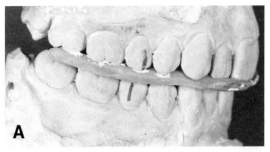
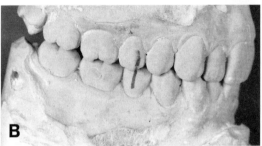

Fig. 14.6 An occlusal deprogrammer. This removes the memory of centric occlusion and, after removal, manipulation onto the retruded arc of closure should be easier

Fig. 14.7 A Articulated models with pre-centric record in place. **B** The record has been removed and the articulator closed. There has been an upward and forward movement, as shown by the marks on the premolars, to reach centric occlusion

surface detail not included on the models and therefore prevent seating of the record.

The wafer is replaced in the mouth and the mandible manipulated again on to the terminal hinge axis and onto the record.

After the zinc oxide–eugenol has set, the record is removed and carefully placed on each model in turn to check for accurate seating (*Fig. 14.5C*). This checks the accuracy of both the record and the models. The accuracy required is seen in *Figure 14.7A*.

To confirm the reproducibility of the record, two further wafers can be taken and the mounting done by a split cast technique. Here, the upper model is grooved and a separating medium applied. It is mounted to the face-bow in the usual way, and the lower model plastered to the first record. When the plaster has set, the record is removed and the upper model separated from its mounting plaster, leaving the locating points. The other two records are then used to orientate the upper model on to the mounted lower model and the articulator closed. If the records are identical, then the location grooves and points will meet exactly. Two matching out of three is an acceptable reproduction.

In the case of patients whose musculature resists the manipulation, a 'deprogrammer' may be needed to remove the short-term memory of CO. The appliance is made at the chairside from cold-cure acrylic and forms a flat bite plane on the incisal edges (*Fig. 14.6*). The record is re-attempted after about 10 minutes, with the deprogrammer out.

The same wax wafer arrangement may be used for lateral and protrusive records for articulator settings in accordance with the manufacturer's directions.

Confirmation of articulated mounting

The articulation should be compared with the patient. This will involve the use of articulating paper and shimstock and general observation of the tooth relationships created by articulator movements.

When the pre-centric record is removed, the articulator should reproduce the retruded arc of closure with the retruded contact position, and then close into centric occlusion via sliding from the prematurities (*Fig. 14.7*). In CO, shimstock should be retained by centric stops on the articulator as it is in the mouth (*Fig. 14.1*). Wear facets should be observed in particular, to see that these approximate to each other on the models as they do clinically.

Comparison of the articulating paper markings made clinically in centric occlusion, retruded contact position, and in eccentric excursions with those on the articulator should show good agreement. The adjustment of the antero-posterior position of the articulator condyles facilitates the closure directly into centric occlusion if a centric relation mounting has been done.

Errors in articulation

These can occur as a result of the compromises made in articulator design and particularly as a result of using an arbitrary hinge axis. It may be possible to compensate for some errors by adjusting the condylar assemblies to bring appropriate teeth into contact, but gross inaccuracies will require remounting to a new occlusal record.

Possible sources of error in articulation are:

- Distortion of the impression
- Air blows on the occlusal surface
- Slippage of the face-bow
- Use of the arbitrary hinge axis
- Expansion of the mounting plaster
- Incorrect occlusal record
- Articulator design compromises
- Compression of the periodontium not reproduced
- Incorrect angles set

Restoration of the occlusion

Conformative and reorganized approaches

As was discussed in Chapter 8, each individual adapts successfully to his or her occlusal irregularities, and will usually continue to adapt as teeth are lost or restored. However, there must clearly be a limit to the capacity of this adaptation and so the golden rule of occlusal restoration is not to create further problems.

This principle is enshrined in the *'conformative approach'* to occlusal restoration. Where centric occlusion and its associated lateral and protrusive movements are functioning satisfactorily, then no procedure must change this. No doctrinaire philosophies of the rights or wrongs of a particular occlusion should intrude on treatment. Each new restoration should blend harmoniously with the functional pattern already present, provided that is satisfactory.

The converse of this is the *'reorganised approach'*. Here changes are made to the existing occlusion following a diagnosis that there is some major occlusal problem present or, of course, when there is no centric occlusion.

An example of when the reorganized approach would be appropriate is the replacement of restorative work that introduces occlusal interferences and/or deviations on mandibular closure that the patient has noticed, usually as discomfort. This type of case requires an articulation in centric relation to make the initial diagnosis followed by careful planning of the new occlusion using diagnostic waxing to develop appropriate tooth relationships.

Occlusal stability

The maintenance of a stable centric occlusion position is important for occlusal harmony. This may be influenced by restorative work and the behaviour of materials.

Intracoronal restorations

The natural cusp/fossa relationship, especially one that is based on tripods, is very difficult to reproduce by freehand carving. The result of inaccurate contacts, or no contacts at all, is tooth movement to seek a stable position (*Fig. 14.8A*).

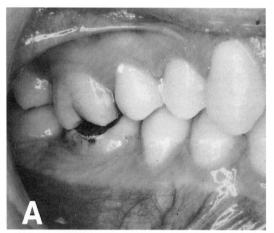

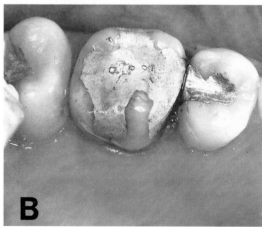

Fig. 14.8 Occlusal stability. **A** Overeruption of the upper molar has been caused by poor reproduction of the occlusal surface of its opponent. To correct this, the upper occlusal plane must be realigned by adjusting the displaced molar, or crowning it, followed by a veneer crown on the lower to maintain the new position. **B** Amalgam restoration with flat plateaux centric stops to provide accurate stability

In moderate to large restorations, the natural fossa should be replaced by a flat plateau (*Fig 14.8B*) that receives the supporting cusp of the opposing tooth. This provides good stability and also directs the occlusal loads axially.

However, the best restoration from the occlusal viewpoint is the small one. Absolutely minimal cutting of the occlusal surface will allow the occlusion to be maintained by enamel in its original state (see *Figs 10.5* and *10.7*).

Choice of materials

The choice of materials to restore occlusal surfaces is equally important. No wholly satisfactory material exists; all direct restorative materials deform under load (creep) or undergo surface loss (see Chapter 9) and, of the indirect materials, ceramic is the most difficult to use efficiently. *Table 14.1* summarizes factors that influence the choice between cast metal and ceramic for the restoration of occlusal surfaces in fixed prosthodontics.

Table 14.1 Factors involved in the selection of materials for occlusal surfaces

Metal	*Ceramic*
Large pulps	Small pulps
Small teeth	Large teeth
Low anterior guidance	High anterior guidance
Average technical support	Excellent technical support
Simple clinical adjustment	Difficult clinical adjustment

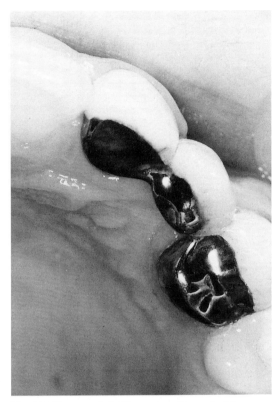

Fig. 14.9 Upper arch bridgework, with most of the functional surfaces reproduced in metal

The relationship of preparations to pulpal and tooth size is discussed in Chapter 15.

A low anterior guidance leads to very little posterior disclusion and therefore the occlusal clearance required to accommodate ceramic may result in a very short preparation. A larger posterior disclusion will permit ceramic coverage.

The average technician is usually skilled in handling wax and will be able to make a functional surface in metal very adequately. However, when firing ceramic it is much more difficult to achieve accurate contacts.

Perhaps the most important veto is provided by the last factor in *Table 14.1*. Marking, adjustment and repolishing of metal is much less time consuming clinically than the procedure for ceramic, which should include reglazing.

Unless aesthetics are of over-riding importance, the better material for occlusal surfaces is cast metal (*Fig. 14.9*).

Bridgework

It is essential that bridgework replaces all the functional contacts in centric occlusion. It used to be suggested that loads on the abutment teeth could be reduced by narrowing the occlusal table of the pontics. This is questionable but, more importantly, such a pontic may not have correct centric contacts.

Figure 14.10 shows a case where occlusal contacts were not provided, leading to considerable problems. The patient was a 45-year-old man, who was complaining that the gap between the lower left lateral incisor and the canine was opening progressively (*Fig. 14.10A*). This, in fact was caused by overeruption of the canine, and the bridge pontic opposing this tooth (*Fig. 14.10B*) had no centric stop.

Orthodontic therapy was provided to realign the canine (*Fig. 14.10C*), and the upper bridge was remade with a positive fossa relationship with the repositioned tooth (*Fig. 14.10D*). This course of treatment took almost two years.

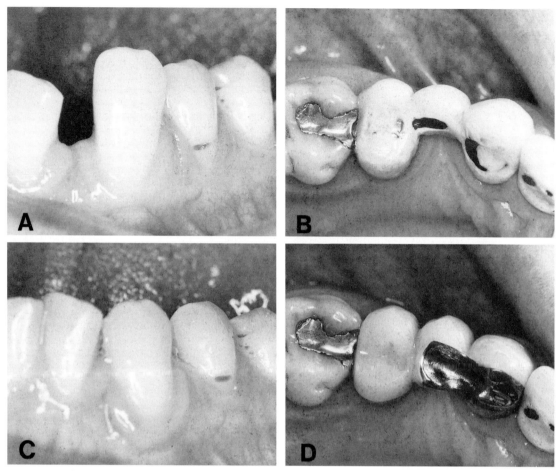

Fig. 14.10 Loss of occlusal stability. The lower canine has overerupted (**A**) because there is no centric stop on the upper bridge pontic (**B**). The tooth was realigned orthodontically (**C**), and a new bridge made with a positive centric stop (**D**)

Anterior guidance

The functional contours of upper anterior teeth are particularly important, and when making crowns or bridges for that region, the articulator must be 'customized' to reproduce conformative movement pathways. This is done at the diagnostic mounting stage and either an adjustable incisal guide can be set to the appropriate angles or, for better accuracy, a customized incisal table can be made (*Fig. 14.11*).

Cold curing acrylic is added to the incisal table and, whilst it is soft, the articulator is moved through the functional pathways dictated by the teeth. When hard, the articulator will reproduce these movements when, say, a series of crowns is being constructed.

A change in the anterior guidance may be indicated when a key functional tooth is being replaced. This problem tends to be centred on the canine. If this tooth is lost in a canine guided occlusion, then consideration must be given to changing the occlusal scheme to group function, so that the prosthetic replacement, whether bridge pontic or denture tooth, is not subjected to unfavourable forces. *Figure 14.12* shows a bridge replacing a canine, in lateral excursion. The pontic receives all the lateral load and transmits rotational forces to the premolar. This latter tooth was mobile and painful. The bridge required replacement and a change in the functional pattern to group function so that the lateral forces could be shared with other posterior teeth.

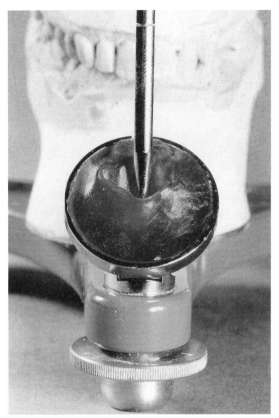

Fig. 14.11 Customized incisal guidance table on the Dentatus ARH articulator

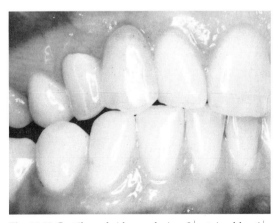

Fig. 14.12 Cantilever bridge replacing 3| retained by 4| only. In lateral excursion, the occlusion is canine guided, and the pontic transmitted rotational forces to the premolar. The occlusal scheme should have been changed to group function to balance the forces on the bridge and the second premolar should have been included in the bridge design

Occlusal equilibration

Indications

This procedure, sometimes referred to as 'selective grinding', involves the recontouring of tooth surfaces so that the occlusion conforms to certain norms. The indications are contentious and there is much disagreement on whether the procedure should be performed.

Various workers have proposed occlusal equilibration:

- To establish occlusal harmony as a preventive measure
- To treat temporomandibular dysfunction syndrome
- As part of periodontal therapy
- As preoperative mouth preparation for crown and bridge work
- Following oral surgery

The doctrinaire 'equilibration for all' is not indicated by the available evidence that suggests that almost all people have occlusal interferences, but only a small proportion are suffering from an occlusal related disorder (see Chapter 26). The use of equilibration for an established disorder is also considered below.

The occlusal imbalance as a primary aetiological agent in periodontal disease is currently discredited. Work from Scandinavia has suggested that occlusal forces are regulated by a feedback mechanism that relates them to the amount of support available. There is evidence though of secondary effects of occlusal irregularities once the primary lesion is established (see Chapter 7).

However, there is some evidence that limited equilibration is of value prior to crown and bridgework. The preparations will remove occlusal surface and in doing so may remove existing prematurities or interferences. This will change the tooth guidance and may also change the centric occlusion position. The practical result might be the loss of occlusal clearance when the restoration is tried in. If the occlusal surface of the lower molar shown in *Figure 8.6D* were reduced, then the condylar guidance would take over the progressive side-shift pathway and no crown could fit in between.

Finally, an excellent indication is following the reduction and healing of maxillofacial fractures or orthognathic surgery, when there may be slight discrepancies in occlusal positions remaining.

Technique

Equilibration must be approached with extreme care – the enamel cannot be put back! Further, the removal of apparently simple and localized

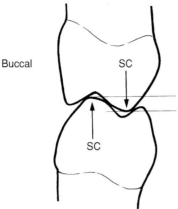

Buccal

SC

SC

A

Fig. 14.13 (see p. 140) Principles of occlusal equilibration, assuming a correct and stable centric occlusion

A Centric occlusion. The contacts between the pairs of centric stops and supporting cusps (SCs) must be maintained for occlusal stability

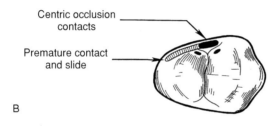

Centric occlusion contacts

Premature contact and slide

B

B Precentric prematurity on an upper premolar. Hollow the mesial slope of the palatal cusp, but do not touch the contacts where the two articulating paper colours will be superimposed from centric occlusion

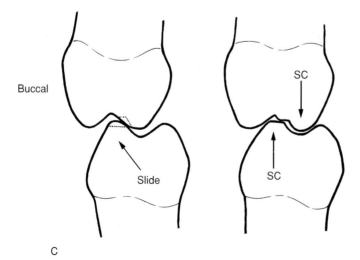

Buccal

Slide

SC

SC

C

C Lateral slide from a precentric prematurity between the palatal cusp of the upper molar and the buccal cusp of the lower molar. The mandible moves to the right after this contact, into centric occlusion. Widen the fossa on the upper, but keep its contact level the same. Reduce the tip of the buccal cusp of the lower, maintaining the same buccal inclined plane contact, and creating a new plateau contact for stability to the palatal aspect

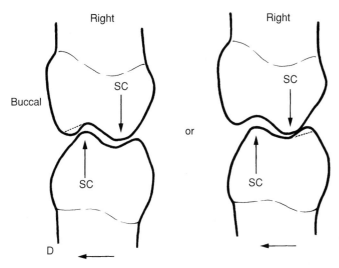

Right   Right

Buccal

SC   SC

or

SC   SC

D ←   ←

Direction of movement to right working side

D Working side interferences: grind non-supporting cusps, i.e. buccal upper, lingual lower, depending on the excursion. The interferences shown will tend to occur only in group function, since canine guidance tends to disclude all the posterior teeth. The adjustment will balance the excursion

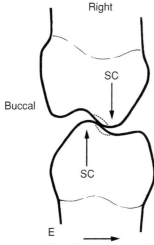

Right

SC

Buccal

SC

E →

Direction of movement to left working side

E Non-working interferences. Hollow the cusp slopes of interfering inclines, without removing cusp tips

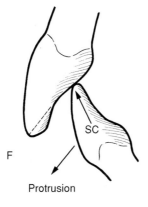

SC

F

Protrusion

F Protrusive interference. Ideally, the lower incisors should have an even path and contacts with the uppers. The diagram shows the adjustment required if the lower incisor has an isolated path, discluding the others. The lower incisor tip must not be reduced – it would then be out of contact in centric, and would overerupt

prematurities can have the knock-on effect of creating more elsewhere.

Full mouth equilibration requires the application of an occlusal 'philosophy'. There are essentially two:

- Freedom in centric
- Centric occlusion coincident with centric relation

Freedom in centric has some sense attached to it, though little scientific support. The basic concept is to allow closure on multiple arcs of closure into a centric occlusion position that has a range of 1 mm or so both anteroposteriorly and bucco-lingually – a 'long centric'. The attainment of any position within long centric can then be achieved without the intrusion of premature contacts. The precise position of centric occlusion is therefore removed, but not occlusal stability. The neuromuscular control of mandibular closure therefore does not have to be so precise and therefore, it is argued, there will be less susceptibility to temporomandibular dysfunction.

In lateral movements, all teeth on the non-working side should be discluded, as should all palatal cusps on the working side. In protrusion, all the posterior teeth should disclude, and the lower anterior teeth should have even and balanced contact with the upper teeth.

The philosophy of CO being made coincident with CR involves the establishment of a precise position based on tripods. Much relies on which CR definition is applied; the posterior–superior position is too far posterior for natural comfort and, in contrast with freedom in centric, the mandibular positioning on closure has to be very accurate. This approach seems to ignore the naturally occurring difference between the condylar positions in CO and CR.

The results of clinical studies of equilibration have been reported but many of these are retrospective and sometimes no more than anecdotal. There have been a few controlled studies and these are inconclusive.

In carrying out an equilibration to freedom in centric, the following rules should be applied:

- Do not remove any supporting cusps from occlusal stability
- Fossae may be widened but must not be deepened
- Prematurities and interferences should be removed by hollowing cusp slopes
- Non-supporting cusps can be reduced in height to remove non-working interferences

These rules are illustrated in the series of diagrams in *Figure 14.13*.

Occlusal management – Summary

The overriding consideration is that most patients are able to tolerate many minor anatomical and technical 'faults' in tooth relationships and restorations. Dentists must avoid being dogmatic about occlusal theory and remember the old saw – 'If it ain't broke, don't fix it!'

Restorations must be constructed to harmonize with an maintain existing tooth relationships where these are satisfactory.

Articulators are essential for the construction of fixed and removable prostheses and there is no substitute for hands-on training with this equipment.

Changes to an occlusion must be planned carefully with proper diagnostic procedures.

15

Fixed prosthodontics: Crowns

Intracoronal restorations are generally satisfactory provided there is sufficient sound tooth tissue to support and retain them and to maintain the occlusion. On the other hand, weakened tooth tissue is vulnerable to fracture and should be protected. Further, large plastic restorations tend not to maintain the occlusion as well as cast metal or ceramic. These are the principal reasons for providing crowns.

Treatment planning

Indications for crowns

The indications for provision of a crown are:

- Protection of remaining tooth tissue
- Maintenance of the occlusion
- Aesthetics

The disadvantages are the possible plaque accumulation at the margins of the crown and the need to remove further sound tooth tissue.

The treatment of a large cavity in a posterior tooth, as discussed in Chapter 11, would be restored in the first instance by a pinned amalgam restoration. This might well give good service for some time, and it is certainly effective as a stabilization measure. However, depending upon its size, there might be remaining enamel and dentine that has become undermined and therefore weakened and the amalgam might not maintain occlusal stability in the long term.

A large cavity in an anterior tooth might be restorable by a composite resin restoration but it is more likely that retention will be compromised by loss of tooth tissue and the aesthetics of a large composite might not be satisfactory.

It is likely that a better long-term result would be achieved in both of the cases described above if a crown was constructed.

Crowns may also be used to improve aesthetics and this is discussed in Chapter 16.

The decision to construct a crown depends not only on the individual tooth factors, as listed above, but on other general factors. These are:

- Patient motivation
- Oral hygiene status
- Periodontal condition
- The restorative state of the tooth
- The occlusion and provision of dentures

Patient motivation

As was stressed in Section I, patient motivation is essential, and any advanced operative work requires a commitment from both the patient and the dentist. The stabilization phase of the treatment plan will give the dentist the opportunity to assess the patient's motivation, and indeed vice versa!

Oral hygiene and periodontal condition

As was discussed in Chapter 13, no matter how accurately made the crown, the junction between it and the tooth will promote plaque accumulation. If this extra plaque is superimposed on already established periodontal disease, this may make the condition worse. Ideally, the periodontium should be stable and the patient's oral hygiene of a high order.

Restorative state of the tooth

Examination of the tooth should ensure that the tooth is either vital or that adequate endodontic treatment has been carried out. An apical assessment with radiographs must be made. If there is doubt about the prognosis of a tooth, it is better not to embark on a complex restoration until the doubt has been removed. Nothing is more frustrating or embarrassing than to find the necessity for endodontics shortly after crown placement.

If the existing restoration has not been placed by the present dentist and is of dubious quality, it should be removed. This is really part of the management of the deep cavity since the dentine can be examined to ensure it is caries free and the periphery may be examined to ensure that there is an adequate base of sound tooth upon which to place a crown margin.

The remaining tooth can also be examined to decide on the techniques of core construction. An assessment of the tooth support likely to remain after crown preparation should be made so that weak undermined walls can be removed. This will influence the type and amount of additional retention to be provided for the core. It is usually best to plan for the worst and for the core to be well retained by an adequate number of pins.

The commonest reason for crown construction is the fracture of one or more cusps. The position of the fracture line may well determine not only the type of restoration but also the fate of the tooth. Subgingival fractures are difficult to treat since the deeper they are, the more inaccessible they are to instruments and impression materials. Gingival surgery is often necessary to expose the margin and assess restorability.

The occlusion and provision of dentures

The ability of an amalgam or composite resin to maintain occlusal stability will depend on the surface area of the restoration in contact with opposing supporting cusps and the accuracy with which the occlusal surface has been carved.

Once cusp or incisal tip loss has occurred, the prognosis for any direct restoration diminishes. While the restoration may not fail catastrophically, the effect of the oral environment on the physical properties of the material will result in slow degradation. The basis for this was discussed in Chapter 9; both amalgam and composite resin undergo creep, and the composite is vulnerable to surface deterioration. Occlusal loading leads to fatigue of both materials.

As a rule of thumb, one cusp can probably be restored reasonably with amalgam, but more than this and crowning should be considered. If an incisal edge is restored with composite resin then not only should the restoration itself be reviewed carefully, but also the opposing teeth in case surface

loss is caused by the hard filler particles of the composite.

The tooth position relative to the adjacent and opposing teeth will influence the type of crown preparation to be used. Imbrication and rotation will alter the design of the preparation and may limit the ability to position its margins satisfactorily. Tilting of the adjacent teeth may limit the path of insertion of the restoration and prevent crown construction unless modifications are made to the approximal surfaces of these teeth as well.

The inter-arch occlusal relationships should be studied prior to preparation. If there has been deterioration in these, there may be opposing cusps which may be intruding beyond the planned occlusal plane and preoperative equilibration of the area must be done (Chapter 14 and see *Fig. 14.8A*).

The *design of a partial denture* that will relate to a new crown must be completed before the crown is made. There may be requirements for guiding planes, rest seats and clasp shoulders that will need to be incorporated into the crown (See Chapter 22).

Principles of preparation

Preparation of any extracoronal restoration depends on planning the following:

● Path of insertion
● Stability of the restoration
● Choice of material
● Margin position and type
● New occlusal relationships

Path of insertion

This is dictated by the approximal surfaces of the adjacent teeth and *not* by the long axis of the tooth to be prepared. Ignoring this may lead to an inability to seat the crown because its margin is obstructed by a tilted adjacent tooth.

The path of insertion is also linked to the stability of the restoration. A long, single path provides maximum retention (*Fig 15.1*) and on tilted teeth, particularly lower molars, a lingually inclined path provides the longest opposing walls.

Stability of the restoration

This is the resistance provided by the preparation to displacing forces. These forces are usually occlusal in origin and give rise to rotational moments. Whilst retention is often considered in

Single path of insertion
Maximum retention

Range of paths of insertion
No retention

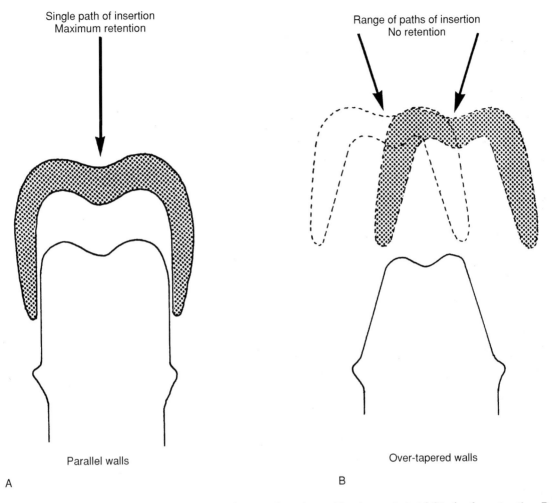

Parallel walls

Over-tapered walls

A   B

Fig. 15.1 The geometry of paths of insertion. **A** A long single path provides the greatest stability for the restoration. **B** An overtapered preparation leads to a range of paths and the restoration will have poor resistance to displacement

relation to the path of insertion, it is unlikely that displacing forces in service act in this direction.

Near-parallelism

Stability is achieved firstly by the principle of opposing parallel walls that need to be based on the same level – parallel walls not on the same base do not provide stability (*Fig. 15.2*).

The preparation of exactly parallel walls is difficult and near-parallelism, with an angle of convergence or taper of about five degrees, is more realistic and achievable. Any increase in taper above this figure leads to a dramatic reduction in stability.

The tapered rotary instruments used in the preparation are manufactured with this taper, and so all that is required is to select the path of insertion and cut the entire periphery of the preparation with the bur held rigidly in this axis. The temptation to angle the bur for apparently easier access, particularly palatally, must be resisted, as this will produce far too much taper.

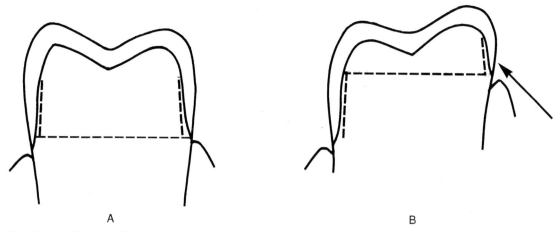

A   B

Fig. 15.2 Stability in a full crown preparation. The parallel walls in preparation **A** are opposite each other on the same base, and provide excellent stability. The parallel walls in **B** are not on the same base, and the crown would be vulnerable to rotational forces

Basic retention will be created by a cervical collar resembling a squashed cylinder, that will occupy one-third to one-half of the crown height. The occlusal third of the buccal and lingual aspects needs to be curved, so that the overall reduction is even, and the final crown is not bulbous (*Fig. 15.3*). Some teeth with short lingual walls have less height bucco-lingually, and so attention must be paid to the approximal areas to create most of the retention.

Cutting the approximal surface can be made difficult by a long and broad contact area. Upper molars are a particular problem in that the contact is frequently wide and can extend down to the cervical margin.

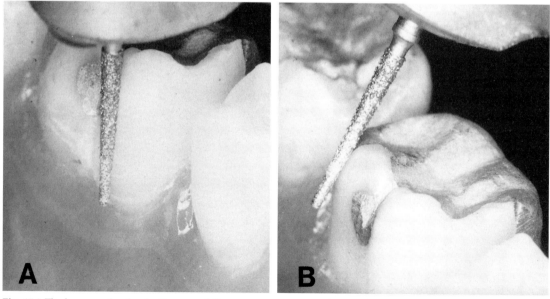

Fig. 15.3 The bucco-occlusal reduction on a full veneer crown preparation. **A** The first stage to create a near-parallel collar in the cervical area for stability. **B** The remainder of the buccal wall must be reduced to conform with the contour of the tooth to avoid the final crown being overcontoured

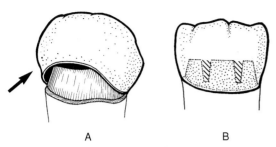

Fig. 15.4 A A short preparation is vulnerable to lateral displacing forces. **B** Incorporation of grooves increases resistance to displacement

Crown height

A short clinical crown will increase the risk of failure by displacement since the path of insertion is very short. Increasing the crown height may be achieved by gingival surgery – *crown lengthening* – but this can produce very unsatisfactory results. Care must be taken to ensure that gross irregularities do not occur in the level of the gingival margin as a result of lengthening a single short wall. There is also danger of the exposure of alveolar bone.

Gingival surgery is probably of most use in the distal segment of the lower arch, where frequently the distal crown height of the last standing tooth is very short; the removal of a wedge of tissue can increase the crown height significantly.

The stability of short preparations can be increased by the use of slots and grooves. These usually need to be placed in the buccal and lingual walls, though approximal grooves are useful where the lingual walls are short (*Fig. 15.4*).

If none of this is possible, then dentine pins incorporated in the casting or the use of dentine bonding agents will be necessary.

Occlusal reduction

Stability is increased by a preparation with a large surface area and having an occlusal surface that follows the proposed cusp outline. A flat topped preparation has less stability and also removes more tooth substance than is necessary.

Margin position and type

The finishing margin of any crown is determined by the gingival contour, the restorative material to be used and the presence of any core.

Where aesthetics is not the primary consideration, the crown margin should be placed supragingivally to prevent plaque accumulation and subsequent gingival inflammation. The margin should therefore follow the sinuous outline of the gingival tissue, with no sharp changes of direction.

The margin should, however, extend beyond the junction of any core, so that it is sited on sound tooth. If the margin is not beyond the core, the core/tooth/crown junction will be vulnerable to recurrent caries.

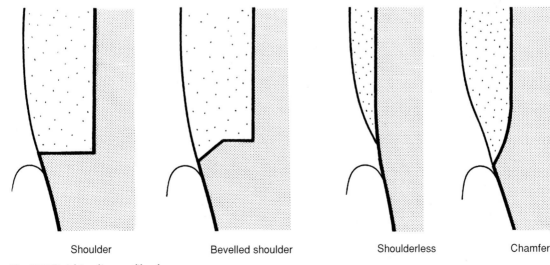

| Shoulder | Bevelled shoulder | Shoulderless | Chamfer |

Fig. 15.5 Finishing line profiles for crowns

The profile of the finishing line (*Fig. 15.5*) is determined by the material from which the crown will be constructed. Ceramic must have a *shoulder* with a minimum width of 1 mm, otherwise the material will be unsupported in thin section. Gold may be finished on a *chamfer* or a *bevelled shoulder*, the object being to achieve a 135° edge to the metal and to create a slip joint that can allow for slight casting shrinkage. This size of margin also allows the gold to be finished without running the risk of distortion.

The bevelled shoulder is used for partial veneer crowns where the supporting cusps require overlaying and the casting may be vulnerable to flexure. It may also be used for metal–ceramic crowns to provide margin strength for the subframe, and to provide a smoother enamel finish. The drawback to the bevelled shoulder is that it sacrifices considerable tooth substance.

The chamfer is the principal finishing line for the veneer crown. It is conservative of tooth structure and provides clear definition of the extent of the preparation for both the clinician when reading the impression and the technician when waxing. It also provides a substantial bulk of metal close to the margin, reducing the risk of flexure under load and the consequential rupture of the cement lute seal.

The *shoulderless* or knife-edge finishing line should not be used, as its definition is poor and can lead to inadequate thickness of metal that may flex under load.

New occlusal relationships

The new crown should harmonize with the existing occlusal relationships where they are satisfactory, but may be required to modify those that are not.

The occlusion should be examined preoperatively for premature contacts and occlusal plane irregularities in the region of the proposed crown. If deterioration of the occlusal surface has occurred, the opposing tooth may have overerupted. If this is not corrected, the new crown will continue the disharmony.

Crowns may also be used to correct rotations or aesthetic malalignments. The new crown position must be stable or the eventual result will be tooth movement and a worse problem subsequently (see also Chapters 16 and 19).

The occlusal clearance provided by the preparation must be sufficient to accommodate the chosen material (see later) and in load-bearing areas there must be an adequate thickness to prevent fracture. The shape of the reduction should indicate the cusp positions to the technician.

Choice of material

The choice is between:

- Gold
- Ceramic
- Ceramic bonded to metal (metal–ceramic)

Gold

Gold is still regarded as the most satisfactory extracoronal restorative material. It has a hardness similar to enamel, does not undergo creep intraorally and may be cast accurately. Creation of the occlusal contour and axial surfaces is relatively straightforward by wax carving. It may be used in thin section and will allow the production of fine margins. It is not, however, regarded as a very aesthetic material.

There are a number of gold types with additions of other metals providing a variety of properties available for use in different parts of the mouth. The clinician should specify the type of gold required for each type of restoration.

The reduction required to accommodate gold is approximately 1 mm throughout, and 1.5 mm, where possible, on the supporting cusps.

Ceramic

Dental porcelain, or ceramic as it now termed, is regarded as the most aesthetic material used in the mouth but is brittle and is liable to fracture in thin section. It is essential to have a minimum thickness of 0.8 mm at the margin and at least 1 to 1.5 mm incisally. It is not strong enough to be used alone for full crowns on posterior teeth or for bridgework. Its weakness is that cracks can originate from micropores on the fit surface, and that these can open catastrophically in tension or bending.

In view of the inherent weaknesses of basic dental ceramic, a number of methods for strengthening it have been developed and most seek to increase the strength and/or translucency of the core; ultimately there is a desire to eliminate metal from aesthetic systems. Strengthening methods are:

- Dispersion strengthening
- Glass infusion
- Crystallization of glasses
- Metal substructure

Dispersion strengthening   The introduction of ceramic crystals of high strength and elasticity into the basic ceramic matrix reinforces the system. The first such system involved the use of alumina crystals and the aluminous crown was introduced in the mid-1960s. This has a high alumina core that is very opaque on to which conventional enamel and dentine ceramics are fired. The improvement of physical properties achieved by this has not really been surpassed until very recently.

Other systems of dispersion strengthening are the inclusion of leucite crystals in either a conventionally-fired material (Optec; Jeneric, Connecticut) or in a castable, heat processed form (Empress; Ivoclar, Liechtenstein). Magnesium–aluminium oxide crystals are incorporated in another castable ceramic, Alceram (Innotek, Colorado).

The disadvantage of the *castable ceramics* is that specialized equipment is required for production of the restoration. Their advantage is that they can be produced by the lost wax process and therefore contouring is easier.

Glass infusion   This produces a denser, stronger core by *slip casting*. In this technique a pure alumina slip cast coping is made on a special gypsum die and partially fired. After shaping, the porous alumina is infused with a low fusing glass of matching thermal expansion that melts and diffuses through the porous alumina by capillary action. The result is a very dense and strong alumina composite. The commercial material is In-Ceram (Vident, California).

Crystallization of glasses   This is the strengthening technique found in another group of castable ceramics. It requires an initial firing process that produces a 'green' ceramic followed by a second firing that converts this material into a dense mass of interlocking crystals. Commercial materials are Dicor (Dentsply, Philadelphia) and Cerapearl (Kyocera, California).

Metal substructure   The use of a cast alloy substructure is the principal and most common method; it is discussed below. A swaged metal substructure, a tin oxide coated, bonded platinum foil, the *twin foil technique* – has the claimed advantage of helping the ceramic resist the static fatigue that occurs as a result of water immersion. However, the clinical and laboratory results of studies on this system are so contradictory that its value remains unproven.

Clinical implications   Whilst the newer systems are of considerable interest, they are as yet unproven clinically and some are not in general use because of the cost of the equipment. Perhaps the most important factor in the acceptance of new ceramics is whether they can be used in the multiple units of fixed bridgework. The majority of current materials has limited application in this field.

The principle of the preparation for an all-ceramic crown of any type is to provide dentine

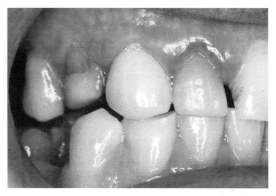

Fig. 15.6 Poorly glazed ceramic on the palatal aspect of 3⌋ has resulted in wear of the 3⌉

support for the ceramic throughout, particularly on the incisal and cingulum areas of anterior teeth. Adequate thickness of material is also essential.

Dental ceramic is harder than enamel and the unglazed surface will abrade tooth surface, and frequently results in considerable wear to the opposing tooth (*Fig. 15.6*).

Metal-ceramic

The most reliable and successful method for strengthening ceramics is the provision of a cast metal subframe to which the ceramic is bonded. This prevents the propagation of cracks from the ceramic inner surface, and the combination provides good aesthetics and excellent strength. Its disadvantage is that it requires considerable tooth reduction to accommodate it.

Ceramic bonding alloys   The alloys intended for ceramic combination should have a:

- Sufficiently high melting point so that they do not deform during firing of the ceramic
- Thermal coefficient compatible with ceramic to avoid fracture on cooling after firing
- Capacity to bond chemically with the ceramic

There are three main categories of alloy:

- Precious
- Semi-precious
- Non-precious

Precious metal alloys contain a large amount of gold and platinum and exhibit good bonding characteristics, are relatively easy to cast, and finish to a high lustre. Their disadvantages are cost and their tendency to sag during firing of the ceramic, particularly when long span bridges are being made.

The semi-precious alloys have better sag resistance and consist principally of silver and palladium, with a variable amount of gold. The silver sometimes leads to 'greening' of the ceramic if the alloy has been overheated during casting and is visible at the metal–ceramic junction.

Both precious and semi-precious alloys have small traces of base metals (iron, indium, tin or zinc), that oxidize on firing to form a surface layer that bonds chemically with the ceramic.

Non-precious, or base metal, bonding alloys are either nickel–chromium or cobalt–chromium. They are cheap but more difficult to cast, and harder to finish. Their high modulus of elasticity gives them the highest sag resistance of all the bonding alloys. The nickel and the chromium oxidize on firing to form the oxide layer for bonding. However, this can be uncontrolled and was one of the major limitations of the early alloys.

Small amounts of beryllium are present in some alloys and this is poisonous. The technician must take care not to inhale the dust whilst grinding the casting. In addition, there are some reservations about the inclusion of nickel, which may induce a sensitivity reaction in patients.

The mechanism for bonding the ceramic depends on three factors:

- *Chemical* – during firing an oxide layer is formed on the metal that bonds with the ceramic
- *Mechanical* – surface irregularities on the casting provide a key for interlocking with the ceramic
- *Compressive* – there is a slight mismatch between the thermal coefficients of expansion of the ceramic and the alloy. That of the ceramic is higher so that on cooling the ceramic shrinks very slightly more and grips the metal. A curved surface is necessary for this to happen effectively

Clinical implications The aesthetics of metal–ceramic restorations present particular problems and these are discussed in Chapter 16. As mentioned above, the clinical preparation requires considerable tooth substance removal to accommodate the metal and ceramic. This particularly applies to the occlusal aspect, where 2 mm clearance is desirable if ceramic is to cover the occlusal surface. Other areas for which ceramic coverage is desired should have a 1.5 mm reduction, which should be removed evenly from the whole surface contour. This means that the final third of the preparation will curve markedly towards the occlusal aspect.

The main clinical fault is under-reduction of the preparation. Two problems follow from this:

1. The technician overbuilds the crown to give adequate thickness of material for aesthetics.

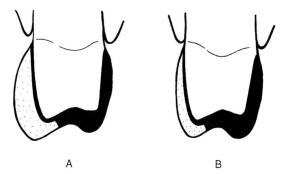

Fig. 15.7 Incorrect preparation for metal–ceramic crowns and the consequences. **A** The crown is made bulbous to reproduce the correct shade. **B** The correct contour is reproduced, but this means that the ceramic is too thin

The crown is then grossly overbuilt (*Fig. 15.7A*)
2. The technician attempts to maintain the original tooth anatomy, which leads to a thinning of the ceramic and metal, with poor aesthetics and the subsequent fracture of the ceramic occlusally (*Fig. 15.7B*)

The choice of material for the functional surfaces must also be considered. Glazed ceramic is usually the patient's choice but it is difficult to produce the anatomical form accurately and adjust it intra-orally. If not reglazed, it will damage the opposing tooth surface. Metal is therefore preferred.

Restoration of root filled teeth

By the time caries and/or trauma has destroyed coronal dentine and the endodontic access cavity has been cut, there is usually little dentine remaining to support a crown. Should a crown be required on a root filled tooth, some form of core needs to be constructed to retain it and provide stability.

The post crown, where the core is itself retained by a post in the root canal, has some limitations. These relate to morphology and size of the roots.

Where the root is very variable and cannot be seen clearly by radiography, the post crown is a real hazard (Chapter 27). This is true of posterior teeth, particularly those which are sometimes one- and sometimes two-rooted. The two-rooted premolar may also have very narrow roots, quite unsuitable for receiving posts.

In these circumstances, it is safer to provide a pin-retained amalgam core, rather than embark on a split cast device. If there is not enough dentine for the pins, then the root canals can be used for retention, but using small cemented preformed posts that only intrude by 3 or so millimetres into the canal.

In the anterior teeth, the post and core is the restoration of choice.

Posts and cores

There is a huge range of post and core systems from which to choose. These may be classified into:

● Cast
● Prefabricated
● Hybrid

Cast post and core

Here the natural shape of the canal is utilized after the elimination of undercuts and irregularities to form a conical preparation. The post shape may either be recorded using the direct technique with inlay wax or a non-residual burnout pattern acrylic, or indirectly by taking an elastomeric impression. The core is waxed to the appropriate shape for the particular tooth and the system has the major advantage that it is made to fit the tooth, rather than the tooth being prepared to fit the system.

The major disadvantage of the cast post is that it is weaker than the equivalent diameter of a wrought post. Therefore, if fracture of the post is to be avoided, the diameter of the canal must be enlarged to ensure an adequate bulk of metal. This means that the technique sacrifices more tooth and weakens the root in comparison with the prefabricated systems.

The cast post is probably the technique of choice for large canals, for difficult alignment problems, and when a cast diaphragm is required to support the root, or make up subgingival deficiencies.

Prefabricated post and core

These posts are factory made in a range of sizes with a matching twist drill system to prepare the root canal to receive the post. The posts may be *parallel sided* or *tapered* and these in turn may be *smooth, serrated, threaded* or *vented*.

The choice is immense and personal preference has a large part to play in selection. Of the various types, the tapered threaded post is the most dangerous, since its insertion can generate enough stress to split the root.

The majority of non-threaded posts are made of stainless steel and are therefore strong in narrow diameters, whilst the threaded systems tend to be brass. Other designs have utilized carbon fibre or composite resins.

Parallel posts are effective in most teeth, but care must be taken with them in small roots, because the danger of perforation of the canal wall is high. Tapered posts are better in narrow canals. The vented posts allow room for the escape of excess cement and are therefore claimed to permit better seating.

Perhaps the biggest drawback of the basic system is that the core position, size and shape is relatively fixed. Some modifications are possible, but are limited in extent. The biggest claimed advantage is that they remove one laboratory stage, and are therefore more economical.

Hybrid – post prefabricated, cast core

This group has prefabricated posts where the core is custom made and cast onto the post. This combines the strength of the wrought post, that is either semi-precious alloy or nickel–chromium, with the advantage of being able to shape the core exactly for the particular tooth.

Figure 15.8 shows the Wiptam technique that utilizes a smooth parallel-sided nickel–cobalt-chromium wire, that fits into a matched preparation. The core is cast gold, and extends into a countersink to reinforce the post and provide resistance to rotation. The shoulder, that receives the crown, is

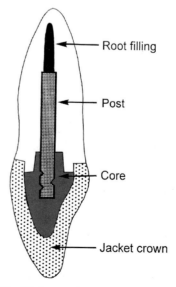

Fig. 15.8 The Wiptam post crown

cut separately and may leave a collar of dentine that effectively lengthens the canal preparation. The collar must have sufficient bulk so that it does not fracture when reproduced on the die.

Some systems provide plastic burnout posts that can be used instead of the metal ones. These create some problems. The narrower posts are flexible and will negotiate curves that the final post will not, and the disadvantages of the cast post mentioned above are reintroduced.

Core waxing may be done either in the mouth or in the laboratory.

Canal preparation

Whatever system is used, there are a number of common features in the preparations. The following aspects are important:

- Root canal morphology
- Length
- Diameter
- Resistance to rotation
- Core characteristics

Root canal morphology

Assessment of the root canal morphology is required before committing the tooth to a post preparation. It is essential to have an adequate apical seal and the root filling material should be removable from the coronal end of the canal. A full length silver point is a considerable impediment and should be replaced with gutta percha if possible. If it cannot be removed, then a post is impossible, and a pinned core has to be considered.

The cross section of the canal and the presence of any curvature should be assessed. A very narrow canal may make preparation difficult and an excessive curvature may limit the extent of the post and reduce retention.

Remember also that the radiograph only shows curves mesially or distally, and not labially or palatally.

Length

The length of the post is one of the most critical features. A short post is capable of exerting enough leverage to split the root when loaded transversely. It also determines in part its retention and, the longer the post, the greater the load-bearing area for dissipation of forces to the surrounding dentine.

As a rule of thumb, the post should be as long as the crown it is expected to retain.

Diameter

The diameter is determined by the anatomy of the canal, the amount of diseased tooth tissue removed and the type of metal used in the post and core construction. In order not to weaken the root, the post should not be more than one-third the total root width for the whole root length. This suggests superiority for the tapered post.

However, if the parallel post obeys the rule in the apical danger zone, it will be narrower coronally. This is how the addition of the custom core adapts the parallel post to fulfil ideal requirements, since the diameter is increased by the cast-on metal. The prefabricated core type does not do this.

The range of post diameters that is successful is 1.2–1.4 mm. Posts of a smaller diameter are vulnerable to bending in the occlusion and those that are larger may jeopardize the root through perforation or splitting.

Resistance to rotation

A cylindrical post will rotate under stress from the occlusion and may not locate accurately when tried in. Some prefabricated systems require cutting of grooves or notches to provide resistance to rotation.

However, the natural shape of the root canal is oval and it seems a pity not to utilize this natural feature and to avoid the stress concentrations and weakness created by antirotational notches.

The canal can be simply enlarged coronally to follow the root contour smoothly and this area can be engaged by a cast-on core.

Core characteristics

The core should provide retention and stability for the final restoration and should be similar to the shape of a conventional crown preparation (*Fig. 15.9A*).

It is possible to realign the position of the crown with the core, which allows derotation or uprighting relative to the root position. However, this option must be used with caution since there is frequently an interplay between the hard and soft tissues, and muscle pressure may well move the altered tooth, producing a bizarre result.

The core can also be smaller than the vital tooth preparation, since there is no pulp to worry about. This gives added bulk to the final crown, which is a considerable advantage for the strength of a ceramic crown, and helps the aesthetics of the metal–ceramic crown.

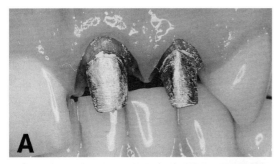

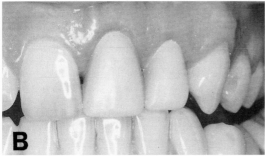

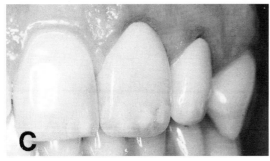

Fig. 15.9 A Two posts and cores in place, showing the basic core shape is similar to the ceramic jacket crown preparation, but is smaller. **B** Provisional restorations. They have been made from transparent crown forms, and provide correct aesthetics, occlusion and gingival contour. **C** The finished crowns. These show the characterization that the skilled ceramist can produce. Note the translucency at the tips and the incorporation of white flecks

Provisional crowns

This aspect of advanced operative work is frequently neglected and little time is devoted to the construction of a good provisional crown.

The functions of a provisional crown are:

● Protection of cut dentine
● Maintenance of the occlusion
● Maintenance of approximal contacts
● Restoration of aesthetics
● Maintenance of gingival health

It is good practice to construct the provisional crown prior to the impression of the preparation, since this will allow proper estimation of the time remaining for this.

Provisionals may be *customized* or made from *prefabricated* crown forms.

Customized crowns

An impression in a putty is taken prior to the start of the preparation and put to one side. On completion of the preparation the putty impression is used to form a mould for a resin-based material. There are currently a number of dimethacrylate polymers, based on the composite technology, that are available for this application. This hardens to the shape of the original crown. Once polymerization is complete, the impression and crown are removed and the polymer trimmed accurately to the margins of the preparation and the occlusion, and polished. The provisional should be cemented with a weak zinc oxide–eugenol (ZOE) cement.

Prefabricated crowns

Anterior crown forms can be tooth coloured, usually polycarbonate, or transparent cellulose acetate. They are available in a range of sizes for each tooth and the size should be chosen to conform to the mesio-distal width. They need to be cut carefully to the cervical margins and then based with a self-curing resin (*Fig. 15.9B*).

The range of sizes can be restrictive; if it fits it is usually good, but if it doesn't it can be terrible. It can be difficult to find one with the correct dimensions both bucco-lingually and mesio-distally.

Posteriorly, the best provisionals are anatomically shaped silver–tin crowns. These are also designed as burn-out patterns for crown waxing. They are soft and can be adapted easily to the occlusion and to the cervical margin. They do not usually require basing with a resin, and can be cemented with a stiff ZOE cement. Their disadvantage is that being soft, they have a limited life.

Shade and impressions

These are considered in Chapters 16 and 17.

Occlusal registration

The construction of a single crown and often a pair of crowns will not require an articulation; hand held models are satisfactory. However, a crown for a strategic tooth, such as the terminal abutment of a bounded saddle, will require articulation to obtain accurate occlusal contours. Occlusal records are discussed in Chapter 14 and, in the absence of a reproducible position of best fit, the technique of using an occlusal registration coping should be used. This technique is described in Chapter 21.

Fitting a crown to an existing denture

This can be a very difficult operation, particularly if a rest seat and two clasp arms are involved as well as the denture base. Clearly the counsel of perfection is to ensure that denture abutment teeth are sound and well restored before a denture is made. However, further caries and loss of tooth substance may happen after a denture has been in service for some time.

The registration of the denture position in relation to the crown preparation must be supplied to the technician. If there is sufficient clearance between the denture and the preparation then the impression can be taken with the denture in place. The technician may cast the denture area immediately next to the crown preparation in acrylic to provide a durable index for guiding the waxing of the crown pattern.

A more accurate method, but one requiring an additional visit, is to take an impression without the denture and ask the technician to construct an acrylic coping on the die. The coping will normally be made of a *pattern acrylic* that burns out of the investment with no residue.

Intraorally, the coping is tried on the preparation and the denture seated. Further pattern acrylic is then added to the coping to register the position of the denture components and the occlusion. The technician uses this as a guide for finalizing the pattern that will be invested and cast.

Try-in and cementation

The sequence is:

1. Check the restoration on the model before the patient arrives ensuring that there are contacts with adjacent teeth and that the occlusion is correct. Examine the die and the adjacent teeth on the model for rub marks which may have introduced errors
2. Do not attempt cementation if the tooth displays any adverse symptoms. If the patient complains of discomfort, diagnose the cause and treat it before cementation
3. Remove the provisional and clean the preparation, ensuring that all cement is removed. If possible this should be done without local analgesic since this can prevent the patient assisting in assessment of the occlusion
4. Try-in the restoration. If it does not seat initially check the *contacts* with floss (*Fig. 15.10A*). If the restoration still does not seat, the fit surface should be examined and, if necessary, a silicone rubber perfecting paste may be used to detect any high spots

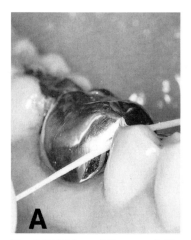 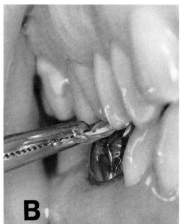 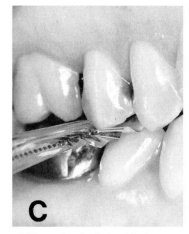

Fig. 15.10 Fitting a full crown. **A** The approximal contacts are checked with floss. **B** The occlusal relationship is checked with shimstock on the crown itself and **C** at the cusp/fossa relationship mesial to the crown. Both contacts should hold shimstock

5. Once the crown has been seated, check the *marginal adaptation*. There should be a smooth transition from the tooth on to the crown. Check the shade in daylight

6. The *occlusal contacts* should be assessed. Premature contacts may be detected using either articulating paper or shimstock (*Fig. 15.10B* and C). The type of articulating paper can affect the results since some are excessively thick and will not allow for differentiation of the high points and normal occlusal stops. Fine articulating paper is preferable and it often advantageous for the occlusal surface of the restoration to have a matt finish in order to detect the minor prematurities that may be present

7. The occlusal contacts must be checked in all excursions. Heavy contacts must be eased but care should be taken that the surface is not over-reduced, as this will take the crown out of occlusion

8. *Choice of cement*. Incorrect selection and manipulation of the cement will affect the life of a crown dramatically.

   The main luting agents are also bases and these were discussed in Chapter 10. There are two choices for cementation. One provides mechanical retention (ZOE or zinc phosphate) and the other provides this and adhesion to tooth and some to the restoration.

   Clearly the second is preferable and zinc polycarboxylate and glass ionomer cements have become popular. The polycarboxylate is the more reliable since there is some concern about the pulpal response to glass ionomers when used as luting materials.

   The cement should be mixed to the manufacturer's specified powder/liquid ratio which should provide a consistency that will allow it to be displaced as the crown is seated and excess will flow away

9. The fit surface of the crown should be coated with cement, placed on the preparation (that has been isolated and dried) and seated home. Considerable pressure should be applied to the seating crown initially to express the excess cement, and pressure should be maintained until the cement has set. For a post crown, the canal should be cleaned and filled with cement prior to seating the post and crown together with the same mix

10. Once the cement has set, excess is fractured away from the margin and the approximal embrasures cleared with floss. It is particularly important that the cement has fully set before removal of excess is attempted. This is especially so with glass ionomer and zinc polycarboxylate cements as these go through a rubbery phase. If these are disturbed at this point the integrity of the marginal seal may be lost

11. After cementation, the occlusal relationship should be rechecked.

Review

The crown should be inspected again a week or so later, since natural occlusal function will have been re-established, and contacts may require further adjustment.

   Radiographic review should be carried out six months later and every two years or so, to check for symptomless development of apical pathology.

Fixed prosthodontics – crowns – Summary

Ensure that the crown is treatment planned in the context of the patient's requirements and the general condition of the mouth.

Important principles in the preparation of a crown are the choice of the path of insertion and features to ensure the stability of the final restoration.

There is a large range of materials available, particularly for the all-ceramic crown. The choice of material affects the preparation design, particularly the shape of the finishing line and the amount of tissue to be removed.

There are many post crown systems. The choice is to a large extent personal, but the hybrid types offer the greatest range of application. Important characteristics in the post preparation are length and diameter. Tooth tissue should be preserved where possible.

Accurately fitting provisional crowns maintain the relationships to adjacent teeth and the health of the dentition.

High standards of acceptance at the fitting stage will lead to long-lasting restorations.

16

Colour and aesthetics

Two of the recurring themes of this book are the requirements for durable tooth-coloured restorative materials and the need to achieve good aesthetics. This is a complex subject and is a mixture of art and science. Advances in both restorative polymers and ceramics have increased the range of techniques available under the broad heading of 'Cosmetic dentistry' and some of these have been described already.

This Chapter considers colour science and shade taking together with the causes and management of poor aesthetics of individual teeth. Section IV considers the aesthetics of fixed bridgework and removable prosthodontics.

Colour

A prerequisite of all aesthetic dentistry is accurate shade taking and matching and, in respect of indirect restorations, good shade communication. The technician rarely sees the patient and is therefore relying on the dentist to describe the shade and its distribution. Perceived colour is highly affected by viewing conditions and it is essential that the shade is taken in the most favourable conditions in order to obtain an accurate result.

Factors affecting perceived colour

Three factors are involved:

- Light source
- Eye response and colour perception
- Environment

Light source

Light is composed of different wavelengths that are dependent upon the source. Incandescent light, such as that provided by normal light bulbs, accentuates the yellow/red range in the spectrum whilst fluorescent light accentuates the blue/green range; both affect colour vision.

Teeth exhibit *metamerism*, that is the property of changing colour in different lighting conditions. Daylight-corrected fluorescent tubes and shade-taking lights with a standard colour spectrum are commercially available and these can help, but they may give rise to more inaccuracies in comparison with good natural daylight. The daylight for shade taking needs to be diffuse, north light; not direct southern sunlight. Teeth also change colour as they become dry; they must be kept wet during shade taking.

Eye response and colour perception

When concentrating on the colour of a tooth, the retinal cones of the eye will fatigue and sensitivity to colour will be reduced. To overcome this, decisions on shade should be made in steps of no more than five seconds. Looking at a pale blue surface, such as a napkin or piece of card, between evaluations of shade can help; this accentuates yellow/orange sensitivity, which is the dominant range of tooth colour. Prolonged viewing of a tooth results in a negative after-image that is the complimentary colour of the original surface viewed.

Colour perception is subjective and varies between people. In addition, colour blindness is quite common and obviously creates problems during shade taking. Using two people to take the shade, dentist and nurse, will even out such inaccuracies. A simple eye test is also useful to discover colour vision acuity.

Environment

Strongly coloured light reflected from furniture, clothing or the walls will influence shade taking, partly from the after-image mentioned above and partly from reflection. Ideally the surgery and its equipment should be of a neutral colour. Strong colours from make-up or clothing should be removed or masked.

Components of colour

In order to communicate subtle variations in colour, it is important to understand the way that a specific colour is measured. Colours may be broken down into three components:

- Hue
- Chroma
- Value

Hue (colour)

This is the description or name given to a colour or family of colours, e.g. blue, red, green, yellow. Dentine is the most important hue within a tooth.

Chroma

This is the intensity or strength of a given hue, e.g. if 10 drops of red dye are added to a glass of water it will become red, and if 100 drops are added the water will still be red, but of a more intense colour. The chroma will have changed but the hue will not. The chroma of dentine is as important as its hue.

Value

This is the total reflectance or luminance, that is related to the brightness of a colour measured on a scale from black to white, e.g. if red is the hue then pink or maroon can be made by changing the value without changing the original hue. The overlying enamel, being essentially colourless, is the principal determinant of value in a tooth, modifying the dentine hue to the observer. The brightness of a colour is probably the most easily perceived characteristic.

Shade guides

The most commonly used shade guide is the Vita-Lumin that allocates a letter for the hue, A,B,C,D, and a number, 1,2,3,4, indicating the chroma. No provision is made for altering or indicating the value.

The basic arrangement is:

- A1–4: browns
- B1–4: yellows
- C1–4: greys
- D2–4: reddish-greys

This means that the observer must make a decision about the combined hue/chroma in almost one step. Selection can therefore be difficult, especially for the novice, as there is a tendency to jump from one group to another, rather than follow a progressive pattern.

If the shade tabs are arranged according to value (degrees of brightness), as in most denture tooth shade guides, selection may be more straightforward. The appropriate sequence is B1, A1, B2, D2, A2, C1, C2, D4, A3, D3, B3, A3.5, B4, C3, A4, C4.

The shade guide has other limitations. An all-ceramic crown will not be the same thickness as a shade tab and, of course, light passes through an all-ceramic crown more readily than one of metal–ceramic.

Construction of the guide may be different from the layering that the ceramist may use. The shade tab has subtle in-built colours and nearly always a neck effect that most ceramists do not include. It is important to ask the ceramist how he or she uses the shades, and it may be necessary to remove the neck colour from the tab to match the ceramist's system. Many laboratories use just core, dentine, enamel and an external stain and it would be useful to ask the laboratory to provide a customized guide of various thicknesses and colours.

Informing the technician

Any time spent accurately obtaining the shade will be wasted unless the information is communicated clearly to the technician. When taking a shade it is essential to include a sketch diagram of the tooth or teeth marking clearly areas of decalcification, internal flecks, lamellae and so on (*Fig. 16.1*).

Work cards, or laboratory prescription forms, can be set out in many ways, but must include the following information:

- Patient's name and sex
- Approximate age: the surface texture of teeth changes with age and the technician can reproduce this effect
- A drawing of the tooth showing the distribution of the various shades, and characterization
- The dentine, enamel and cervical shades
- Amount of glaze: high, as guide, or low
- Amount of translucency: high, as guide, or low
- Type of restoration required
- If a metalwork try-in stage is required

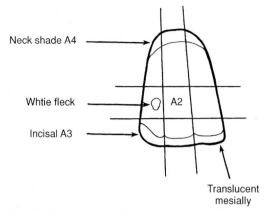

Neck shade A4

Whtie fleck

Incisal A3

A2

Translucent
mesially

Fig. 16.1 Sketch made at the chairside to provide instructions for the laboratory for shade reproduction

- If a biscuit bake (unglazed) try-in stage is required
- Ceramic or metal occlusal surface

Discoloured teeth

Discoloration of the teeth may be due to intrinsic or extrinsic stains.

Extrinsic staining results from:

- Plaque and calculus
- Mouth washes
- Diet
- Discoloured restorations
- Smoking

Intrinsic staining results from:

- Caries
- Erosion
- Chemical ingestion, including fluoride and tetracycline
- Trauma
- Non-vitality and root filling
- Neonatal jaundice
- Genetic and developmental malformations

Extrinsic staining

This is very common and patients may not appreciate the effects of tea, coffee, smoking, red wine and chlorhexidine mouth washes. The misinformed patient may resort to home-bleaching kits when all that is required is a scale and polish and instruction in oral hygiene.

The discoloration and microleakage associated with polymeric restorations has been discussed in Chapter 9. Corrosion products from amalgam diffuse into the surrounding dentine, causing a greyish-black stain.

Intrinsic staining

Developmental disorders vary in intensity from case to case. Enamel hypoplasia may be seen as localized insignificant white spots or more extensive areas of poorly formed tissue that are very liable to take up extrinsic stains. Other more serious conditions, amelogenesis imperfecta and dentinogenesis imperfecta may lead to badly discoloured teeth; these are considered in Chapter 25.

Chemicals may be incorporated in dentine and enamel during their formation. The most dramatic of these is tetracycline. Different effects are produced by different members of the tetracycline family, by the dosage and duration of treatment and the age of the patient at treatment. Effects range from mild grey bands to total blackness. It is surprising, in view of this problem being common knowledge, that tetracycline is still prescribed for children by the medical profession.

The dental profession, on the other hand, in its keenness to prevent caries has caused a somewhat similar problem with fluoride. Systemic fluoride supplements, perhaps with their dosage not monitored accurately by parents, coupled with ingestion by children of fluoride toothpaste, has led to a high incidence of fluorosis in the more dentally aware population. This may be seen as grey or white patches in the enamel.

Neonatal jaundice may lead to incorporation of the yellow pigment of bilirubin in the dentine.

Discoloration caused by caries is discussed in Chapter 2 and erosion is discussed in Chapter 25.

Trauma, particularly that resulting in loss of vitality, may induce dentinal changes. Blood may pass from the pulp into the dentine and the breakdown products of haemoglobin will appear as black or brown stains. Non-vital dentine can lose its translucency, probably as a result of mineral deposition in response to the trauma, and become more yellow.

Root canal therapy may cause three staining problems. If all the pulp is not removed from the crown, particularly from the pulpal cornua, this will undergo breakdown and cause staining. The older silver-containing root canal sealers have to be handled carefully so as not to leave residues in the access cavity, because these can stain the dentine. Finally, the access cavity of an anterior tooth should be sealed with a tooth-coloured material and not amalgam; amalgam may interfere with the translucency of the crown, making it look darker.

Management of discoloration

The remedies for *extrinsic stains* and discoloured restorations are straightforward – polishing of both or replacement of the restoration. A stained restoration may not be a functional failure but, if the patient is aware of it, it is an aesthetic failure. In respect of root canal access discoloration, remove the access seal, remove stained dentine within the coronal area and restore it with a lighter shade composite

Intrinsic stains may be more difficult to treat. The possibilities, depending upon the cause and the severity, are:

- Microabrasion
- Bleaching
- Ceramic veneer
- Crown

Microabrasion

Staining or a developmental problem that is fairly superficial in the enamel can be eliminated by removing the stained enamel. Here, 'fairly superficial' means to the depth of several hundred micrometres only. The removal must be carefully controlled and very conservative. It is important to maintain the overall enamel surface character.

This procedure may be done using a combination of abrasive and dilute acid. Commercial products are available that use hydrochloric acid together with abrasive impregnated wheels. An effective substitute is dry pumice mixed with phosphoric acid etching gel and applied by hand with a composite polishing rubber (*Fig. 16.2*).

The technique removes superficial stains only and must be abandoned if the stain turns out to be deeper than originally estimated.

Bleaching

The intrinsic pigments of the stained dentine may be bleached by chemical action. The technique uses 35% hydrogen peroxide or similar agents and these may require activation with white light. The technique is usually used on teeth that have discoloured after root canal therapy. The access cavity is reopened under rubber dam and a pledget of cotton wool soaked in the bleach inserted. The cotton wool is sealed in place for a week and 'refreshed' as necessary. Yellow stains respond better than brown or orange. However, the changes are not permanent and relapse is common.

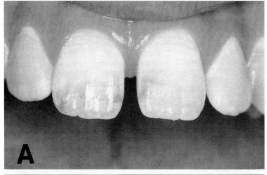
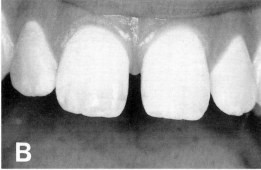

Fig. 16.2 Enamel hypoplasia that is superficial and amenable to microabrasion. **A** Before treatment. **B** After treatment

External bleaching of vital teeth is possible but the procedure is only effective for some extrinsic and superficial stains and is very temporary.

Ceramic veneers

These are effective for masking more substantial hypoplastic defects of enamel, intrinsic staining and mild malformations. They utilize a half-enamel thickness reduction of the labial surface and the acid etch technique to bond a thin layer of ceramic to the tooth. They are a valuable conservative alternative to the ceramic jacket crown.

The cementing agents are similar to those used to cement resin retained bridges (see Chapter 19), ceramic and composite inlays. To complete the technique, 'opaquers' that are fluid composite resins can be used to mask strong underlying colours or modify the shade of the veneer. The mode of adhesion to the ceramic relies on etching or sand blasting and then coating the fit surface with a silane coupling agent.

Adhesion is much better to enamel than to dentine and the best results are obtained with either complete attachment to enamel or, where enamel has been lost, with at least 2 mm of enamel present around the periphery of the restoration. If

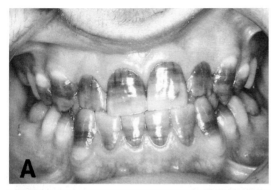

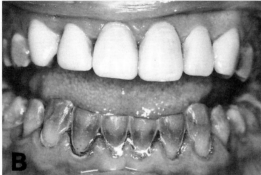

Fig. 16.3 Tetracycline staining. A A severe case of blackish-yellow staining. B Ceramic veneers on 321│123 and the preparations for the lowers. The ceramic must be opaque to mask such deep stain

too much dentine is present, then crowns are a better alternative.

Indications
If the stain or anomaly is deep within enamel or in dentine then the choice is between a veneer and a crown.

A suitable checklist is:

- Is the discoloration severe enough to warrant treatment?
- Is there enough crown left to support a veneer?
- Is the discoloration minor enough to be masked by thin ceramic?
- Is there any occlusal restriction?

The first point is to consider whether the patient is being excessively conscious of a minor defect. Some people naturally have teeth of a slightly odd colour and these often fall into the shade guide range of C and D. A careful and sympathetic explanation of natural tooth colour and the disadvantages of operative treatment may dissuade such patients from sacrificing structurally normal enamel to correct a minor problem.

The second question is whether the tooth is too heavily restored to support a veneer. For example, a veneer preparation on a tooth with large mesial and distal class III restorations plus an endodontic access cavity might not be supported by much sound tissue.

Very dark staining, such as that of tetracycline staining, may not be masked by veneers. Notwithstanding this, even opaque veneers can achieve a very acceptable change, often appreciated by patients, from gross staining (*Fig. 16.3*).

Ceramic in thin section is very vulnerable to chipping. If there is parafunction or evidence of excessive tooth wear, veneers may fail.

Preparation The preparation (*Figs 16.4A and B*) involves the reduction of a one-half enamel thickness over the whole surface, which means that there is a variable thickness of enamel removal. The reduction is extended into the approximal embrasures but not through the contact area, and should, if at all possible, remain on enamel.

Defects, such as acid erosion, should be made good with glass ionomer cement and the finishing margin should be a narrow shoulder or chamfer prepared at the level of the free gingivae and not placed in the gingival crevice.

The incisal edge should be reduced, utilizing a reverse bevel onto the palatal surface. The thickness of the incisal reduction should be at least 1 mm.

Provisional restorations are not successful as their retention would be by adhesives which might interfere with the cementation of the final restoration.

Laboratory stages The impression is cast first in divestment refractory stone, i.e. stone that can be heated in the ceramic furnace without breaking up, and then in die stone. The veneer is built and fired on the divestment and adjusted finally on the die stone model. The ceramic that is used must be translucent; the glass cores referred to in Chapter 15 cannot be used because they are opaque. Standard dentine and enamel ceramics, or the newer leucite-reinforced ceramics, are satisfactory and their translucency enables minor colour correction to be achieved by varying the shade of the underlying cement.

After adjustment of the margins and the occlusion, the fit surface is treated. This is better done, if possible, after clinical try-in because contamination from the mouth may interfere with adhesion.

Techniques for fit surface preparation are:

- Etching
- Sand blasting

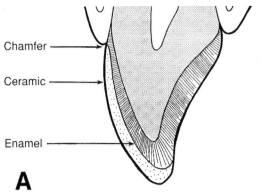

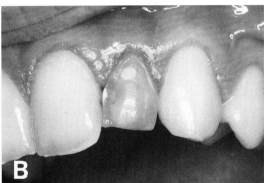

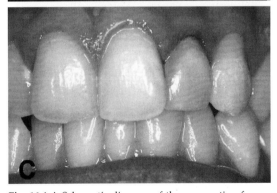

Fig. 16.4 A Schematic diagram of the preparation for a ceramic veneer on a central incisor. Note the incisal reduction and the palatal reverse bevel. **B** Preparation on a lateral incisor. Note that the approximal contacts are maintained. **C** Completed ceramic veneer on 2

Etching is very technique sensitive. The glazed surface of the veneer is first protected with wax and the fitting surface etched with 30–40% hydrofluoric acid for no more than three minutes. The etched surface must be neutralized by placing it in a furnace at 600°C for five minutes, followed by ultrasonic cleaning in distilled water for three minutes after cooling.

Because of the dangers of hydrofluoric acid, substitutes are available, but the safest way is to avoid etching altogether and grit blast the surface instead with 50 μm grit. This grit blasting may be done using a small unit in the dental practice.

Try-in and cementation
The tooth is cleaned with dry pumice and a slowly rotating brush to remove plaque and pellicle that might otherwise contaminate the veneer. The veneer is placed carefully on to the tooth and the margins and the occlusion checked. If necessary these may be adjusted by fine diamond points followed by a diamond paste.

The shade is observed in natural light in order to decide whether the 'universal' cement will be satisfactory or whether a lighter or darker shade is required.

The lightly filled composite cements or luting agents may be dual-cured or light cured. Whilst the dual-cure type may provide better polymerization if the activating light is attenuated by the veneer, their colour stability is poorer because there is an increased amine concentration for the self-cure system.

Depending upon the product, it will come with the basic shades grouped into whites, yellows, browns and perhaps greys. There will be a separate opaquing agent. There may be either individual syringes of each colour or a base colour and containers of add-in colours – *tinters*.

The base paste may be tried first without mixing in the activator. Additions may be made as desired to change the colour, keeping some on the mixing pad, until the effect under the veneer is correct. The underside of the veneer must be cleaned for each application – the reserve on the pad will become the final cement in due course.

When the correct effect has been obtained, rubber dam is applied, the underside of the veneer is cleaned with isopropyl alcohol and, if this has not been done already, grit blasted. (Wax must be applied to the glazed surface first to protect it.) A silane coating is then applied to the veneer and air dried. The bonding resin comes next; this is air dispersed to prevent pooling. Then apply the luting cement and position the veneer.

'Tack' cure for 10 seconds with the activating light and check the orientation of the veneer. If this is correct, the cement can be fully cured by exposure to the light from several angles.

If the orientation is incorrect, the veneer can be removed gently and cleaned to repeat the cementation.

After curing, check and remove excess from the margins, check the occlusion both in centric occlusion and lateral and protrusive excursions and show the patient (*Fig. 16.4C*).

Aesthetics

Incorporation of colour and characterization

Careful selection and use of colour can create illusions to apparently change the position or size of a crown. This can be used for a malaligned or poorly shaped tooth to give it the appearance of being wider or shorter than it really is. By lightening or darkening selected teeth in a full arch, the illusions of flatness or more rounded appearance can be created. Wide teeth can be apparently narrowed by the placement of shaders or stains mesially or distally that highlight the central area.

The contour and texture of a crown should mirror its neighbour, enabling the reflection of light to be equal to that of the natural tooth. A roughened labial surface should be left on the core of a crown so that light entering through the more translucent layers of ceramic will be reflected in different directions, adding vitality.

If the technician has been asked to make six anterior crowns with just the shade and the sex of the patient to guide him, he can make the crowns take on a definite masculine or feminine appearance by attention to detail and careful shaping. Labial surfaces may be made to look flat and therefore wider and more masculine, or, alternatively they can be rounded, smaller and feminine with greater vitality due to the reflected light from the curved surface coming at a variety of angles.

Artificial ageing can be achieved by creating flat worn incisal edges, loss of lamellae and thin enamel.

Colour may be imparted to a crown by the application of internal colourant ceramic effect powders. When building colour into the crown, the ceramist will remove unfired body ceramic almost to the opaque layer, hollowing and cutting an angle so as to achieve a blend and carefully introducing either gingival effect or dilute stain into the depression. Upon firing, the colour will show through the more translucent body ceramic. Traces of orange on the incisal edge, decalcifications, and so on may all be incorporated in the same way.

Colour may also be included by cutting back a previously fired crown. A cut is made into the crown with a diamond disc, the selected colour applied, airdried, and then overlaid and refired. Similarly, the blue effect sometimes present on mesial and distal corners can be obtained by grinding ceramic away to the desired depth and painting the prepared surface with a blue wash, overlaying with a clear ceramic and refiring.

The use of clear ceramic and inlaid colours is particularly effective, and imparts a very natural appearance. Surface staining is less effective and does not give the three dimensional effect achieved with internal segmented building. It is also vulnerable to abrasion during intraoral service, thus losing its effects.

However, surface stain can be added quickly and easily, being mixed with a liquid binder and painted on to the fired crown before glazing, and is therefore popular.

Aesthetic problems

Dark line at gingival margin

This was common with earlier metal–ceramic systems but has now been eliminated by the use of a ceramic margin. Until recently ceramic margins were very difficult for the ceramist to construct because the ceramic shrinks by approximately 15% upon firing, leading to a rounding off and loss of adaptation at the critical natural tooth/crown margin. To overcome this problem a shoulder ceramic has been developed that exhibits far better stability during firing. This material enables crowns and bridges to be made that have no metal margins and an accurate marginal finish with good biocompatibility.

Core shine

This usually occurs in cases where insufficient labial reduction has taken place during clinical preparation. The technician, in an attempt to bring the crown into line with the adjacent teeth, exposes the underlying core by grinding or is forced to cover it by insufficient dentine build-up. This results in an area of the crown that looks lifeless. Opaque ceramic must be covered by at least 0.5 mm of dentine ceramic to diffuse the reflected light from the opaque. Doing this, though, in the underprepared tooth results in a bulbous over-contoured crown with poor aesthetics.

The correct treatment is to ensure that a minimum of 1.5 mm is removed from the labial surface during preparation to allow enough depth of ceramic to create a life-like aesthetic restoration. The metal substructure needs to be a minimum of 0.3 mm thick, the opaque needs a minimum of 0.4 mm, which leaves only 0.8 mm for the dentine and enamel ceramics to create an acceptable result.

Shadowed regions

Shadowing occurs in areas where there is an excessive amount of dentine ceramic or in areas where there is not an opaque backing. Typically, in bridges these occur interstitially or at the cervical margin of pontics. In order to compensate for these darker areas of lower chroma, ceramics that have an increased opacity and chroma have been developed – these are known as *opacious dentines*. The opacious dentines can either be blended with conventional dentine powders or applied in layers.

These new ceramics can help considerably to increase chroma and to diffuse reflected light, hence improving the aesthetic result.

Conclusion

With the advent of these new ceramics and by using a layered build-up technique it is now possible for the ceramist to control the reflection and scattering of light in a similar manner to natural teeth. With the use of opacious dentines, control over value and chroma is possible and life-like aesthetic restorations are now far more easily achieved. However, when patients move from one type of light to another, changes in apparent shade are inevitable. The most dramatic of these is the sight of metal–ceramic crowns in television arc lights!

Malformed or missing teeth

The most common problems are:

- Peg-shaped upper lateral incisors
- Missing upper lateral incisors
- Central incisors lost through trauma

More extensive *hypodontia* and dental problems associated with *cleft palate* are considered in Chapter 20.

Peg-shaped lateral incisors

The management options are:

- Persuade the patient that it is better to do nothing
- Reshape by veneers or crowns
- Extract and either open or close the space

No treatment Some individuals, particularly females, may become very concerned that their appearance is not 'conventional'. This was mentioned above in relation to shade. Slightly malformed teeth may not be noticed by the casual observer but are glaringly obvious to the patient who grimaces at herself close to the make-up mirror.

Minor discrepancies in tooth shape need to be put into perspective (tactfully) together with an explanation of the possibly deleterious effects of restorations and their need for periodic replacement. Often, patients will be reassured and elect to having nothing done.

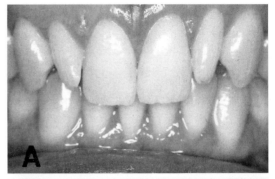

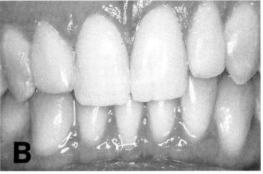

Fig. 16.5 Peg-shaped lateral incisors. The appearance has been improved by the addition of acid etch retained composite. **A** Before treatment. **B** After treatment

Reshaping The amount of natural tooth will have a bearing on the choice of treatment. Very small teeth are impossible to prepare with sufficient remaining tissue to support a crown or a veneer. It is also problematic to increase the size of a tooth, because this usually results in an unfavourable gingival contour.

Here the best solution will often be the use of acid-etch retained composite resin to increase the incisal length and width of the tooth without encroaching on the gingival margin (*Fig. 16.5*). Some commercial products are supplied in a range of shades equivalent to the Vita shade guide together with opaque shades. This may mean a range of at least eighteen shades, providing a comprehensive colour matching system. The possible disadvantage is that the material may need replacing in five to six years due to discoloration.

Larger pegs can be veneered successfully to increase their size but again the gingival relationship would not be ideal and the patient must be taught careful flossing and brushing techniques.

Extraction This would be the last resort and would be reserved for badly formed and displaced pegs. Orthodontics should be considered to either open or close the space. Space closure is probably more desirable, since this avoids a prosthesis to replace the lateral incisor. However, the disadvantage is that the canine may be moved into a more prominent position and may require reshaping (see below).

Missing upper lateral incisors

Absent upper lateral incisors may result in retention of the deciduous canines and eruption of the permanent canines into the lateral incisor position. Alternatively, the deciduous canines may be shed as normal and spacing may result between the central incisors and the permanent canines.

Management options are:

● Reshaping the permanent canines to resemble lateral incisors
● Orthodontic treatment to retract the canines, and bridges or implants to replace the lateral incisors
● Veneers/bridgework to correct aesthetics without orthodontic treatment

Reshaping   This is the simplest option but carries with it the problem of making a large tooth look small. The incisal edge can be made square and level by either composite resin addition or ceramic veneer, or in some cases by simply grinding the tooth.

This type of reshaping will remove the 'Dracula' appearance but will not change the bulk or prominence of the tooth which can be a problem if the canines are labially placed. Here, to reduce the prominence of the tooth, a radical crown preparation is required to provide a flatter labial surface. Ideally, a post crown would provide the best appearance, but elective devitalization should not be prescribed without a strong indication. Even with a large labial reduction the ceramist would have considerable difficulty with shade control (*Fig. 16.6*).

The case shown in *Figure 16.7* had retained deciduous canines and the upper permanent canines had erupted into the lateral incisor position. The deciduous canines had to be extracted because of caries and root resorption. Two bridges were made to replace the missing teeth and the permanent canines were reshaped by crowns to resemble lateral incisors. Inevitably, the size of 'new' lateral incisors is dictated by the underlying canine teeth, which cannot be prepared extensively to allow smaller crowns to be constructed.

Orthodontics   In certain respects this is an ideal treatment because the canines will be moved bodily into their correct positions. Lateral incisors of the

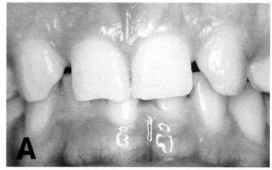

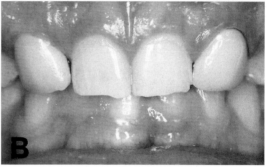

Fig. 16.6 Prominent canines in the lateral incisor position that cannot be corrected effectively by veneering. Crowns are necessary to create less prominent teeth of the correct shape. **A** Before treatment. **B** After treatment

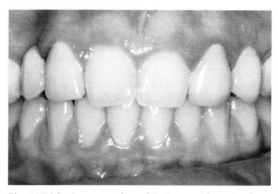

Fig. 16.7 Missing upper lateral incisors with retained c|c and the permanent canines in the lateral incisor position. The c|c have been replaced with bridges and the 3|3 have been converted to resemble lateral incisors by crowning. The underlying size of canines restricts the reduction in width

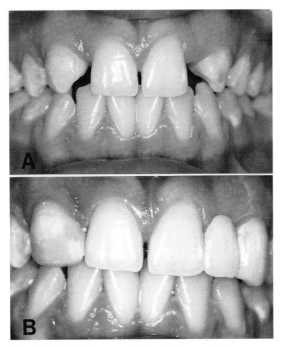

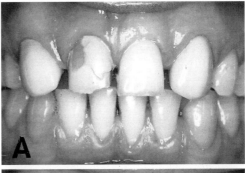

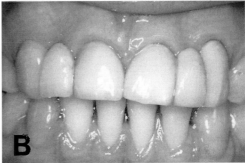

Fig. 16.8 A Missing upper lateral incisors with uneven spacing. **B** The 3| has been recontoured with acid-etch retained composite and |2 has been replaced by a bridge retained by a ceramic veneer on |3.

Fig. 16.9 A Missing lateral incisors where there is restricted space for their replacement. **B** Two three-unit fixed–fixed conventional bridges 3–1|1–3 where the 2|2 have been made to overlap the retainers to achieve extra width

correct shape can then made as bridge pontics, usually as resin retained bridges (see Chapter 19). However, the disadvantages are that space is needed for the canine retraction, usually by extraction of posterior teeth, and fixed appliance therapy will be needed, perhaps taking at least a year.

Veneers/bridges without orthodontics
This approach removes the need for prolonged treatment and loss of more teeth. However, it will almost always be a compromise because of the limited space available for extra teeth. *Figure 16.8* shows a case where there was enough space for a reasonable lateral incisor on the left side but the space available on the right was much smaller. The upper right canine was enlarged by means of acid-etch retained composite whilst a veneer bridge (see Chapter 19) was made on the left.

Figure 16.9, on the other hand, shows a much more difficult case because the lateral incisor spaces were neither small enough to allow enlargement of the canines, nor big enough to allow full-sized lateral incisors to be made. The case was complicated by previous attempts to veneer the incisors and canines.

The lateral incisors have been made as wide as possible on two fixed prostheses by overlapping the central incisor and canine retainers. The preparation of the four teeth for crown retainers provided more flexibility in the final mesiodistal diameters of the new teeth.

Missing central incisors

If the space has been maintained then these will fall under the treatment planning decisions discussed in Section IV. However, in a young patient it may be possible to move the adjacent lateral incisor into the space or, if the case has been neglected, the lateral incisor may drift forward. The conversion of the lateral incisor to look like a central incisor may be done by either a veneer or a crown. The disadvantage is the gingival contour and its relationship where the larger crown or veneer joins the smaller root.

Malocclusion

Whilst many malocclusions are corrected orthodontically in childhood, it is still common for adults to request the correction of crowding and other malocclusions. These patients often request rapid treatment and may not wish to wear orthodontic appliances. They usually expect their appearance to be corrected by crown and bridgework.

Notwithstanding their preferences, these patients need to be persuaded that orthodontic therapy will provide the better results in most cases. Irregular incisors are difficult to crown or veneer and such treatment results in teeth that have thick incisal edges and create periodontal problems.

Colour and aesthetics – Summary

Modern materials and techniques offer much scope for cosmetic dentistry. The artistic aspects of tooth colour and shape are more difficult to teach and come with experience.

Shade taking must be done in good natural light without the influence of strong colours.

Liaison with the technician must be good in respect of shade communication and reproduction.

Composite additions, ceramic veneers and bridgework each has its place in correcting aesthetics. Each is accompanied by its advantages and disadvantages and sometimes the treatment plan is a compromise between tooth conservation, the patient's aspirations and technical possibilities.

17

Impression materials and techniques

The long chain of positive and negative dimensional pitfalls between completion of the preparation and the cementation of a cast restoration begins with the impression.

Choice of impression material, management of gingival tissues and clinical technique all contribute to the accuracy of the final restoration.

An impression material should be:

- Accurate and dimensionally stable
- Easy to handle
- Pleasant tasting
- Compatible with blood and saliva
- Non-irritant and non-allergenic
- Tear resistant
- Compatible with model materials

The patient would like the material to taste pleasant and have a short setting time. Impression taking can be a messy procedure so the material should be easy to remove from tissues and clothes. It should not damage the oral tissues or the tooth and, very importantly, the material should not contain constituents likely to produce sensitivity reactions.

The operator's requirements are somewhat different. The material should be easy to mix, with a working time that is long enough to allow it to be placed around a number of preparations before setting starts. In order to reproduce the details of the preparation, it should flow well and have a low surface tension, so that it will wet the surfaces of the preparations. This is essential in order that the restoration will fit well and not fail due to leakage or plaque accumulation.

Impression taking would be very easy if the materials were miscible with saliva and tissue fluid. A number of the more recently available materials are claimed to be hydrophilic, but currently the only material that is truly hydrophilic is the reversible hydrocolloid.

After removal from tooth undercuts the material must have a high elastic recovery to reproduce these areas and the rate of this recovery from deformation must be rapid (Chapter 9). Also, the material should not be excessively rigid. If it lacks elasticity, it may well be difficult to disengage from undercuts and could traumatize the soft tissues. A stiff material would also be difficult to remove from its model and stone dies may be damaged.

Perhaps the most significant properties for clinical success are dimensional accuracy and dimensional stability. All the elastomers set by a polymerization reaction that results in shrinkage; this varies with the type of material. The result is a contraction towards the internal surface of the impression tray, assuming that the tray adhesive is strong enough to resist the forces.

With simple extracoronal preparations this contraction does not present major problems since the die produced from the preparation will be slightly larger than the original preparation. Therefore, the restoration will seat on that preparation, but the width of the cement lute will be increased.

Greater problems exist with complex intracoronal features, such as slots and grooves. Here, the dimensional changes are much more complex and consequent variations result in either difficulty or failure of the restoration to seat completely.

The material should also have a high tear resistance, since once the impression has entered a gingival crevice, a thin area of material might well be damaged on removal.

Table 17.1 Types of indirect impression materials

Rigid			Elastomeric			
Composition	Hydrocolloids		Polysulphides	Polyethers	Silicones	
	Irreversible Alginate	Reversible Agar-agar			Type I Condensation cured	Type II Addition cured

Impression materials

A general classification of impression materials is given in *Table 17.1.* With the development of elastomers, the rigid materials, often used within a copper ring, have fallen from grace almost completely, as have the techniques of direct wax pattern-making in the mouth.

The irreversible hydrocolloids, the alginates, are excellent for preliminary impressions, but because of their dimensional instability, have no place as final impressions for crown and bridgework, though they are satisfactory for partial and complete dentures. The reversible hydrocolloids, agar–agar, on the other hand, are excellent for the reproduction of detail and mix well with intraoral fluids. However, they require specialized equipment and must be cast immediately upon removal from the mouth.

The principal materials now used for fixed prosthodontics are the rubber based *elastomers.* The currently available materials fall into three main groups:

- Silicones (polysiloxanes)
- Polyethers
- Polysulphides

The elastomers are generally available in one of four forms described as *putty, heavy bodied, regular* and *light bodied,* the basic difference between the four forms being the filler loading.

The silicone materials are divided into two separate subgroups:

- Condensation curing (type I)
- Addition curing (type II)

Condensation silicones

Until the general acceptance of addition cured materials, the condensation curing materials were very popular in general dental practice because of their clean handling and rapid set. They may come in all four consistencies, but the most popular are the putty and wash materials, the wash being light bodied. The active constituents are shown in *Table 17.2.*

The elastomer sets by a condensation polymerization reaction with the formation of ethyl alcohol as a byproduct. The alcohol subsequently evaporates, causing further shrinkage over and above that of the polymerization reaction. Shrinkage continues for several days with 0.5% occurring in the first 24 hours. This is significant if the technical laboratory is some distance from the practice. The greater setting contraction occurs in the light bodied materials where the polymer is the largest component.

The light bodied material has the ability to reproduce the surface detail well, but has a relatively low tear resistance and many of the materials are difficult to handle.

Table 17.2 Components of elastomeric impression materials

Type	Base	Catalyst	Filler
Type I Silicone	Dimethyl siloxane	Stannous octoate Alkyl silicate	Copper carbonate or silica 2-8 µm
Type II Silicone	Dimethyl siloxane	Chloroplatinic acid	Silica
Polyether	Polyether - ethylene imine terminated	Dichlorobenzene sulphonate	Silica
Polysulphide	Polysulphide (Thiokol)	Lead dioxide Dibutyl phthalate	Titanium dioxide, silica or copper carbonate

The setting reaction is temperature dependent with a marked reduction in both working and setting times in the presence of a relatively small increase in ambient temperature, particularly when the humidity is high. This can result in a material being manipulated at a time when it has already commenced its setting phase, causing development of setting stresses in the material that are relieved after removal of the impression. This, in turn, leads to a restoration that, whilst fitting the die, will not seat satisfactorily in the mouth. Failures with these materials are more commonly associated with complex intracoronal preparations and bridgework.

Addition silicones

These are now the most popular of the elastomers and their active constituents are shown in *Table 17.2*. The setting reaction here has no low molecular weight byproduct and this results in a material that shows little or no dimensional change. The shrinkage figures quoted are in the range 0.05–0.07% at 24 hours.

However, a secondary reaction does take place if incomplete polymerization has occurred, with the liberation of hydrogen gas. A number of the materials have finely divided palladium added that is supposed to absorb the hydrogen. Because of this, impressions should not be poured immediately, otherwise the liberation of hydrogen will result in a roughened die stone surface

The material has low tear resistance and is prone to tear if engaged in deep undercuts or the gingival crevice; care is required on removal of the impression. It is also particularly temperature sensitive.

The other main disadvantage is that the tray adhesive is not strong and is relatively unreliable. This can result in the impression material pulling away from the tray in places. This is not necessarily always visible and consequently it is only when the restoration is tried-in and does not fit that the problem is seen.

The addition silicones have poor wetting characteristics and are also hydrophobic; this may lead to poor reproduction of detail and may also make model pouring troublesome. Wetting agents have been developed for both intraoral and laboratory use to overcome this problem.

The excellent dimensional stability often results in very accurately fitting castings that may prove difficult to seat, and the master die should be treated with the appropriate die spacer (see below).

Polyethers

These materials have a small but enthusiastic following and when used with care produce very satisfactory results. Their components are shown in *Table 17.2*. They are usually purchased as a two-paste system of a regular consistency.

The original materials, whilst apparently being very dimensionally stable, were affected by humidity and showed variable unpredictable shrinkage when a diluent paste was added. Modifications in formulation have improved this, but at the expense of the handling properties.

There have been a number of cases of allergic reactions to the material, causing a burning sensation in the tissues covered by the impression and, in severe cases, marked erythema. Reformulation has reduced this, although some patients still comment on the burning sensation when the impression is being taken.

The tear resistance of the material is similar to that of the silicones but its stiffness is considerably higher. This stiffness can result in problems during removal of the impression from the mouth which can also be impeded by the hydrophilic character of the material; it tends to 'stick' to the mucosa. It is advisable to have a double-spaced special tray so that there is more material to flex to facilitate removal of the impression. If a stock tray is used, then this should have sufficient rigidity to prevent distortion during removal of the impression from the mouth.

The stiffness may also cause difficulty in the laboratory, since it is relatively easy to damage the dies on removal of the impression, particularly if they are narrow. Lower incisor crown preparations can be a particular problem.

The material is quite temperature sensitive and may set rapidly on a hot day. This may be critical as the working and setting times of these materials are the shortest of all the elastomers.

Polysulphides

These are the oldest of the elastomers, and in spite of their smell and dirty handling continued in use because of their reliability and strength. However, they have, to a great extent, been displaced by the addition silicones.

The components are shown in *Table 17.2*. The material is usually used as a combination of heavy and light consistencies, with the heavy bodied version being particularly difficult to mix. There is also a regular consistency material. It is the lead dioxide that makes the material unpleasant to use.

The setting reaction is condensation polymerization with the formation of water as the byproduct. Impressions should be kept in a sealed moist bag to reduce the shrinkage that would be caused by the evaporation of the water. There is a small setting contraction of 0.13–0.25% at 24 hours, with little further shrinkage after this.

On the plus side, the material has a much higher tear resistance than the other three elastomers, but it does not show such good recovery from deformation. The working and setting times are the longest of all the elastomers and it appears to be the least sensitive to temperature changes.

Impression techniques

Management of gingival tissues

This and excellent control of saliva are the keys to successful impression taking.

The first requirement is that the tissues should be in good health and undamaged. Careless preparation, with abraded gingivae, will repay the operator with a poor impression. Poorly fitting provisional restorations will accumulate plaque and cause gingival enlargement and bleeding.

In the interests of periodontal health, crown margins should be at the level of the gingival margin and not be placed in the gingival crevice unless aesthetics will be improved by such location. Gingival margins should be recontoured if the preparation has to enter the crevice by more than 0.5 mm, perhaps where there is a deep core. Impression taking is made easy by supragingival margins.

If there are problems with bleeding tissues the impression should be abandoned. Accurately fitting provisional restorations should be placed, perhaps cemented with a periodontal dressing material, and the impression taken on a subsequent visit when the gingivae have recovered.

Gingival retraction

To provide clear definition of the finishing line, the gingival tissues must be displaced from the preparation and any exudate from the crevice controlled. There are several types of material which may be used for this.

Mechanical displacement using a variety of cord is probably the most popular. Cords come in two forms: *braided* and *twisted*. The braided form is easier to place and may be supplied in several sizes. The twisted type has a tendency to become untwisted during placement. There are also a number of elasticated rings that may be pushed over the preparation and into the crevice.

All the proprietary brands may be impregnated with agents to control oozing from the crevice; these may be vasoconstrictors or styptics. Epinephrine (adrenaline) hydrochloride is the most common of the first group, but must be avoided in certain patients who have either cardiovascular problems or are sensitive to it. Aluminium trichlo-

ride, alum, is a common styptic, as is ferrous sulphate. As well as being impregnated in the cord, retraction solutions may be purchased separately. Care must be exercised in their use, since excess application can cause irreversible damage to the tissues, particularly gingival recession.

Cord placement   Care must be taken in placement of the cord to avoid damage to the epithelial attachment. Teeth must be isolated by cotton wool rolls and a saliva ejector and blown dry. The cord is laid around the gingival margins of the prepared tooth. The width of the cord should match the depth of the crevice and, if necessary, a multi-stranded cord can be split into several thin strands. It is better, though, to have cords of different diameters available.

The cord is pressed gently into the gingival crevice using a small flat plastic instrument, keeping the cord between the blade and the tissue (*Fig. 17.1*). A local analgesic is often advisable as the procedure can be uncomfortable.

The cord should not be left *in situ* too long as permanent recession may be caused. About five minutes is necessary to provide optimum retraction, maintaining saliva control all the time. If the cord does not obstruct the margins of the preparation, it can be left in place whilst the impression is taken. If this technique is used, it is most important to remember to remove the cord before the patient leaves the surgery! To remove the cord after the impression has been taken, it should be first moistened with water to avoid damaging the friable gingival tissue.

It is more common, though, to remove the cord when the impression material is ready to syringe around the preparation. The cord must be removed very gently to prevent the initiation of bleeding or oozing.

It is sometimes possible to dispense with retraction and blow the light bodied material into the gingival crevice with compressed air. This is quite effective, but may result in a very thin section of rubber because of the lack of retraction, and this is liable to distort or tear.

Electro-surgery

This technique involves the use of a high frequency electric current that may be used to either coagulate bleeding tissues or fulgurate (spark drying by ionization). When used carefully, it can produce a very clearly defined margin.

There is a risk, however, that the misuse of this technique will result in serious gingival tissue damage, particularly if the tissues are inflamed and oedematous at the time of surgery. Its main advantage is the haemostasis obtained.

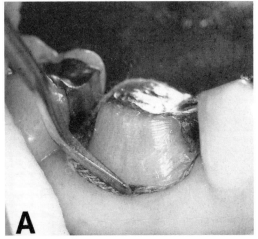

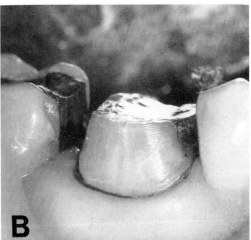

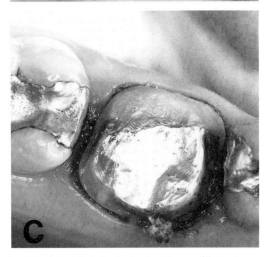

Fig. 17.1 A Braided gingival retraction cord being inserted into a gingival crevice. **B** and **C** Insertion completed. Note the lack of gingival trauma following preparation of the full crown

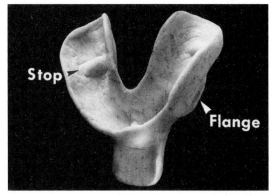

Fig. 17.2 Special tray with posterior flanges to aid removal and occlusal stops to locate it on the teeth

Special trays

The main advantage of a correctly made special tray is that it ensures a uniform thickness of the impression material, thereby reducing risk of uneven distortion. The tray also confines the material, assists in its adaptation to the teeth and prevents it escaping into the rest of the mouth. The thickness of the tray material can be controlled to give good rigidity, thus avoiding flexing and distortion of the impression on removal from the mouth. This last characteristic is an important factor in the choice of stock/disposable trays.

Adequate spacing should be provided between the tray and the teeth to accommodate a reasonable volume of impression material and stops should be placed around the arch to ensure that the tray locates accurately on to the teeth. It should be extended to about 2 mm below the gingival margin of all teeth and should wrap around the end of the alveolar ridge to confine the material to the tray (*Fig. 17.2*).

The weak link may be the tray adhesive. Those used for the polysulphides are very good, but those provided for the addition silicones are poor and perforations should be incorporated in the tray to assist retention. Whichever type is used, it must be given adequate time to dry before the material is mixed; this may be as much as 15 minutes.

Full arch, rather than sectional, impressions are desirable for accuracy of occlusal contacts.

Handling the materials

There are three main ways in which impression materials may be used:

- Putty and wash
- Regular/universal single mix
- Light and heavy bodied double mix

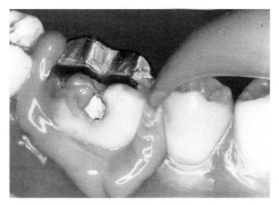

Fig. 17.3 Syringing the light bodied material around the gingival margin. Care must be taken to apply the material to the tooth surface so that air does not become trapped

Putty and wash technique

This technique uses a very high consistency putty within a stock tray instead of a special tray, together with a fluid, light bodied perfecting wash.

Condensation and addition silicones are the only successful materials that have been produced for this technique. The technique has the possible advantage that no special tray is required, but there are dangers of uneven shrinkage setting up stresses within the material. The later release of the stresses leads to dimensional inaccuracies.

Putty and wash materials may be used in one-stage or two-stage techniques.

One stage   Here, both the putty and wash materials are fluid at the same time. Following mixing, the wash is syringed around the preparation, ensuring that the nozzle of the syringe remains within the exuding material to reduce the risk of air blows. Syringing should start at the distal margin of the preparation and be brought forward (*Fig. 17.3*). It is necessary to cover the preparation and the occlusal surfaces of the adjacent teeth with a thin film, the latter being recorded for occlusal registration.

The putty is loaded into a rigid stock tray as soon as the syringe has been filled, and is inserted into the mouth immediately the wash is in place. All these materials are very rapid setting and working time is exceptionally short.

Considerable pressure is required to seat the tray because of the stiffness of the putty. It is also important to insert the tray in the long axis of the preparations. An oblique seating direction will displace the putty away from the teeth and because of its high viscosity it will not flow back around the teeth. The result is referred to (incorrectly) as *drag marks* (*Fig 17.4A*). The tray and impression material must be supported under moderate pressure until the materials have set, since disturbances will result in distortion.

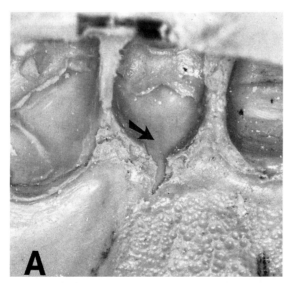

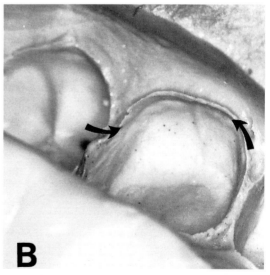

Fig. 17.4 A 'Drag' marks; these have resulted from the incorrect insertion of the tray. **B** An impression of a chamfer finishing line (arrowed). Clarity here is essential for the technician to be able to see where to finish the waxing. There should be registration of uncut tooth beyond the finishing line

Two stage Here a putty 'tray' is prepared before the wash is mixed. The stock tray is first filled with the putty and seated home. A polyester sheet may be placed as a spacer on the surface of the putty before insertion or, alternatively, the tray may be rocked to provide the space necessary for the wash.

Once the putty has set it is removed, washed and dried and sluice ways cut in the buccal and lingual aspects in the areas adjacent to the preparation. Any material remaining approximally is also removed. These modifications allow escape of excess wash material in the second stage of the technique. The putty must be clean and dry and uncontaminated with saliva.

The perfecting wash is syringed around the preparation and all occlusal fissures to form a thin film over the area where fine detail is required. The putty 'tray' is then reseated and the wash and putty will unite chemically as the wash sets.

Results using this technique can be good but a number of problems may arise:

- Saliva interposed between the putty and wash
- Build-up of wash in certain parts of the occlusal section of the impression that results in an incorrect occlusal relationship. This usually follows inadequate sluice way preparation in the primary putty impression
- Displacement and distortion of the tray during its second seating. This can result in uneven distribution of the wash and, worse, distortion of the tray itself

Special tray technique

The putty/wash techniques involve production of a close fitting 'tray' in putty, but this is bulky and can introduce errors with incorrect seating. A special tray saves impression material and is easier to handle.

Two mix technique The materials used are light and heavy bodied, with the heavy bodied material acting as a support for the fine detail reproducing light bodied material. The light bodied material is syringed around the preparation and on to the occlusal surfaces of the other teeth, and the heavy bodied material is loaded into the special tray that is seated, again, in a direction parallel to the long axes of the teeth. The tray must be located accurately and held immobile until the material has set.

If the tray is not placed as soon as the light bodied material has been syringed, there is a risk of saliva contamination between the materials, and impression failure. Impressions of the lower molars are the most vulnerable, with the tongue often becoming interposed at the crucial stage. This

problem may be reduced by not introducing the light bodied material until the heavy bodied material is almost mixed. However, too much delay may mean handling the material beyond the point when it has commenced its setting phase.

Quite heavy pressure should be applied for about the first 15 seconds after insertion to ensure that the material flows and, at the same time, it is important to ensure that the stops on the fit surface of the special tray locate accurately on the surfaces of the teeth. Without the stops, the tray will come into contact with tooth surface over a large area, and even in the area of the preparation, with a consequent failure of the impression.

Single mix technique The special tray technique may be used with materials of a single, regular, or medium bodied consistency using the same mix in both the tray and the syringe. Whilst this can be successful, it is sometimes difficult to syringe the material because it is stiffer than the light-bodied type, and the tray portion can flow rather freely because it is more fluid than the heavy bodied type. This technique is commonly used for impressions for partial dentures.

Removal of the impression

It is always tempting to remove the impression as soon as the outer aspect of the material has set. This may have disastrous consequences, since the light bodied materials set at a slower rate than the heavy bodied materials. Early disturbance of the materials will result in distortion of the impression and dragging of the material at the margins of the preparation.

The best indication that the material has set in the mouth is when the material has set on the mixing pad, and a timer may give some guidance. Ambient temperature and humidity cause large deviations from the manufacturers' predicted behaviour, and it is better to leave the material in place for as long as possible.

The impression should be removed without rocking or shaking. One sharp pull in the line of insertion of the preparations is the ideal. This is assisted by having flanges at the side of the special tray, rather than using the handle.

Assessment of impressions

After removal, the impression should be thoroughly washed to remove all contaminants and then dried. Careful examination should be made in good light, using a hand lens if necessary. The operating light or fibre optic illumination is usually suitable. A clear outline of the finishing margin all

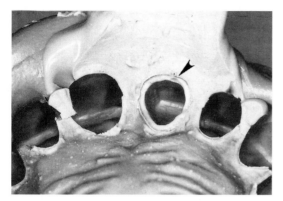

Fig. 17.5 An impression of a shoulder. The air-blow (arrowed) does not obstruct the edge of the finishing line, and therefore the impression can be used. The technician will have to trim the defect away on the die

round the preparation should be visible, with a small extent of impression material beyond it (*Fig. 17.4B*).

There should be no air blows on the margin but sometimes small air blows on the fit surface may be accepted (*Fig. 17.5*). Subsurface air voids may not be seen and a special check is necessary (*Fig. 17.6A*). This may be done by gently pushing the surface of the material with a round ended instrument. Any areas where the surface is deflected indicate that there are large air voids beneath, which would only become apparent on pouring the model (*Fig. 17.6B*).

It is important to ensure that the material has not pulled away from the tray. This should be apparent at the periphery of the impression where it is easy to see.

If there is any doubt about the accuracy of the impression, it may be possible to pour it immediately and examine the preparations. This may save time and money, but should be done in liaison with the technician to ensure that the appropriate casting technique is used.

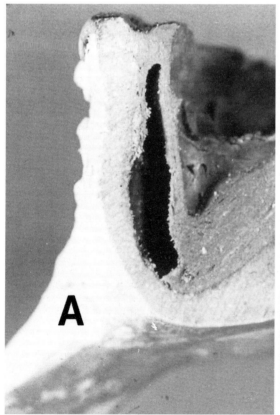

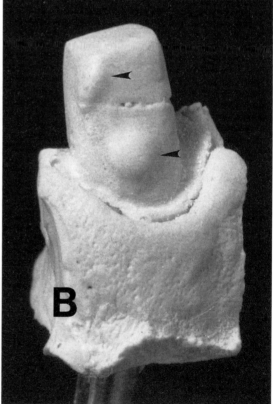

Fig. 17.6 A Large subsurface air void under the impression of the preparation. On casting, the die stone displaced the thin layer, and the die had a surface bulge on it. The fault arose due to poor loading of the tray. **B** Two die artefacts (arrowed) caused by stone displacing light-bodied material into subsurface voids

Decontamination

The dentist has responsibility for ensuring that impressions, models and other equipment passing to the laboratory are not contaminated with body fluids or bacteria from the patient. This is one of the principles that should be enshrined in the dentist's *prevention of cross infection* protocols.

Several agents have been recommended and some lead to dimensional changes in the impression material; others, such as glutaraldehyde, present risks to the dentist and his or her team.

Currently, the recommendation is for immersion of the impression, etc. in a 1% sodium hypochlorite solution for 20 minutes. Items coming from the laboratory also need decontamination.

Model construction

The laboratory should always be informed as to which type of impression material has been used so that production of the working die may be done correctly. As mentioned earlier, addition cured silicones may release hydrogen if cast too soon and this affects the model surface. If metal plated models are required, the process will be affected by the impression type. Both types of hydrocolloid material are adversely affected by water loss, and therefore must be cast as soon as possible or kept in a humidifier.

In order to improve the abrasion resistance of the model, stone die and plaster *hardeners* may be used. These are resins in solution that are simply painted directly on to the die and surrounding areas. They harden, seal and waterproof the surface, and protect the definition of margins without altering dimensions of the die.

Die relief or *spacer* solutions can be used to increase the size of the die by a controlled amount. Claimed advantages are:

- Surface roughness is reduced, making pattern removal easier
- Space is created to accommodate the cement lute
- Adjustment can be made for dimensional problems in the investment (this applies to ceramic bonding alloy investments)
- The casting is larger in the case of a crown or smaller in the case of an inlay therefore it seats more easily clinically

The decision to use die spacers should be made jointly between the clinician and technician, since the amount of relief required has to match the dimensional changes of the impression material. A very accurate material, such as addition cured silicone, ought to have die relief used on its models.

With higher shrinkage materials, such as condensation silicones, die relief would create a very loose restoration.

Two thicknesses are available, coloured gold or silver, and the application of four alternate coats increases the die by 25 μm. The die spacer should not be used within 0.5 mm of the margins of the preparation.

Dimensional changes associated with indirect restoration construction

Each stage in the construction of an indirect restoration is accompanied by dimensional changes, either expansion or contraction. Each of the changes must be controlled or counterbalanced such that when the restoration is fitted, the interfacial gap between tooth and restoration is of the order of 25–50 μm.

The stages and their dimensional changes are as follows:

- *Impression* – polymerization shrinkage of elastomer
- *Casting model* – hygroscopic expansion of model plaster
- *Waxing* – expansion and contraction of the wax on heating and cooling
- *Investment* - hygroscopic expansion on setting and thermal expansion on heating in the furnace
- *Alloy* – expansion on heating, contraction on cooling
- *Ceramic* – contraction on firing

The major predicted and counterbalanced process is alloy casting. The alloy expands on heating and will contract after casting. Since the casting is done at a high temperature, the investment mould will have expanded already. The casting shrinks on cooling to what will be its final dimensions. Dimensional changes of the investment must balance the behaviour of the alloy and may be altered by:

- Hygroscopic expansion – mould placed in warm water on initial set
- Thermal expansion – gradual heating increases this
- Alteration of the powder/liquid ratio
- Lining (non-asbestos) of casting ring to permit free expansion

Alloy manufacturers recommend appropriate investments and how these should be treated to produce an accurate casting with their particular alloy.

If used correctly, die relief offers an opportunity to balance impression material changes with those that result finally from casting the alloy or firing the ceramic.

Impression materials – Summary

The material of choice for one or two preparations is addition cured silicone in a putty/wash technique. Polyethers are satisfactory as heavy/light bodied or regular bodied in a stock tray

For multiple preparations, consider a special tray with a heavy-bodied/light-bodied technique

Gingival management should involve supragingival margins wherever possible, no trauma during preparation and careful use of retraction cord and solution

Complete moisture control is essential

Syringe the light-bodied material with the nozzle close to the preparation to avoid air inclusions

Insert the tray in the long axis of the preparations to avoid 'drags'

Remove with a single short, sharp tug and avoid rocking

Check that the impression is free from air-blows, drag marks and material discontinuities

Decontaminate the impression before it leaves the surgery

FIXED AND REMOVABLE PROSTHODONTICS: THE REPLACEMENT OF MISSING TEETH

18

Diagnosis and treatment planning for fixed and removable prosthodontics

Here we consider the possible consequences on the remaining dentition of the loss of teeth, whether to replace them or not, and the general approach to the choice of a prosthetic replacement.

Consequences of tooth loss

No matter how good our preventive programmes and conservation skills, teeth will still be lost as a result of caries, periodontal disease and traumatic injuries. Consequences of the loss of a tooth or several teeth will vary from patient to patient, but in general the following are possible:

- Tilting, drifting and rotation of adjacent teeth
- Overeruption of opposing teeth – loss of occlusal stability
- Increased plaque accumulation and periodontal disease
- Abnormal sites for carious lesions
- Damage to remaining teeth due to increased function – tooth wear
- Loss of masticatory efficiency
- Loss of aesthetics
- Speech problems
- Alveolar resorption
- Loss of support for soft tissues

The principal effects are summarised in *Figure 18.1*.

Loss of occlusal stability

The extent to which this may occur depends upon the original tooth relationships. The teeth around a single unit space may well have stable contacts such that no deterioration occurs (*Fig. 18.2*). In other cases, there may be slight changes in tooth position resulting in less than perfect relationships but not necessarily requiring restoration of the missing teeth (*Fig. 18.3*).

However, overeruption and drifting may be dramatic (*Fig. 18.4*). The changes in tooth positions may lead to abnormal functional relationships such as non-working interferences in protrusion and lateral excursions, and pre-centric prematurities.

Loss of masticatory efficiency

Whilst the loss of a single tooth is unlikely to have any significant effect on mastication, the loss of two or more in the same quadrant would probably require the patient to modify his chewing pattern to maintain effective function. It is unlikely that this would be noticed and, even with many missing posterior teeth, the vast majority of patients continue with a normal diet.

However, once a substantial amount of posterior support is lost, mastication is transferred to the anterior teeth which have a narrow occlusal table, making them unsuitable for grinding. The consequence will often be tooth wear or *tooth surface loss* (see Chapter 25). A typical case of anterior tooth surface loss following loss of posterior teeth is shown in *Figure 18.5*.

Increased plaque accumulation – caries and periodontal disease

The opening of contacts by tilting, drifting and rotation into an edentulous space may encourage

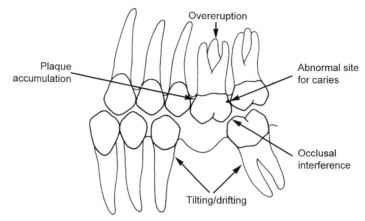

Fig 18.1 The consequences of tooth loss.

food packing and plaque accumulation that in turn may initiate or increase the progress of periodontal inflammation. The same applies to the overerupted tooth, where embrasures and contact relations are changed to an unfavourable relationship for natural plaque control.

Tilted teeth may be more vulnerable to periodontal breakdown due to unfavourable loading from the occlusion.

Caries too may be initiated by plaque accumulation in poorly accessible areas, but of course this disease also requires a carbohydrate substrate. Therefore the overall caries rate is of importance in predicting the initiation of new carious lesions. In the event of new caries, because the contact area of an overerupted tooth will be resited to an area of thinner enamel, the tooth can be more vulnerable to carious spread.

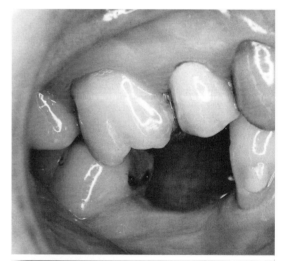

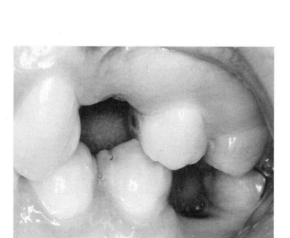

Fig. 18.2 Edentulous spaces at |4 and |6 where tooth relationships have remained stable

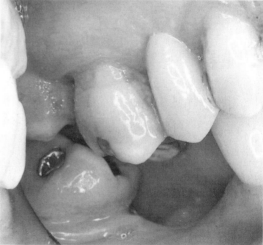

Fig. 18.3 Slight deterioration of occlusal relationships around missing molars but not indicating tooth replacement

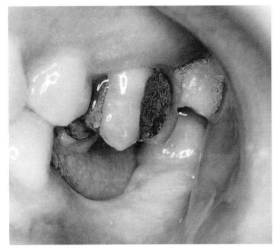

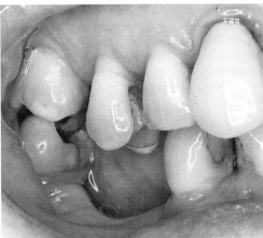

Fig. 18.4 Edentulous spaces with associated deterioration of occlusal stability. In the upper picture $\underline{6}$ has overerupted, in the lower picture $\underline{4|}$ has overerupted

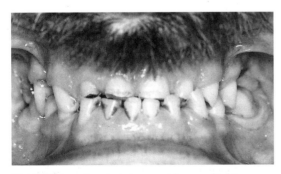

Fig. 18.5 Loss of posterior support has resulted in anterior tooth surface loss due to changes in chewing pattern

These effects are not absolutely certain and other factors such as the patient's diet and plaque control effectiveness will be important. In a mouth with a low caries rate and good oral hygiene the effects of tilting, rotation and drifting may be minimal.

Aesthetics, speech, alveolar resorption and soft tissue collapse

Losing a front tooth clearly affects aesthetics but a posterior tooth is not usually considered essential for good looks. This of course varies according to the social perceptions of the patient's social group or occupation. Perhaps an actor or public speaker may be more concerned about the loss of a premolar or molar.

Speech may be affected, particularly in respect of anterior tooth loss. There may be lisping or spitting on speaking. However, these effects are not often noticeable because of the general ability of the patient to adapt to such changes.

Alveolar resorption is a natural consequence of tooth loss, there being no need for the bone if there is no tooth and periodontium to support. Both intra- and extra-oral soft tissues may collapse or spread into the space. The tongue will spread laterally and the perioral soft tissues may collapse inwards. This latter effect may affect aesthetics considerably, particularly in middle age and after, when muscle tone is reduced.

Summary

As with many other biological processes the effects of tooth loss are often unpredictable. Though the list of possible problems is large, many patients do not exhibit any of these and in others the effects may be minimal. Clearly, the more teeth that are lost, the greater the possibility of problems. The most important are those that could induce further pathology and deterioration of the remaining dentition.

The two principal problems are probably periodontal disease and damage to the remaining teeth from altered masticatory patterns.

Replacement of missing teeth

This section must open with the statement that *not every missing tooth needs to be replaced*. This might come as a shock to a well motivated patient who has invested much time and trouble in attending for prolonged but ultimately unsuccessful endodontic therapy, only to learn that the resulting space will remain unfilled! Such a patient needs to be informed that all methods of replacing missing teeth carry with them the possibility of causing further damage to the dentition and other problems.

On the other hand, there are obviously several potential benefits to be gained from tooth replacement:

- Restored aesthetics
- Restored function
- Prevention of deterioration of the remaining dentition

Of these, the patient will be highly motivated to the restoration of aesthetics but might need some convincing as to the value of the other two, particularly the last. From the treatment planning viewpoint, the restoration of function and the maintenance of the remaining dentition will need to be balanced against the possible harm that may be induced by the provision of a prosthesis (see below).

Missing teeth may be replaced by:

- *Fixed prostheses – bridgework*, which may be:
  Resin retained (adhesive)
  Crown retained (conventional)
  Endosseous implant retained

- *Removable prostheses – partial or complete dentures*, which may be:
  Tooth borne
  Tissue borne
  Combination of the two

Detailed indications, contraindications, design and construction aspects of the above are considered in subsequent chapters (19–24), but the general aspects of each are considered here.

Choice of prosthesis

Once the decision to replace a missing tooth or teeth has been made, many factors will be involved in choosing the appropriate prosthesis:

General factors

- Patient aspirations and motivation
- Ability and training of the dentist
- Ability and training of the technician
- Clinical and laboratory facilities available
- Economic factors
- Age and general health of the patient

Intraoral factors

- Restorative condition of the dentition, in particular the abutment teeth
- Number of missing teeth and their location
- Tooth relationships – the occlusion
- Periodontal condition, caries and oral hygiene
- Presence of an existing partial denture
- Alveolar bone dimensions and position

General factors

The patient

The patient's prime position in the formulation of a treatment plan was discussed in Chapter 1 and these same principles apply here. A patient with low motivation, who is unable to attend regularly or who cannot for whatever reason be treated 'normally' should have a simple treatment plan. In the context of choice of prosthesis, this will usually mean a partial denture.

There should be no general upper age limit affecting the choice between a bridge and a partial denture but age may bring with it some restrictions that affect the delivery of dental care. The influence of the medical history in the drafting of a treatment plan and its delivery was discussed in Chapter 4.

Young patients will have immature dentitions with large pulps and unstable gingival margin position and are not usually suitable for bridgework. Also, they may be involved in contact sports that again would contraindicate bridgework.

The dentist, the technician and their facilities

The construction of fixed prostheses requires excellent clinical and technical skills and appropriate facilities. Whilst some aspects of the construction of partial dentures require similar skills, in general this line of treatment is usually simpler and less demanding. It may also be that the consequences of a poorly constructed partial denture will be less harmful to the dentition than those of a poorly constructed bridge. At least the partial denture can be removed for cleaning, and the tooth preparation for it is usually minimal.

Economic factors

Economic factors, including state or private insurance schemes, influence the delivery of advanced restorative care to a large degree. Endosseous implant retained prostheses are outside the scope of some schemes and are outside the financial resources of many patients. Fixed bridgework is also affected, though to a lesser extent, whilst partial dentures sometimes seem to be regarded as the bargain basement treatment; this attitude somewhat devalues the skills and techniques required for their proper construction.

Intraoral factors

Restorative condition of the dentition, in particular the abutment teeth

The provision of any prosthesis should be against a background of a stable and well-restored dentition. The presence of active caries or periodontal disease ought to preclude the construction of a prosthesis that should wait until intraoral conditions are suitable. A prosthesis may aggravate a pre-existing condition and make things worse.

However, delaying the construction of a prosthesis may not always be possible, for example when the patient requires the restoration of aesthetics. In these circumstances it is necessary to make a prediction of the outcome of the pre-prosthetic periodontal and restorative therapy. If this prediction is guarded it would be acceptable to construct a simple intermediate partial denture whilst the mouth is being stabilized. If the dentist has more confidence in the outcome, then provisional bridgework could be constructed pending stabilization of the rest of the mouth.

The condition of the abutment teeth is a major consideration in choice of prosthesis. Bridgework requires biologically and structurally sound teeth of good prognosis to support and retain it. Each tooth should have a healthy periodontium, even though this can be reduced through previous periodontal disease. The pulp should be unquestionably vital or the tooth should be properly root filled with no apical pathology. There should be enough sound dentine or enamel to support the chosen retainer.

Whilst the abutment teeth are also important in the support and retention of a partial denture, the alveolar ridge can often be used to supplement them. Their condition, therefore, is not as critical as for bridgework.

Number of missing teeth and their location

In general, a single missing tooth is best replaced by means of a bridge, all other factors being equal. Even in the presence of moderate periodontal disease there is evidence to suggest that a bridge creates less unfavourable conditions for plaque control than does a partial denture. There is also evidence to support the use of single tooth endosseous implants but economic factors are likely to prevent their general use.

An edentulous space resulting from two missing adjacent teeth bounded by remaining teeth can be restored by bridgework. Where the space is of three or more teeth, the partial denture becomes the more reliable option. Here there may be insufficient adjacent teeth to support a bridge adequately, or technical difficulties in construction may limit the treatment plan.

Where the edentulous space is unbounded at one end, i.e. a free end saddle, the restorative options are further limited. A bridge may be used to restore one tooth as a distal cantilever design, but to restore more will inevitably require a partial denture.

Several missing teeth, each in different areas of the dental arch, could be replaced by several independent bridges, but usually the most cost effective and simple option is to make a partial denture.

Tooth relationships, the occlusion

As discussed in Chapter 20, the design of a simple bridge involving two or more abutments requires that these teeth be aligned roughly parallel. The construction of a bridge on malaligned teeth is not impossible, but is more difficult technically. The greater the disruption to normal tooth relationships, the more a partial denture is indicated. Irregularities of the occlusal plane will also compromise the design of a bridge and if these are difficult or impossible to correct then usually a partial denture is preferable.

Periodontal condition, caries and oral hygiene

As was stated above, all prostheses should be placed into stable and pathology-free mouths. In the face of poor oral hygiene, all types of prosthesis are likely to fail. It is a matter of some clinical judgement as to whether intraoral conditions will deteriorate more where there is a dirty bridge compared to a dirty partial denture present. The counsel of perfection is to place a prosthesis only in a mouth that is properly maintained by both the patient and by the dentist and where active caries and periodontal disease have been eliminated.

In relation to implant retained prostheses, the presence of periodontal disease is a significant contraindication. There is considerable potential for periodontal infection to spread to the implant sites and cause problems.

Presence of an existing partial denture

When a further tooth is lost in close association to an existing denture, the simplest approach is to add another artificial tooth to the denture. The mixing of a denture and bridgework in the same arch may lead the patient to dispense with the denture and rely on the bridgework alone. This is true particularly of an anterior bridge combined with a partial denture replacing posterior teeth; having an anterior tooth on the denture is a great motivator to proper denture wearing.

Alveolar bone dimensions and position

These will be affected by the extent of postextraction resorption. Placement of bridge pontics on to the alveolar ridge may be complicated if there is extensive resorption, and a denture base may be more appropriate.

The amount of bone remaining is of crucial importance in the provision of endosseous implants. A detailed consideration of implants is outside the scope of this book but restricted alveolar bone would limit the siting of implants, making vital structures such as nerves, blood vessels and the maxillary antrum vulnerable to damage.

Deleterious effects of dental prostheses

There is no doubt that the placement of a prosthesis, whether fixed or removable, brings with it certain disadvantages. Principal amongst these is the possibility of causing further deterioration of the dentition. Possible deleterious effects are:

- Recurrent caries
- Loss of pulp vitality
- Tooth wear
- Periodontal disease
- Soft tissue infection and damage
- Alveolar bone infection

These effects will vary in incidence and magnitude according to the type and design of the prosthesis. Their management is discussed in Chapters 27 and 28.

Fixed bridgework

The construction of a bridge requires tooth preparation to accommodate the retainers. In the case of resin retained bridgework this preparation is minimal and this type of bridge is likely to have less untoward effects on the dentition. Where conventional bridges are made, the retainers are usually full crowns and here there is the potential for loss of vitality as a result of the trauma of the preparation. If the abutment tooth has already been carious and restored, this potential is increased.

Retainer margins, no matter how well fitting, and the pontic/retainer embrasure spaces introduce plaque traps that require special oral hygiene measures to be performed by the patient. The consequences of plaque accumulation may be periodontal disease and, in the presence of a substrate, recurrent caries.

Damage to opposing teeth is possible if ceramic on the bridge is in functional contact with them. The ceramic is harder than enamel and, if poorly glazed or rough, will cause rapid tooth surface loss.

Bridge abutment teeth may transmit unfavourable twisting forces to the periodontium. If the periodontium is already inflamed, these forces may accelerate periodontal breakdown. On the other hand, if the periodontium is healthy, it appears that

supporting a bridge does not bring any untoward effects (see Chapter 20).

Implant retained prostheses

Damage to local vital structures (nerves, blood vessels, antrum) is possible during placement. The endosseous implant is also a potential entry point for bacteria and 'periodontal' infection of the soft tissues and bone is possible.

Partial dentures

The contact areas of clasps and denture base to the surrounding teeth are sites for plaque accumulation and its consequences of caries and periodontal disease. Movement of the denture base, particularly tipping and rotation, may accelerate periodontal breakdown in the presence of active periodontal disease.

Stagnation under a denture base may create conditions favourable to establishment of infection by *Candida albicans* (thrush), leading to denture-induced stomatitis.

Continuing care and replacement

All restorative work brings the requirements of continued maintenance and monitoring by the dentist and scrupulous oral hygiene by the patient.

Perhaps of even greater importance is the realization that eventually repair and replacement will be necessary for most restorations. This does not reflect upon the standards of care, but a realistic appreciation to be conveyed to the patient that nothing lasts forever. General wear and tear and changes in the oral cavity may lead to local or general failure of restorations.

All other things being equal, i.e. that no pre-existing problem, such as a questionable root filling, exists then the life expectancy for a bridge would be between 10 and 15 years and a removable partial denture perhaps 10 years. Even during that time minor problems such as the fracture of a component or even major repairs such as root canal therapy through a retainer may be necessary.

Because of their complexity of construction, implant-retained prostheses require even more intense maintenance. Failure of joints and superstructure components is possible as well as the basic failure of the implant itself

A very positive commitment to continuing care in relation to any prosthesis is required by both patient and dentist. Effective oral hygiene and attendance for regular review is the patient's role in this.

Shortened dental arch

Bearing in mind the above description of the deleterious effects of dental prostheses, a philosophy of non-replacement of lost posterior teeth has evolved, known as the *shortened dental arch*. Whilst this concept could be applied to any missing molar teeth, it has come to refer to dentitions that have no teeth distal to the second premolars in all four quadrants, i.e. all the molar teeth have been lost and deliberately not replaced. This arrangement has also been termed a *premolar dental arch* or a *premolarized occlusion*.

There is some evidence to support the concept in that patients have been observed to function adequately with such a reduced occlusal table and the possible deleterious effects of a prosthesis on the premolar teeth, in particular tipping and periodontal problems, are prevented.

Loss of occlusal stability of the premolars due to distal drifting and wear has been shown to be small and the poorer aesthetics of missing molars has not been considered a problem.

The concept may also be applied if the premolar arch is not intact, particularly if the second premolars are missing. These teeth may be replaced, all other factors being equal, by distally cantilevered units attached to the remaining teeth or endosseous implants. The biomechanics of this type of arrangement must be considered. It is suggested that the distally cantilevered unit be restricted to one premolar only to reduce tipping forces and if several teeth are involved in the prosthesis that it is constructed from gold alloy and acrylic resin to allow flexure without fracture. A long metal-ceramic structure would be more likely to lose ceramic through cracking if subjected to flexure.

Treatment planning for prosthodontics – Summary

The loss of natural teeth may result in deterioration of the remaining dentition and affect the patient adversely.

The provision of a prosthesis will restore aesthetics and function, as well as playing a part in maintaining the dentition.

The prosthesis, however, may cause deterioration in its own right and the decision to restore the edentulous space must take into account both the advantages and the disadvantages of treatment.

The choice of prosthesis is based on a complete assessment of both the patient and the intra-oral conditions and many factors must be considered, with the condition of the mouth itself being of principal concern.

The active co-operation of the patient in both provision of the prosthesis and its subsequent maintenance is of paramount importance to its success.

19

Fixed prosthodontics: Resin retained bridgework

The next three chapters consider fixed prosthodontics. In this chapter there are the basic definitions for bridgework. The history, design, treatment planning and techniques of resin retained or adhesive bridgework are described, together with the materials involved in their construction.

General definitions for bridgework

A bridge, also referred to as a *fixed prosthesis*, is a false tooth, or teeth, permanently attached to natural teeth. The false tooth, the *pontic*, is joined by *connectors* to *retainers* that are cemented to the *abutment teeth*. The retainers may be either wings (*resin retained* or *adhesive bridgework*) or inlays or crowns – (*conventional bridgework*) (Fig. 19.1)

The pontic may be fixed to the retainer by a *rigid connector*, or it may have a movable joint (*non-rigid connector*). Bridges may be classified according to the type of connectors either side of the pontic, as either *fixed–fixed* or *fixed–movable*.

In addition, the pontic may have only one connector and be free at the other end – a *cantilever bridge*. If the pontic is some distance away from the retainer, and the connector is a metal bar, this is a *spring cantilever bridge*.

Bridges are also referred to by the total number of retainers and pontics, for example a *five unit bridge*.

Resin retained bridgework

History

The concept of the resin retained bridge (RRB) is that metal 'wings' are retained by the acid etch technique to enamel surfaces adjacent to the edentulous space. The wings are part of a metal subframe that also supports a resin or ceramic tooth. The use of metal and resin in this way was first reported by Rochette (1973) who described a perforated metal periodontal splint that was adapted to retain a false tooth. Metalwork covered the whole of the lingual enamel surface and retention to the cementing composite resin was achieved through small holes in the metal. Other workers developed alternative ways of obtaining macromechanical retention to the metal but these and the Rochette system have now been superseded.

In the late 1970s, Livaditis and Thompson at the University of Maryland developed an electro-etching procedure for non-precious ceramic bonding alloys to produce a microporous surface that provided a micromechanical interlock with the cement. This gave rise to the 'Maryland' bridge that had the advantages of thinner wings and no perforations compared the Rochette type.

Electro-etching, however, was a demanding technique and two other techniques, acid etching and grit blasting, were developed. Grit blasting was the most simple and reliable and the other two have been largely superseded. This has not stopped incorrect use of the term 'Maryland bridge' for all RRBs.

Further improvements in longevity have been obtained by the development of specific affinity cements and by metal primer systems that increase the bonding of the cement to the metal.

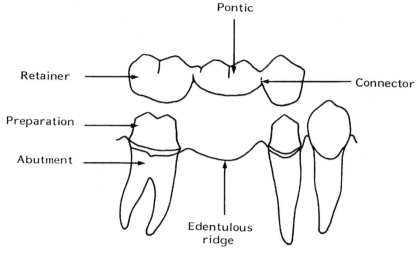

Fig. 19.1 The components of a bridge

Design

The original bridges and splints were made with no tooth preparation, but now considerable enamel preparation is required to promote long-term success; the technique is also referred to as *minimal preparation bridgework*. The objectives of the preparation are to create features that will enhance the stability of the bridge and, to as great extent as possible, to accommodate the casting within the original tooth contour. Other aspects of RRBs have evolved empirically with clinical experience. Perhaps the most interesting of these has been the reduction in the number of wings used; most single tooth RRBs are now retained by a single wing to a single abutment. This is the result of an appreciation of the twisting forces applied during function that translate to peel forces across the adhesive.

Clinical experience showed that two-wing RRBs often failed by debonding of one wing. The problem was managed by removing the debonded wing intraorally to leave a single wing bridge. These single wing bridges were surprisingly successful and this led to the current design concepts. This observation of the biomechanics of this bridge system has implications for the design of conventional bridgework (see Chapter 20).

Tooth preparation

The objectives of tooth preparation are to:

- Accommodate the metal within the original contour of the tooth
- Provide occlusal clearance if necessary
- Direct stress away from the adhesive
- Provide as great a surface area of enamel for bonding as possible
- Achieve clear finishing lines

To achieve this it is necessary to:

- Identify a single path of insertion
- Remove the bulbosity from as wide an area of enamel as possible without exposing dentine – half enamel thickness preparation
- Extend the preparation to as much of the buccal and lingual surfaces as possible to create 'wrap around'
- Avoid the incisal one-third of anterior teeth to maintain translucency
- Incorporate rest seats, slots and grooves as appropriate, to increase stability and accurate location of the casting for cementation

The typical anterior tooth preparation, that is shown on an incisor (*Fig. 19.2A*), requires clearance from the occlusion to enable correct reproduction of the anterior guidance, an internal cingulum rest for location and stress bearing, approximal reduction in the path of insertion and a supragingival chamfer finishing line palatally. If the cingulum area is small, slots or grooves should be cut to enhance stability (*Fig 19.2B*).

There is a danger of producing greyness of incisal edges if the metalwork extends too far incisally. For this reason, the preparation should be confined to the cervical two-thirds of the crown. Care should be taken also to avoid bringing the approximal reduction into the line of sight and a

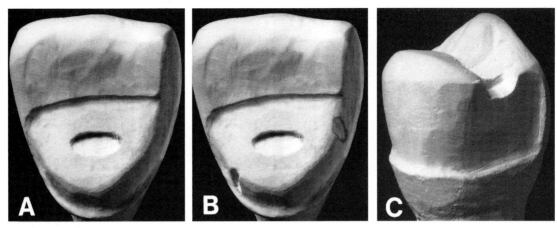

Fig. 19.2 A Anterior resin retained bridge preparation; **B** Incorporation of grooves in the anterior preparation to increase stability. **C** Posterior resin retained bridge preparation

'fade out' of the reduction should be done to maintain enamel in the labial region.

The posterior tooth preparation is shown on a premolar (*Fig. 19.2C*). Again approximal bulbosity is eliminated and a lingual/palatal wrap around, extending as far as possible into the distal embrasure, is cut. Rest seats are cut on the occlusal surface and must be at least 1 mm deep to be effective.

Treatment planning

Table 19.1 summarizes the indications and contra-indications for resin retained bridgework.

The occlusion

The resin retained bridge is useful for short spans and where unfavourable tipping forces are absent. Potential displacing forces from the occlusion are difficult to predict, but patients with a clenching or grinding habit or an edge-to-edge incisor relationship may create unfavourable conditions. A further

occlusal problem may be variations in the level of the occlusal plane caused by tilting or overeruption into the edentulous space. It is preferable to correct this before making the bridge, as the irregularity may be another source of unfavourable displacing forces.

Abutment teeth

These should have sound and well supported enamel. Whilst small restorations are acceptable, more extensive cavities are likely to have weakened cusps. If there is any doubt about the integrity of the chosen abutment, then the existing restoration(s) should be removed and the enamel inspected. Ideally the abutment tooth restoration should be composite resin or glass ionomer cement because of the better bonding of the adhesives to these materials (see below). However, small amalgam restorations are acceptable.

The precise choice of abutment is somewhat empirical, but as a general rule the more posterior tooth of a bounded space is more suitable. The rationale for this is that the more posterior the

Table 19.1 Indications and advantages for resin retained bridgework

Indications	Contraindications	Advantages	Disadvantages
Short spans (one or two teeth)	Long spans	Technically simple	Metal visible through tooth
Sound enamel available	Heavily restored teeth	Cheaper than conventional	Debonding problems
Favourable occlusion	Multiple upper anterior teeth		

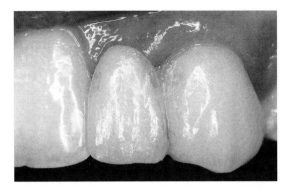

Fig. 19.3 Ceramic veneer retained bridge replacing |2 cantilevered from |3

tooth, usually the larger and less visible it is. The exception is the upper lateral incisor, and this tooth should be avoided as the sole abutment because of its small crown and reduced root support.

The amount of etchable surface and potential wrap around varies from tooth to tooth because of variation in size and position. The size is of particular significance in the lower arch, where the lingual surfaces of the anterior teeth are relatively small, and in the posterior region, where the lingual crown height is often low. Similarly, very severely tilted or rotated teeth might be difficult to use as abutments. All incisor and canine teeth have short palatal or lingual walls, and here slots or grooves are useful to increase stability.

Bridge span

While it is possible to replace more than one tooth with an adhesive bridge, more failures appear to occur with multiple replacements. The use of more than one abutment on either side of the space is also rather risky since the differential stresses are applied to bonds of varying areas, and debonding is likely. A single molar should be regarded as two tooth 'elements' and two wings, one at each end, are usually prescribed for retention.

The upper central incisor may be replaced by a single wing cantilever from the other central incisor or as a cantilever from two wings on the upper lateral incisor and canine. In this latter design it is important to incorporate slots, grooves and rests in the preparations to increase stability.

Design variations

The introduction and development of adhesive techniques has lead to many variations in design as dentists attempt to establish the limits of the techniques.

For example, buccal wings could be used if enamel is better there and the aesthetics are acceptable. The bridge could be constructed completely in ceramic with the wings being veneer preparations (*Fig 19.3*). This is useful if the adjacent tooth is to be veneered anyway.

Spacing is difficult to reproduce but connectors can be constructed to lie below the space, out of sight. However, stresses on the wings may be increased by this design.

Hybrid designs are also in use where a conventional crown is used on one side of the pontic with a bonded wing on the other (*Fig. 19.4A*). However, there is a retention/stability differential between these retainers which might result in cementation failure.

A further refinement that has been proposed to 'balance' the retention differential is the incorporation of a 'stress breaking' joint in the design (*Fig. 19.4B*). The biomechanics of this type of system have not been fully explored and this is discussed in more detail in the next chapter. However, the jointed system does offer the advantage of being able to use gold for the full crown whilst making the wing in base metal. This provides a better resin bonding system (see below).

Cementation

Cementation must be carried out in a dry field and the application of rubber dam is essential, particularly in the lower arch because of the potential for contamination of the etched tooth and the fit surface of the metalwork.

Before the dam is placed, the following must be checked:

- Shade
- Seating of the metalwork
- Occlusion (if possible)

These cannot be checked with the dam on.

The cementing sequence is as follows:

1. Try in and check margins and the occlusion. If the casting is not stable the occlusion cannot be checked easily until after cementation
2. Place the rubber dam
3. Clean the abutment teeth using a slurry of pumice and water. Non-oil based prophylaxis pastes may be used but they may contain fluoride, which reduces the effectiveness of the etching
4. Grit-blast the bridge wings or, if there is no access to a grit-blaster, clean the laboratory-blasted bridge wings with absolute alcohol or a proprietary cleaning agent

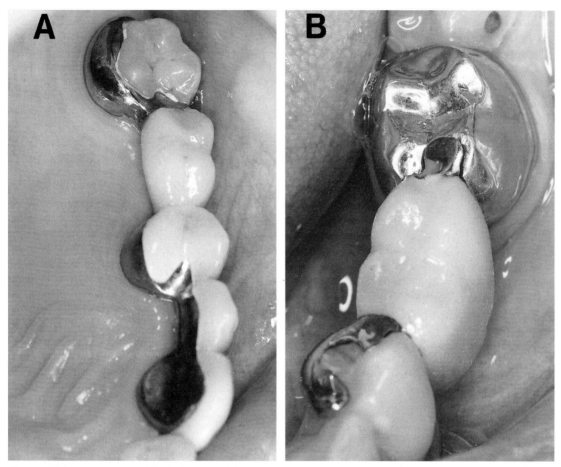

Fig. 19.4 Hybrid resin retained bridges. **A** Fixed–fixed design using a wing on the 7⌋ and full crowns on the 53⌋. **B** Fixed–'movable' design with a wing on ⌊5 and a full crown on ⌊7 including a joint within it

5. Prime the metal, if required
6. Acid etch the area of the tooth preparations
7. Mix and place the cement on the bridge and seat home
8. Remove excess prior to setting and place oxygen barrier, if required
9. Remove the dam, clean the margins and adjust the occlusion
10. Check that the embrasures are clear for oral hygiene measures

Dental materials aspects

Metal subframe and pontic

The choice of metal alloy relates particularly to the method of adhesion of the retaining wings. The electro-etched (Maryland) system is particularly affected by the alloy composition and the principal alloy used in this technique was a nickel–chromium–beryllium ceramic bonding alloy. (Non-beryllium alloys did not electro-etch well.) However, the beryllium content of such alloys represents a health hazard on inhalation of the grinding dust, therefore these are not recommended.

The more universal use of grit blasting has lead to the use of nickel–chromium ceramic bonding alloys. There is some concern about the nickel sensitivity that might be induced by these alloys, particularly as more metal is exposed to the mouth by a wing than in a conventional crown or bridge.

The nickel–chromium alloys are harder, denser and more difficult to cast than the semi-precious alloys and also more time consuming to adjust and finish clinically. However, they have the advantage of being stronger in thin section and therefore the retaining wings can be thinner – of the order of 0.3–0.4 mm.

Pontics may be made from ceramic or polymers. Ceramic is the most durable with oven-processed composites being a second choice.

Adhesive cements

There are two basic types:

- Fine particle composite resin luting cements
- Dual affinity resin cements

These are mostly two component autopolymerizing systems but there are also a number of 'dual cure' materials available that are initiated by visible light, but also have a slow autopolymerizing component. This means that polymerization takes place even when the curing light does not reach the full thickness of the material.

The formulation of the first group is based on restorative composites with less filler of smaller particle size diluted with lower molecular weight resins. They rely on micromechanical interlocking to both the etched enamel and the metal wing for their retention.

The second group has a similar basic formulation but also has a chemical agent present to aid adhesion, particularly to the metal. The individual materials are based on 4-methacryloxyethyl trimellitic acid anhydride (4-meta), 4-meta with methyl methacrylate, 4-meta with bis-GMA or the halogenated phosphate ester of bis-GMA. Some of these have shown very high bond strengths to enamel and apparently offer advantages over the purely mechanical retention of the other types of cement. Their chemical bonding to the metal is dependent on there being a metal oxide layer present.

The setting reaction of some cements is inhibited by oxygen and air must be excluded from the bridge margins to permit polymerization. Vaseline is effective and similar compounds are supplied with the materials.

Metal surface conditioning

The success of resin retained bridgework depends to a great extent on the adhesive bond between the metal, cement and tooth. Therefore, an understanding of the various methods for conditioning the metal fit surface is crucial.

The electro-etching technique creates a surface that enables the resin cement to make a micro-mechanical interlock with it. Surface contamination with water, saliva or organic debris will prevent the interlocks from forming, explaining the care that must be taken with the bridge once it has been etched. The electro-etched surface does not allow the chemical affinity cements to use this aspect of their formulation.

Grit-blasting of a nickel–chromium or chromium–cobalt ceramic bonding alloy with 40–50 μm aluminium oxide grit creates a surface disruption of the metal that allows similar micromechanical interlocking but also leaves a well-bonded oxide rich layer. The dual affinity cements react with this oxide layer to enhance their adhesion.

Semi-precious ceramic bonding alloys, on the other hand, do not form this oxide layer on grit blasting and to obtain the reactive oxide surface they must be tin plated and then heated in a ceramic furnace to oxidize the tin.

A further treatment method is the deposition of silicon and silane compounds on to the metal surface. This requires special equipment but bonding is only moderately improved.

Debonding

Catastrophic failure of resin retained bridges by sudden debonding is the major drawback of the technique. It is now more dramatic, with the use of single wings being more common. A two-wing bridge might fail on one wing first, allowing the patient a little warning of disaster. One way of providing reassurance is to supply the patient with an emergency stand-by partial denture.

Debonding may occur either almost immediately after placement or much later. The immediate type occurs in the first 48 hours after cementation and the debond is likely to be caused by contamination during cementation and failure of the tooth–adhesive interface. The later failures can occur at either of the two interfaces but, increasingly, evidence of failure within the cements has been found; this is presumed to be the result of fatigue.

Debonding appears to be more common in cases where multiple abutments have been used. When partial debonding occurs, it is essential that the bridge is removed and recemented, otherwise there is a high risk of recurrent caries under the loose wing. Alternatively, the loose wing can be cut off and the bridge thereby converted to a cantilever type.

Resin retained bridgework – Summary

The development of the technique and materials has proceeded rapidly. It is now the treatment of choice for single tooth replacement.

Unfavourable occlusal factors and heavily restored abutment teeth may contraindicate the technique.

Minimal tooth preparation is required to enhance mechanical stability.

Retention is achieved through a dual affinity polymer-based luting cement via the acid-etch technique to enamel, and grit-blasting to the bridge alloy. Base metal bonding alloys are preferred.

Patients should be warned of the possibility of catastrophic failure and perhaps supplied with an emergency partial denture to have in reserve.

20

Fixed prosthodontics:
Design and planning of conventional bridgework

Here, replacement of teeth by conventional bridgework is considered. The principles underlying the choice of design and treatment plan are described. Of particular importance are the condition of the abutment teeth and their periodontal support. The problems of hypodontia, changes in appearance and cleft palate are discussed.

Introduction

The more routine use of adhesive bridgework of various designs, and its long-term success, has lead to considerable reduction in the indications for bridgework retained by inlays and crowns. In sound mouths, the resin retained bridge is now the treatment of choice for a single tooth, with conventional bridges being used for more extensive cases.

Design considerations

There is very little scientific evidence to support many of the principles of conventional bridgework. These principles have evolved empirically through clinical experience and some documentation of failures. Experience in the biomechanics of resin retained bridgework has called into question some of the previously accepted tenets of conventional bridgework.

The design of conventional bridgework depends upon:

● Biological factors
● Mechanical factors
● Aesthetic factors

Biological factors

The longevity of conventional bridgework depends firstly on the biological integrity and prognosis of each of the abutment teeth chosen in the provisional design. The crown must be caries free and the pulp must either be healthy, or be replaced by a sound root filling with no apical pathology. The periodontium must also be healthy and well maintained.

Teeth that have suffered previous periodontal breakdown are not excluded from being abutments, but the disease must have been stabilized and the plaque control maintained at a high level.

The number of abutments required to support the proposed pontics is often a matter of opinion. Ante proposed that the combined surface area of the periodontium of the abutment teeth should be equal to or greater than that of the teeth to be replaced. This seems to assume that the abutments will be subjected to greater loading, possibly up to one-and-a-half times more.

However, work from Scandinavia, where extensive bridges were provided for periodontally dubious teeth, together with clinical experience, suggests that Ante's law is overcautious, and that occlusal loading is reduced by a biofeedback mechanism to a level appropriate to the support available. This concept is also supported by experience with resin retained bridgework where the single wing cantilever design has been found to be successful. For the case shown in *Figure 20.1* the 'older' conventional bridge design would almost certainly have involved two abutments.

Rather than looking at the axial occlusal loads on abutments, it seems more important to consider the possible leverage and torque that may be applied. This will arise during function and parafunction in lateral excursions and protrusion, and the assessment of the occlusion is crucial in bridge design. For example, in a canine guided occlusion, lateral stresses on other teeth are small, and perhaps this is more favourable when they are used for abutments.

This is not to say that a large number of pontics can be supported by a few abutments, because the retention of the bridge is also important. Rather, bridges made with less than the traditionally ideal level of support can be clinically successful.

The *periodontal surface area* of the abutment teeth is clearly important, though. The upper canine and upper first molar have the largest areas making them ideal for bridge support, whilst at the other end of the scale, the upper lateral incisor has a very small root and is often unsuitable as a terminal abutment. Pragmatically, then, it would seem sensible to adopt designs that utilize the teeth with the largest periodontal surface areas available in the particular circumstances.

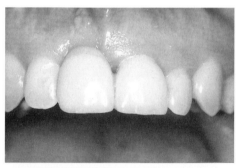
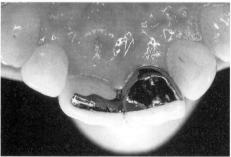

Fig. 20.1 Single retainer cantilever bridge replacing 1̲. This design would not have been used prior to the experience with single wing resin retained bridges.

Mechanical factors

Each abutment tooth must also be structurally sound. It must either have dentine of sufficient quality and quantity to allow the preparation of a retentive crown, or it must be capable of being restored, depending upon its position, by a pinned core or a post and core.

Each preparation should provide excellent mechanical retention, achieved by near-parallelism of walls (Chapter 15). In a multi-abutment bridge each of the preparations must provide proper stability individually. If, for example, a short preparation is included, this will be a site for stress concentration and subsequent cementation failure.

The most retentive retainer is a full crown, with the partial veneer crown being a close second. For simplicity of preparation and reliability of fit, the full crown has become the most used retainer. The use of inlays as bridge retainers has largely died out – mainly because a tooth that is suitable for an inlay would also be suitable for a resin retained wing and therefore the conventional bridge would be contraindicated. Partial veneer crowns leave the buccal surface uncut and can therefore be aesthetically better and are more conservative of tooth tissue. However, the preparation is more technically demanding.

Parallel preparations

Abutment preparations for a fixed–fixed bridge must be parallel. The bridge will eventually be inserted in one piece and this will not be possible if each preparation has a different path of insertion, caused usually by abutment tooth tilting. This aspect of each case must be assessed using a model surveyor. The problem of non-parallel alignment of abutment teeth may be solved by:

- Preoperative orthodontics
- Compromises in preparation angulation
- Assembly joints
- Telescopic retainers or copings

Orthodontics may be used to upright the malaligned tooth or teeth. However, this may not always be practical due to the length of time required or the reluctance of the patient to undergo the treatment that usually requires fixed appliances.

Preparation angulation may be changed from the ideal for each abutment to a compromise in keeping with that required for the bridge design. However, such alterations may result in:

- Loss of retention of individual retainers
- Inability to seat the bridge

Figure 20.2 shows this diagramatically. It is possible to cut parallel preparations on tilted teeth but

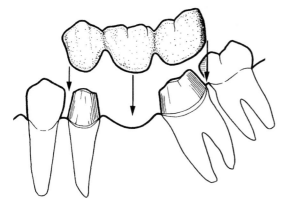

Fig. 20.2 Tilted teeth – the problem of a fixed–fixed bridge. The seating of the bridge is prevented by the mesial aspect of the last molar, even though the preparations have been cut with a common path of insertion. Also, retention of the prepared molar is reduced by the angulation

adjacent teeth may prevent the bridge being inserted. Also, changing the path of insertion may reduce preparation height and extent of preparation walls that are parallel to each other, thus reducing the retention.

Assembly joints

To overcome this loss of retention, the paths of insertion of each retainer can be made in the long axis of each abutment crown. The bridge can be assembled in the mouth at cementation by means of a joint in one of the connectors parallel to the path of insertion of the other bridge element (*Fig 20.3*). The dovetail slot may either be milled in the casting or be a preformed precision retainer (*Fig 20.4*).

Non-rigid connectors/movable joints   In addition to permitting the assembly of individual elements of bridges, joints have been used for many years as *non-rigid connectors*, also referred to as *movable joints*. The concept is that even when a bridge may be made fixed–fixed from the angulation of the abutments, empirical biomechanical considerations suggest that one retainer may either take more stress than another or that one is less retentive than another. The design factor of *stress breaking* has been applied to these circumstances.

Stress analysis suggests that this concept is flawed. The type of joint shown in *Figures 20.3* and *20.4* is capable of very little freedom of movement. Loading in the long axis of the joint might allow some independent movement of the

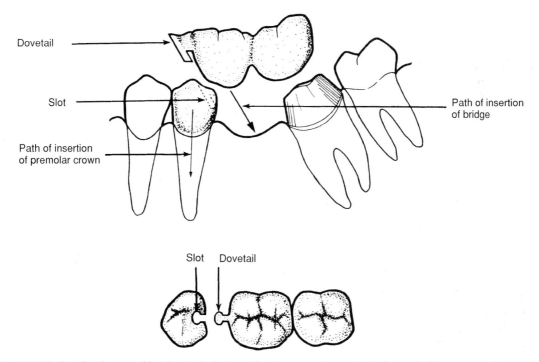

Fig. 20.3 Tilted teeth – the assembly joint. Each abutment has its preparation cut in its long axis. The crown on the premolar has a dovetail-shaped slot cut in its distal aspect (the preparation must be reduced to accommodate it) and the pontic has the dovetail-shaped piece to fit the slot. The line of the dovetail is the path of insertion of the molar preparation

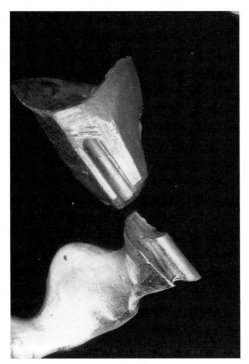

Fig. 20.4 A precision retainer that can be used as an assembly joint

bridge elements but, of course, most masticatory movement would cause lateral and shear forces on the bridge. In the face of these forces the joint would, in effect, be a rigid connector and not break stresses at all.

This concept is a very good example of scientifically unsubstantiated clinical opinion.

Telescopic crowns or copings

An alternative way of overcoming discrepancies in paths of insertion is to use telescopic crowns based on metal copings (*Fig. 20.5*). Each abutment is prepared to receive a casting in whatever path of insertion is appropriate for that abutment. Each casting or *coping* has its outer aspect shaped to the common path of insertion for the bridge and slots/grooves may be incorporated to increase retention.

This structural system, whilst solving the angulation problem, also has the advantage that the individual abutments are capable of being treated separately in the event of failure. Very often the overlying bridge is cemented with a temporary cement that allows easy removal of the bridge if problems arise.

Aesthetic factors

This may well be one of the major reasons for providing bridgework and a decision must be made about which teeth should have tooth-coloured components and which can remain all metal. The all metal retainer utilizes a minimal preparation and is technically less demanding than an aesthetic one.

The aesthetic component has to have space in the preparation to accommodate it and requires higher technical skills for its construction, particularly if it is to function in the occlusion. Aesthetic materials tend to be applied directly to a metal subframe and

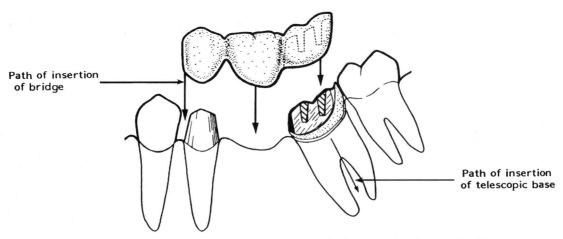

Path of insertion of bridge

Path of insertion of telescopic base

Fig. 20.5 Tilted teeth – the telescopic crown. The preparations are in the long axis of each tooth. A gold coping is made for the molar, which is milled to receive a partial veneer crown with slots and grooves. The path of insertion of the bridge is then aligned with the premolar preparation

may be ceramics or polymer-based composites. Pre-formed cemented facings are no longer used.

Wherever possible, and with the agreement of the patient, the occlusal surfaces should be reproduced in metal (Chapter 14).

If the purpose of the bridge is to alter the aesthetics, then this must be planned carefully at the diagnostic stage (see below).

Pontic design

Pontics may require a functional component as well as an aesthetic one.

For its functional aspects, the pontic should provide occlusal stability by the inclusion of centric stops and supporting cusps as appropriate. Its participation in the new occlusal scheme should be decided (see below) and it should not create any interferences.

Pontic function could be fulfilled by a flat 'plate' of metal, and the *wash-through* or *sanitary* pontics

are useful from the periodontal viewpoint, in that the tissues around the pontic are readily accessible for cleaning. However, their use is usually confined to the molar region, and is now rare because of their aesthetic limitations.

The majority of pontics need to be aesthetic and this means the inclusion of a tooth-coloured facing in conjunction with the metal functional surface. The aesthetic component must reproduce the embrasure spaces and contact the soft tissue of the alveolar ridge. This tissue contact must be firm, but not intrusive, to reduce plaque accumulation under the pontic. Contact should be confined to the buccal or labial aspect of the ridge, with the remainder accessible to the tongue for natural cleansing (*Fig. 20.6*).

If alveolar resorption has been extensive, pink ceramic may be incorporated at the neck of the pontic or, alternatively, a removable pontic with gumwork should be considered (See below).

Special oral hygiene techniques are required to maintain the undersurface of the pontics and

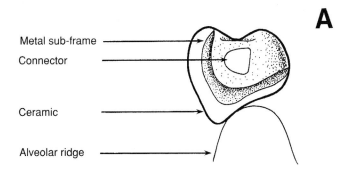

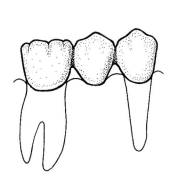

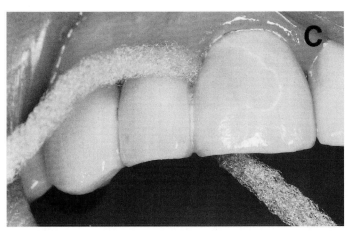

Fig. 20.6 Features of bridge pontics. **A** The ridge contact of a premolar pontic. Ceramic covers the soft tissue. **B** The embrasure spaces are made wide enough to allow cleaning. **C** Superfloss being used to clean the embrasures and fitting surface of an anterior pontic.

connectors in a plaque-free condition, and the most useful aid is Superfloss (*Fig. 20.6C*).

Preoperative considerations for conventional bridgework

The patient

The patient must be well motivated, clearly informed of his or her responsibilities in maintaining the proposed restoration and understand the sequence of appointments and what is to be achieved at each. The patient must be capable of

maintaining good plaque control and any caries, periodontal disease and poor restorations must have been stabilized.

The occlusion

A preoperative occlusal analysis should have been performed (Chapter 14) and consideration given to possible tooth movement in order to achieve more favourable tooth relationships.

Orthodontics has an important role to play in mouth preparation where there are malposed teeth or uneven spacing, particularly anteriorly. Uneven spacing is illustrated in *Figure 20.7*. The case has

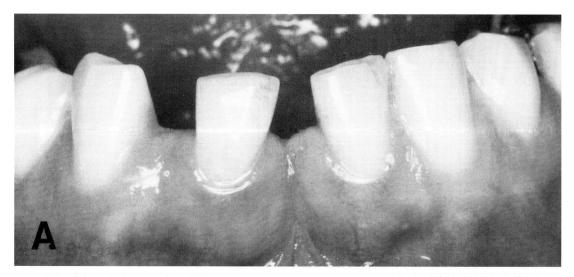

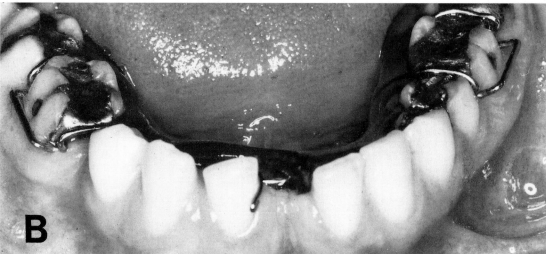

Fig. 20.7 Pre-bridge orthodontics. **A** The uneven spacing caused by the loss of one central incisor would make bridgework difficult. **B** The lateral incisor has been retracted by a simple appliance and the single tooth space can now be restored with a cantilever bridge

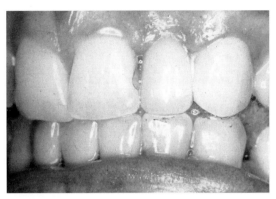

Fig. 20.8 The |2 has been replaced as a cantilever bridge from the |3. In left lateral excursion, the pontic takes all the load and transmits this as rotational forces to the canine, which was painful. The bridge should have been made to maintain canine guidance

TREATMENT OF POTENTIAL ABUTMENT TEETH

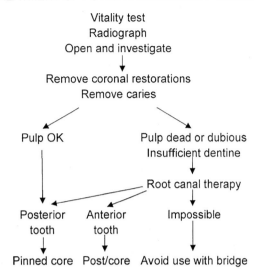

Fig. 20.9 The treatment of potential abutment teeth

been converted from a difficult four or five-unit bridge to a simple two-unit bridge.

Equilibration of precentric prematurities is desirable on those teeth destined for preparation. If a prematurity is removed by the preparation without knowledge of its relationship, the occlusal pattern can be changed, leading to loss of occlusal clearance of the preparation (Chapter 14).

The pattern and strength of occlusal function in lateral and protrusive excursions is of great importance in anterior bridgework. For example, an upper lateral incisor can be replaced as a cantilever bridge from the canine in favourable cases. But this design should not be used if the pontic will receive lateral stresses from the lower incisors in lateral excursions. This would result in unfavourable rotational forces being applied to the canine. In these circumstances, the bridge should either have positive canine guidance, thereby discluding the lateral incisor pontic, or it should involve the central incisor as well in a fixed–fixed design (*Fig. 20.8*).

partial denture before bridgework was contemplated, there may be gingival complications if the denture was tissue borne. This is discussed in Chapter 13.

These points, then, imply that a very thorough examination of the mouth aided by vitality tests and radiographs (Chapter 2) is essential prior to the prescription of bridgework.

Teeth that are provisionally designated for retainers should have any restorations of unknown origin or quality removed, and the remaining tooth examined to determine its physical and biological state (*Fig. 20.9*). Even if the natural history of the restoration is well known, it must be assessed for its possible durability under a retainer when prepared: a simple example is the replacement of a non-pinned amalgam by a pinned core, because the tooth substance providing the retention of the former might well be removed during preparation.

Abutment tooth assessment

The biological integrity of all the teeth must be clear from the start. Those teeth to be included in the bridge should not have pulps of dubious vitality, nor have any root fillings of questionable prognosis.

Loss of periodontal support does not in itself preclude the use of particular teeth as retainers, but the disease must be controlled and stable. This will involve a thorough periodontal assessment and associated therapy. If the patient has worn a

Aesthetics

The provision of good aesthetics is clearly an important goal for both the patient and the continuing reputation of the clinician!

The basic design outline will detail those areas to be tooth-coloured and those to be constructed in metal. The patient should be aware of and approve such recommendations. Now further consideration must be given to the particular characteristics of tooth colour and position. The technician must be involved at this stage so that he or she can give advice about any shade matching problems that might dictate a change in design or might require special techniques.

If the existing tooth shape and position is satisfactory for appearance and function, then this must be copied exactly. This original blueprint may be in the form of an existing denture or bridge. However, if a change in aesthetics is proposed, then this needs to be defined clearly at the planning stage.

Small changes, such as the closure of a diastema, can be easily accomplished, but major changes, such as reduction of overjet, are far more complicated. This may involve elective devitalization of teeth outside the proposed arch line, together with post and cores and, worse still, the positioning of retainers or pontics in zones where tongue activity may make them unstable. This type of major cosmetic change should be attempted only when the patient's objectives and motivation are clearly established, and the clinician is clear in his own mind that these can be satisfied. Additional abutments will need to be included in the design to withstand the unfavourable muscle forces. In other words, it is a permanent splint that is being constructed.

The provisional restoration needs to be very accurate, and considerable time must be spent in assessing its stability. The patient must also be in absolute agreement that the new teeth are what were envisaged. *Figure 20.10* shows a case where the overjet and incisor irregularity have been reduced by means of a splint. This involved devitalization of the central incisors and crown preparations on the lateral incisors and canines. The extent of the change, particularly in overjet, was quite small and the amount of work involved was large, but the end result was patient satisfaction.

A word of warning – dentists and plastic surgeons are prone to the attention of perfection seeking individuals. If the patient appears to be making unreasonable or strange demands, the dentist should be suspicious. It is better to refuse to provide treatment, tactfully.

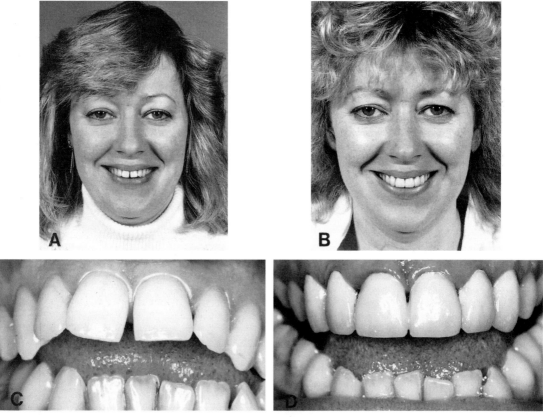

Fig. 20.10 The change in aesthetics provided by a splint on 321|123 **A** and **C** Before. **B** and **D** After

Basic bridge designs

Much (if not all) bridge design is empirical, based on the accumulated, acquired wisdom of clinical experience, or simple personal prejudice! As has already been stated, very little objective work has been carried out on the biomechanics of the subject and it is doubtful as to how much in the way of physical laws would be appropriate in an area that is so dependent on biological status and response. It is a truism to say that every case is different.

A few basic guidelines can be advanced, such as:

- Keep designs as simple as possible. For example, if two upper incisors are being replaced, make two three-unit bridges, rather than one six unit
- Use canine or molar teeth as abutments wherever possible
- Avoid upper lateral incisors as strategic abutments

The diagrams in *Figure 20.11* show a series of 'standard' designs that will work in favourable cases. Unfavourable factors, such as short roots, loss of periodontal support, 'heavy' occlusion and so on might cause the empirical addition of a further retainer to each design. Full crowns are shown as the retainers, but partial veneer crowns could be substituted.

Precision retainers

Simply, precision retainers are connectors that retain dentures without the use of externally visible clasps. The denture may be a complete denture or partial, unilateral or bilateral. The unilateral partial denture is sometimes called a *removable bridge*. This is considered to have an advantage over a conventional bridge in that it is partly tissue borne, and therefore larger spans can be contemplated. Again, this is an empirical decision.

Precision retainers consist of two precisely interlocking parts, male and female, one of which is soldered into the retaining crown and the other which is processed into the denture. The part fitting the retaining crown may be intra- or extracoronal. The intracoronal type requires a more extensive tooth preparation to accommodate it within the crown profile.

There are many designs, most named after their inventors. Some include internal springs and stress breaking devices, and others fix the denture permanently by means of minute screws. They are expensive and technically demanding to use, but do have advantages in a few particular cases. It is

worth being familiar with two or three types of basic design.

Where there has been extensive alveolar loss, a denture base is often necessary to make up the deficiency. In this type of case, a pair of extracoronal retainers, such as the Mini-Dalbo (see manufacturers' list on p. 281), can be used (*Fig 20.12*).

Larger partial dentures may be aesthetically more pleasing in the absence of clasps, but teeth having the precision retainers on them must be splinted for support to other teeth, thus making the overall treatment plan complicated, costly and technically demanding.

The use of precision retainers in complete dentures is discussed in Chapter 24.

Special problems

Cleft palate

With modern orthodontic and plastic surgical management of the cleft palate, cases with massive crown work to retain obturators are a thing of the past. The cases treated by modern techniques, though, may require crowning of teeth which are malaligned in the cleft, or bridges to replace missing teeth in the cleft area, particularly the lateral incisor.

Bridgework design must be modified so that the bridge is not fixed on either side of the cleft. This applies equally to resin retained bridges and conventional bridges. The cleft may be stabilized by fibrous tissue only, and movement between the maxilla and premaxilla is possible. The forces generated by such movement are easily sufficient to debond a resin retained bridge of a fixed–fixed design, and cantilever types are more reliable.

Hypodontia

Congenitally absent teeth can present considerable restorative problems. The common occurrence of missing upper lateral incisors and retained deciduous canines is discussed in Chapter 16.

Cases with several missing teeth are usually associated with considerable drifting of the other teeth and these usually have small crowns. These cases must be treatment planned with the orthodontist to discuss tooth movement into more favourable positions to support bridgework. If each missing tooth can have a natural tooth on each side, and these natural teeth have reasonably sized crowns, then bridgework is possible. Larger spaces coupled with small crowns usually commits the patient to partial dentures.

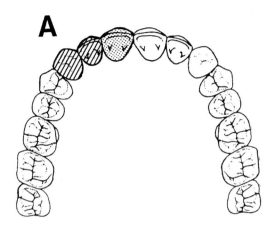

Fig. 20.11 Some basic bridge designs

A Cantilever
Pontic: 1|
Retainers: 32|
Uses canine as major support; useful if the adjacent central incisor cannot be used in a single crown cantilever

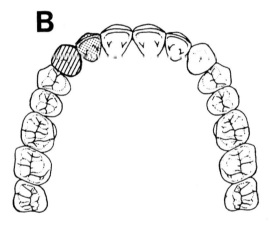

B Cantilever
Pontic: 2|
Retainer: 3|
Must be no lateral stress on pontic in excursions

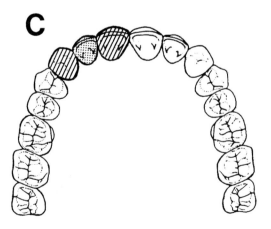

C Fixed–fixed
Pontic: 2|
Retainers: 31|
If the occlusion causes lateral stress on the pontic in **B**, use the central incisor as well

Design of conventional bridgework – Summary

Much bridge design is empirical.

The important considerations are choosing abutment teeth that are biologically and structurally sound and have healthy periodontia.

Full assessment of the occlusion and tooth alignment using a diagnostic mounting is essential.

Full crown retainers of gold or ceramic fused to metal are the simplest and most reliable retainers.

Malaligned teeth may be incorporated in bridgework after re-alignment by preoperative orthodontics or by using assembly joints or copings.

21

Fixed prosthodontics: Clinical procedures for conventional bridgework

> The decision to construct a bridge has been made and its design decided. The abutment teeth are stable with appropriate foundations in place. This chapter discusses the clinical, practical stages in bridge construction.

The sequence of clinical stages in constructing a bridge is:

1. Preoperative diagnostic mounting and model surveying
2. Shade registration and provisional bridge planning
3. Preparations
4. Working impression
5. Occlusal registration
6. Try-in and trial cementation
7. Permanent cementation
8. Review and recall

Preoperative diagnostic mounting

The original diagnostic mounting may be adequate for this stage, but, if any teeth have been equilibrated, or major changes in tooth contours have been made by cores, then new impressions should be taken and a new mounting made.

The mounting should be in centric occlusion unless this position cannot be defined accurately. In this case centric relation is used (see Chapter 14).

The occlusal registration for a centric occlusion mounting should be without an interocclusal record if at all possible. Orientation of the models to the position of best fit, together with checking this position against the patient, marking it and

mounting, should be satisfactory for most patients.

If missing teeth prevent the accurate orientation of the models, then occlusal rims will be necessary, but these should be adjusted carefully to ensure that centric occlusion is being recorded, and not a position influenced by the presence of the rims in the occlusion.

If there are enough teeth, but the position is imprecise, two 'islands' of cold-curing pattern resin, one in each quadrant of the lower arch, will provide the minimum interference with closure, and will locate the models accurately for mounting with tooth-to-tooth contact.

The incisal table should be customized to the protrusive and lateral excursions (Chapter 14).

The mounting will provide a record of centric occlusion before it is destroyed by tooth preparation, and will be the basis for the provisional bridge. Accurate surveying to decide the path of insertion will be done and a duplicate mounting will allow trial preparations to be carried out as a rehearsal to predict problems of angulation and paralleling.

Shade and provisional bridge

The shade and tooth characteristics should be recorded at the planning stage, particularly before teeth are cut.

The provisional bridge must also be planned before the teeth are cut. Its functions are:

- Protection of cut dentine
- Maintenance of the occlusion
- Maintenance of gingival health
- Restoration of aesthetics
- Maintenance of abutment position

and in some cases

- Diagnosis of changes to the occlusion and/or aesthetics

The provisional bridge may be made at the *chairside* after the preparations have been completed or in the *laboratory* either before or after the preparation stage. The majority are made of synthetic resin, but spans of more than four units need a metal subframe and resin facings for durability. The provisional may be in use for as long as six weeks and therefore needs to be constructed carefully.

Chairside construction of provisionals is appropriate for short spans of uncomplicated bridgework. These may only be in place for a matter of a couple of weeks and, for this relatively short period, the inferior aesthetics and lower strength are not usually a problem.

Chairside construction technique

The preoperative model is used as a template with the shape of the pontics and retainers being provided either from the diagnostic waxing or from the addition of denture teeth to the model. The areas of the buccal and palatal surfaces that will have minimal reduction should be overcontoured by adding wax, so that eventually this will be reproduced in the provisional as thicker walls. Without this, the overlying resin would be too thin for adequate strength.

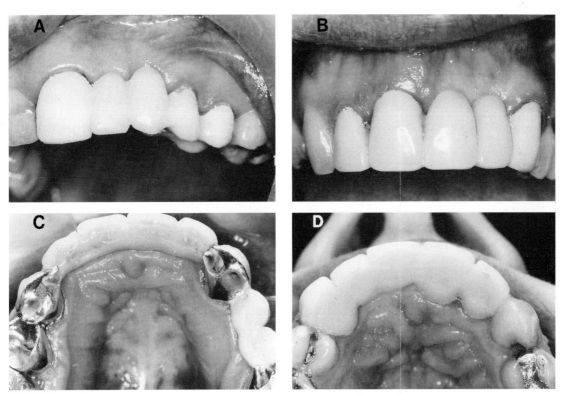

Fig. 21.1 Provisional bridges. **A** Cold curing resin, chairside made type. This has very bland aesthetics and has to be overcontoured for strength. It is satisfactory for short spans, or for a few days whilst a more accurate provisional is made. **B** All resin, laboratory constructed type. The labial aspects are made from denture tooth facings and the remainder is made from a waxing and hydroflask cured acrylic. This is suitable for trying new occlusal schemes and changes in aesthetics. If it is made from trial preparations on the diagnostic mounting, the retainers must be rebased in the mouth with the addition of cold curing resin. **C** Cast silver/resin type. This is necessary for long spans. The incisors are denture tooth facings, retained to the metal by hydroflasked acrylic. The occlusion and aesthetics can be checked accurately on this type of provisional. **D** As for **B**

An impression is made of the area of the bridge in silicone putty. Only a sectional impression is required, but this must extend by at least one tooth either side of the abutment teeth so that the impression, or mould as it is to become, can be stabilized in the mouth. A refinement of the putty impression is to use a vacuum-formed resin sheet that is moulded to the preoperative model or diagnostic waxing.

At the chairside, following the completion of the preparations, the seating of the mould is checked for accuracy, gingival retraction cord is placed to protect the gingival tissues, a smear of petroleum jelly is applied to the dentine surfaces and a self-curing resin, preferably one designed for provisional bridges, is mixed and syringed around the necks of the prepared teeth and into the mould. The filled mould is seated on to the teeth, located correctly and left in place until the initial set of the resin has occurred. The mould is then removed, together with the new bridge and its excess. The excess is trimmed carefully back to the preparation margins and the pontic gingival margins rounded. The embrasures, particularly at the cervical margins, must be cleared carefully.

The bridge is replaced on to the teeth, and the marginal adaptation checked. The occlusion is then corrected using abrasive points following identification of inaccuracies with shimstock and articulating paper. Additions can be made easily to the resin as necessary (*Fig. 21.1A*).

Laboratory construction technique

The all-resin bridge can be made by flasking the waxed trial preparations model, perhaps having incorporated denture tooth facings as appropriate, and processing in the same way as a denture. At the chairside, the fit of the bridge is likely to be inaccurate because the free-hand cutting of the teeth is unlikely to match the free-hand cutting of the model. Therefore the bridge must be relined in resin on the preparations to achieve accuracy (*Figs. 21.1B* and *D*).

The metal based bridge, whether cast in silver, student's alloy or even bonding alloy, requires exactly the same technique as that required for the final restoration. It must be made from an impression of the finished preparations as quickly as possible, with an all-resin bridge made at the chairside as a very temporary intermediate restoration (*Fig. 21.1C*).

If the provisional has been used to verify a new occlusal scheme and has been adjusted for this or for tooth shape and position, an impression of the arch including the bridge must be taken and remounted to the existing mounted opposing model. The incisal table should then be recustomized.

Preparations

Whilst each abutment will be prepared in accordance with the basic principles discussed in Chapter 15, the major consideration in most bridgework is achieving a single path of insertion for the bridge.

The desired path of insertion should be decided from the diagnostic mounting using a model surveyor and the path should be marked on the model abutments. If an assembly joint is to be used with different paths for each abutment, these paths can again be marked on the model.

In short span bridges, with two or three abutments, the path can usually be transferred to the mouth by eye, with extreme care being taken to keep the burs in this single path whilst cutting.

For longer spans and multiple abutments, some additional help will be necessary. Proprietary parallelometers can be purchased, the simplest being a pair of parallel pins on an extending arm.

This approach may not be sufficient for cross-arch work and some reference device can be made for the particular patient in the laboratory. A flat sheet of 4 mm acrylic sheet is trimmed to fit the arch to be prepared, and modified with cold curing acrylic to locate accurately to the occlusal surfaces. It should extend laterally beyond the buccal surfaces of the abutment teeth by about 2 mm.

The model is mounted on a surveyor whose survey rod is aligned with the chosen path of insertion. The acrylic sheet is placed on the model and holes are drilled by a surveyor mounted handpiece to locate pins at the side of each abutment. The pins can be screwed in, or glued by cyanoacrylate cement. This device locates in the mouth to indicate the desired paths for each abutment.

Additional help can be provided during the tooth preparation by cutting the teeth roughly and then taking an alginate impression. This is cast in plaster mixed with hot water for a rapid set, and the resulting model is checked with a surveyor for accuracy of paralleling whilst the patient remains in the chair. Afterwards, the preparations are finally defined.

The presence of posts and cores in the design can be used to assist paralleling. Preparation for the posts is the first stage and an impression is taken of the post holes. The cores can then be waxed parallel to the predicted path of insertion (*Fig. 21.2A*) and, when cemented, provide a very accurate guide for preparation of the other abutments (*Fig 21.2B*).

Modification to the basic design of abutment preparations is also necessary in the connector region. Tooth removal should be increased here to

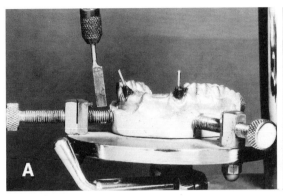
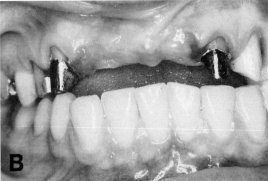

Fig. 21.2 A Waxing the cores for an anterior bridge. The model has been mounted on a surveyor to align the cores precisely with the chosen path of insertion. **B** The cores cemented. The bridge is to replace 21│1 from 43│23, and the preparations have been completed using the cores as alignment guides. Note the shape of the vital tooth preparations giving good retention and the contour allowing correct thickness of ceramic. Note also the lack of gingival trauma after preparation

provide additional strength in the subsequent casting. Where precision retainers or other non-rigid connectors are to be used, box preparations will usually be necessary to accommodate them.

Impression and shade

These have been dealt with in Chapters 16 and 17.

Occlusal registration

Centric occlusion is required, with clear tooth-to-tooth contacts. If a position of 'best fit' is still present, in spite of occlusal reductions, this should be used without an interocclusal record; reproduction of the position from the preoperative mounting is possible.

If centric occlusion has been lost by the tooth preparation, then the most accurate method of registration is by *registration copings*. These are shells of acrylic or metal that fit the prepared teeth accurately and on to which cold curing resin is added to register the tooth relationships (*Fig. 21.3*). The coping can be made on the master die and used to check that the preparation margins have been accurately reproduced. Metal, such as cast silver, is better than resin for this purpose if the margins are really questionable.

Alternatively, copings can be made intraorally on lubricated preparations by freehand application of resin and the occlusion registered at the same time. Clearly, these cannot be used to check margins.

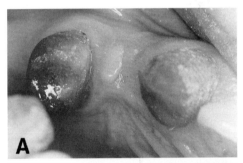
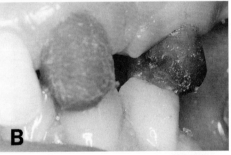
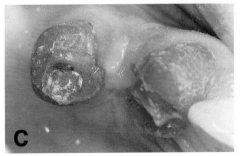

Fig. 21.3 Laboratory made copings of pattern resin for occlusal registration. **A** Occlusal view. **B** Buccal view in occlusion. **C** Occlusal view of registration imprints

The master model, when completed, is mounted to the untouched opposing arch of the preoperative mounting. A further face-bow registration is therefore not necessary.

Articulator angles will have been determined from the diagnostic mounting and can be set again for the master models. However, when constructing crowns and bridges, it is common to use condylar angles that are slightly lower than average. This has the effect of making cusp heights lower, cusp slopes shallower and fossae more open. Therefore the likelihood of introducing occlusal interferences unwittingly is much reduced.

Upon completion of the impression and registration, the provisional bridge should be cemented with a weak zinc oxide–eugenol (ZOE) cement, or a proprietary temporary cement.

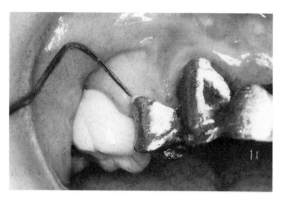

Fig. 21.4 Metalwork try-in showing examination of the margins

Try-in

This is possibly the most critical stage, wherein the established errors are either seen and accepted, or completely missed. It depends on the level of perfection and perception of both the dentist and the technician as to what passes and what is rejected. Only the obvious needs stating – the larger the errors, the less chances of success for the restoration.

Metal subframe

The try-in of the metal subframe before addition of ceramic has several advantages:

- Accuracy of the casting can be checked. If there are errors, then the time and cost of adding ceramic to a deficient base are avoided
- The localization between abutments can be checked and changed if necessary without jeopardizing the ceramic by resoldering
- The occlusion can be checked and adjusted without damaging the ceramic glaze

For short spans, where the dentist and technician are confident in the impression, then a metalwork try-in could be omitted. For longer spans there should always be one (*Fig 21.4*). Now that the use of shoulder ceramics is common, the metal subframe does not need to extend to the outer edge of the shoulder. However, for the purposes of a metal try-in the technician should provide this aspect so that fit can be checked. This excess metal will be cut back before the ceramic is added.

Where one retainer fits and the other(s) does not seat fully, there can be a localization error. The bridge should be sectioned carefully into individual pieces, with one connector being maintained to hold each pontic. Each retainer should be tried on its abutment individually (*Fig. 21.5A*). If each seats accurately, the new arrangement should be fixed by addition of cold-curing acrylic in the mouth.

To stabilize the retainers for this procedure, a small amount of non-setting paste, e.g. zinc oxide in Vaseline, should be applied to the retainers' fit surface (*Fig 21.5B*). A non-residue, burn out pattern resin is then carefully applied to the sectioned joint to stabilize it rigidly (*Fig. 21.5C*). The relocalized bridge is then removed, cleaned and returned to the laboratory for soldering.

Failure of a sectioned retainer to seat requires a new impression after the preparation has been inspected carefully for undercuts. These may have created an impression fault not seen on the die.

If the dentist is at some distance from his laboratory, relocalization may be impractical and it is then more common for a complete new impression to be taken.

Final bridge

The bridge should be examined carefully with the teeth dried and isolated and, where possible, a pack in place to prevent loss of the bridge into the pharynx. The following must be checked:

- Marginal adaptation of retainers
- Retention and stability
- Integrity of contact areas with adjacent uncut teeth
- Adaptation of the pontics to the soft tissues
- Occlusal relationships in centric occlusion, centric relation and excursions
- Aesthetics – colour, shape and tooth position
- Speech
- Patient approval

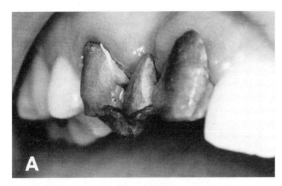

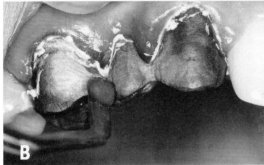

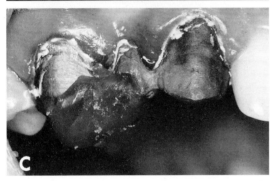

Fig. 21.5 Relocalization of a metal sub-frame. **A** The try-in did not seat on the premolar. The bridge has been sectioned between the pontic and the premolar retainer, and now seats correctly. **B** Zinc oxide–Vaseline paste has been applied to the fitting surfaces to stabilize the bridge during application of the fluid acrylic. **C** The acrylic must be extensive to make sure that there is no movement upon removal of the bridge and during its journey to the laboratory

Marginal adaptation

A probe should traverse all the margins smoothly from tooth to retainer without catching. Positive edges can be trimmed back, but negative edges are a deficiency and the retainer must be modified or remade. If the master die does not reproduce the defective margins, then a new impression of the problem abutment is needed. The new die can be relocated alongside the satisfactory dies in a new model and the new retainer soldered into the new restoration.

If the margin was reproduced on the original die, then ceramic can be added to the retainer. Soldering, though, to build out a deficient metal margin is not usually acceptable.

If a retainer is not seating onto the abutment margin, then the following should be checked:

- Fit surface of preparation – temporary cement remaining
- Fit surface of retainer – ceramic present, casting excess from airblow in investment
- Contact areas – tight, preventing seating
- Movement of abutments under provisional bridge
- Localization of retainers – one seats and the other(s) lifts off

The first four are fairly easy to overcome. Careful inspection will reveal extraneous material and use of floss will demonstrate tight contacts.

Small tooth movements may have occurred whilst the provisional bridge was in place. This may be due to occlusal forces or due to slight displacement by the temporary cement. Not every bridge seats home exactly at the first attempt, and small discrepancies can be overcome by 'stressing' the periodontal ligament by alternate loading and releasing.

Cotton wool rolls or a tongue spatula may be placed on the occlusal surface of the bridge, and by alternate clenching and relaxing, the patient can induce minor movements of the abutments. This works only for small seating problems.

Retention and stability

The bridge should not be dependent on its cement lute for retention. Looseness may be caused by over-tapered preparations or poor adaptation of castings. The fit of the individual dies on their retainers should be checked and if these are loose, the bridge should be remade. If the dies are tight, then an impression fault is possible; the impression will need to be retaken after checking the parallelism of the preparations.

The bridge should not rock when pressure is applied to each retainer and if it does, there is likely to be a casting error on an individual retainer, or seating problems referred to earlier.

Contact areas

Check these with floss. A correct contact allows floss to 'click' through on pressure. Slack contacts will require the addition of solder or more ceramic to correct them. Tight contacts should be eased and repolished.

Adaptation of pontics

The pontic should touch the underlying soft tissue lightly on insertion of the bridge. The neck of the pontic should blend smoothly with the alveolar ridge to promote natural cleaning during function.

Occlusal relationships

Occlusal stability should be checked by marking each new cusp/fossa relationship with articulating paper and checking that each holds shimstock on light closure. The natural cusp/fossa relationships should also be checked with shimstock to ensure that the bridge is not preventing even occlusion elsewhere.

Check mandibular closure on the retruded arc of closure to centric relation to ensure that the bridge is not introducing new precentric premature contacts.

Adjust cusp slopes or fossa width but not supporting cusp height, as the removal of the cusp tip will also remove occlusal stability

Check lateral and protrusive excursions for freedom of movement and for the presence of non-working interferences. If the bridge is reproducing canine guidance, this must be steep enough to disclude the non-working side. If interferences are introduced, the bridge must be modified, rather than equilibrating other teeth. Similarly, incisal length should provide enough depth of incisal guidance to disclude the posterior teeth (*Fig 21.6*).

Aesthetics

The patient should be the final arbiter of appearance. Aesthetics were discussed in Chapter 16.

Speech

A standard passage of prose to be read by the patient can be used, but it is better for natural speech to be the deciding factor. This means a period of trial cementation.

Trial cementation

Once a bridge is cemented permanently, the modifications that can be done subsequently are very limited. Therefore, it is better to fit the bridge with a weak temporary cement and allow the patient to try it for about four weeks for speech and function, and for the other members of the family to approve the appearance.

The patient must be warned, though, of the weakness of the cement, and to return immediately if there are any symptoms; this usually means cement failure in a retainer.

Permanent cementation

The patient's opinion and experience are discussed after the trial cementation, and the occlusal

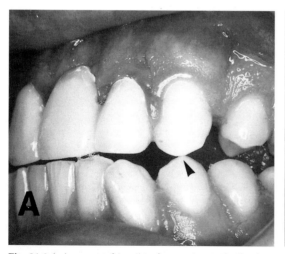
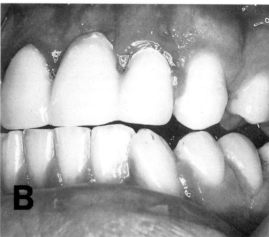

Fig. 21.6 A A non-working interference in protrusion (arrowed). The patient has a provisional bridge at 21|1. In protrusion the incisal edges are not in contact because of the interaction between |3 and |4. The choice is either to lengthen the incisors to disclude the interference, or to equilibrate. **B** In this case, the appearance was satisfactory therefore the interference was equilibrated

relationships rechecked. Modifications to tooth shape, colour and size are possible by refiring the ceramic. This may mean refitting the provisional bridge whilst the permanent one is away in the laboratory.

If further modifications are made or the patient has any reservations, another period of trial cementation is indicated.

Only when all are satisfied should the bridge be cemented permanently. After the cement has set, check the marginal adaptation again and clean excess cement from the embrasures and from under the pontics.

Teach the patient appropriate oral hygiene procedures (Chapter 20).

Review and recall

Finally, check the bridge again a week or two after cementation and make sure the patient is performing the oral hygiene required and that there are no problems with this. Routine six-monthly recall should be arranged and the apical condition of all the abutments reviewed radiographically at this time. Further radiographs should be taken routinely every two years or so. Silent pulp death and apical infection of abutment teeth are possible.

Anterior bridgework

This presents the dual problems of combining aesthetics with function. It is an important part of bridgework, since the cosmetic aspect is a strong motivating factor for the patient. This, coupled with the desire to be rid of the intrusion of a partial denture, provides a demand which can only be satisfied by the highest clinical and technical standards. The ability to make good anterior bridgework is a good practice builder; the converse is also true.

The patient will either have an existing partial denture or bridge and there are two possible lines of treatment. The existing prosthetic teeth may be satisfactory from the aesthetic and functional viewpoint, in which case they should be copied exactly in combination with the new retainers.

On the other hand, one or both aspects may be unsatisfactory and this will necessitate more in the way of diagnosis and planning and a longer stage with the provisional bridge.

Replacement of existing aesthetics and function

Where the patient is to have a denture or bridge replaced that has *satisfactory* aesthetics and function, the sequence following stabilization is:

1. Diagnostic mounting and examination of the occlusion
2. Customize the incisal guidance table of the articulator
3. Provisional bridge, preparations
4. Provisional bridge approval
5. Final bridge – trial cementation and permanent cementation

Changing aesthetics and/or function

Where existing teeth and/or function are *unsatisfactory*, the sequence is:

1. Diagnostic mounting and examination of the occlusion
2. Diagnostic waxing to establish new aesthetics and/or function
3. Customize incisal guidance table to diagnostic waxing
4. Preparations and impression; chairside provisional
5. Construct provisional bridge on master model to diagnostic waxing
6. Check function and aesthetics of provisional and modify if necessary
7. Approval of provisional
8. If modifications have been made, impression of provisional *in situ*
9. Articulate model of approved provisional and recustomize incisal guide
10. Mount master model, construct final bridge
11. Trial cementation
12. Permanent cementation

Case report 1

The re-establishment of original aesthetics when these have been changed by a poor bridge or partial denture will be greatly helped by old photographs of the patient. *Figure 21.7A* shows a case where the upper central incisors were originally replaced by a partial denture following trauma. Some years later, the patient's general dental practitioner offered her a bridge instead of the denture.

The bridge design was a six-unit fixed–fixed bridge from the upper lateral incisors and canines. The bridge was fitted, apparently without the patient's agreement, and this is shown in *Figures 21.7 B* and *C*. The patient was unhappy with the

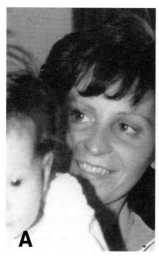
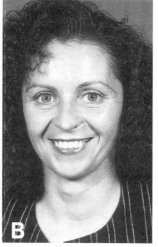
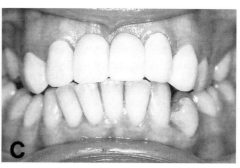

Fig. 21.7 Replacement of a partial denture by bridgework 1. **A** The patient with a partial denture replacing 1|1. **B** and **C** The first bridge showing poor contour and shade

appearance and if this is compared with the old photograph reproduced in *Figure 21.7A*, it can be seen that the incisor angulation has been changed. The shade was also incorrect; the new bridge was Vita A1 in comparison with the shade of the adjacent teeth that was C2.

The sequence for the management of the case was that described earlier for changing aesthetics and function. Following the visit for the diagnostic mounting, the old bridge was removed by cutting each retainer with a serrated tungsten carbide bur (Beaver Jet, see manufacturers' list on p. 281). The underlying preparations were inspected and checked for vitality and were found to be satisfactory. An impression was taken and a 'temporary' provisional bridge made at the chairside.

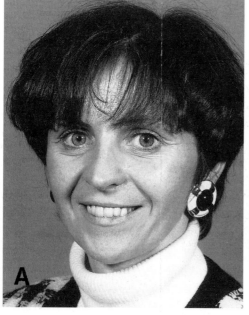
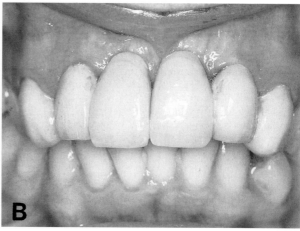

Fig. 21.8A and B Cemented bridge replacing that shown in *Figure 21.7*

With the aid of the old photograph a provisional bridge was made in the laboratory on the master model. It was fitted at the next visit with temporary cement. The patient wore this for four weeks and returned with the approval of her family and herself.

An impression was taken of the provisional bridge in place and the model from this provided the guide for the technician for the tooth shape and position. The bridge design was changed for simplicity from a single six-unit bridge to two three-unit cantilever bridges. The trial cementation was uneventful and the bridges were cemented permanently four weeks later (*Fig. 21.8*).

Case report 2

Figure 21.9A shows a patient who had the four upper incisors replaced by an acrylic partial denture after an accident when she was 13 years old. The denture teeth are small and set centrally over the edentulous ridge. The tooth size is probably the result of the denture being made in the patient's early teens and subsequent growth and development of the dentition over the subsequent 13 years has left the denture behind.

The teeth are now to be replaced with a bridge and to improve the aesthetics they need to be larger and set anterior to the ridge. This repositioning is complicated by alveolar resorption. To disguise this and to fill in the embrasure spaces, which would appear black to the casual observer, pink ceramic has been incorporated (*Fig. 21.9B*). The facial appearance has been improved by the lip support provided by the anterior setting of the pontics.

This new appearance and function was assessed using a provisional bridge. When the bridge was considered satisfactory by the patient, a model was mounted on the articulator and the incisal guide customized. To customize the incisal guide, cold-curing acrylic was placed on the incisal table, and whilst soft, the incisal pin was moved in it with the tooth-to-tooth contacts being maintained in protrusion and lateral excursions. When hard, the table reproduced the movement paths that were guided by the provisional bridge contours (see Chapter 14).

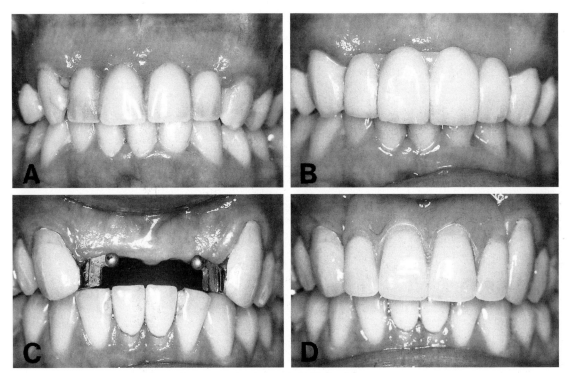

Fig. 21.9 Replacement of a partial denture by bridgework 2. **A** The denture teeth are too small and are set palatally. **B** Bridge with pontics set more anteriorly to support the upper lip. Pink ceramic has been incorporated in the embrasures to hide minor alveolar resorption. **C** This case has extensive alveolar resorption and requires a denture base to replace 21|12. It is retained by Mini-Dalbo precision retainers attached to crowns on 43|34. **D** The removable bridge in place

Alveolar resorption

The two cases described above show two methods of adapting the pontics for anterior bridges. The first case (*Fig. 21.8*) has the pontics touching the edentulous ridge directly and because there has been little resorption the mucosa appears as natural gingival tissue in the pontic embrasures.

The second case (*Fig. 21.9B*) shows more resorption, and without the filling of the embrasures with pink ceramic, dark spaces would be seen between the pontics. These spaces might also lead to air bubbles being formed during speech and accumulation of debris.

If there is even more resorption then the use of simple pontics would be difficult. Then it is better to use a denture base to make up the tissue loss and this could be incorporated in a precision retained removable bridge (*Fig. 21.9C* and D).

Spring cantilever bridge

In this design, the anterior pontic is retained by an abutment tooth in the posterior region and the connector is a long metal bar that is supported by the palate (see *Fig. 20.11F*).

The advantages of the design are that sound anterior teeth can remain uncut and that natural spacing of the anterior teeth can be reproduced. The disadvantage is the presence of the bar in the palate, which requires regular cleaning to avoid it initiating inflammation.

It is another design that has been largely superseded by resin retained bridgework, though there are still a few cases for which it is indicated.

The choice of abutment is important, as is shape of the vault of the palate. A single premolar, usually the first, is sufficient to retain the bridge, since the bar provides a tissue-borne element to the design and is also a stress breaker.

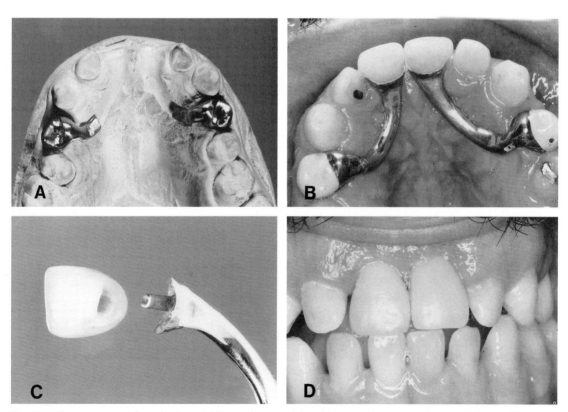

Fig. 21.10 Two spring cantilever bridges. **A** The working model with the metal–ceramic retainer subframes. The paths for the bars have been gouged from the palate at a depth appropriate to the tissue compressibility. The area for the soldered joints on the retainers is some way from them, so that the ceramic will not crack when soldering takes place. **B** and **D** The completed bridges in centric occlusion. The anterior spacing and short crown length made this an ideal case for cantilevers. **C** Porcelain jacket crown pontic, made on an aluminous tube.

The retainer can either be a partial veneer or a full crown, depending on the aesthetics and the skill of the operator.

The palate must be shallow so that the bar is well supported. A steep vault will not support the bar and it will lie vertically, rather than horizontally, and more stress will pass to the abutment. The palate must also be 'mapped' by testing compressibility of the tissues in the path of the bar with a ball-ended instrument.

The bar should be embedded to an appropriate depth, and in the more compressible areas it should be to about 2 mm, whilst in the more fibrous areas, 0.5 mm would be possible (*Fig. 21.10A*).

Figure 21.10A also shows the arrangement of two metal–ceramic crowns to link with a pair of bars. The soldered joint, which should be some distance from the ceramic, is applied prior to soldering. Trying to solder the bar at the crown margin would almost certainly result in cracking of the ceramic.

The final bridge requires time at the fitting stage to compress the tissues under the bar before cementation. The tissue will blanch initially and tissue fluid is displaced as the bar embeds itself. This is aided by alternate pressure and relaxation applied by the patient's masticatory muscles.

The pontic is a separate jacket crown that can be replaced independently of the bridge if necessary in the future (*Fig. 21.10C*). At the fitting stage it should be left slightly long to allow for further embedding of the bar during the first week and adjusted at the review visit (*Fig. 21.10D*).

The patient must be shown how to clean under the bar with floss, and this procedure must be done at least once a day.

Clinical procedures for conventional bridgework – Summary

Detailed planning on an accurate diagnostic mounting is essential.

Planning will involve choice of the path of insertion, retainer and pontic design.

A provisional bridge will be needed to stabilize the abutments and restore aesthetics and function.

Retentive preparations parallel to the path of insertion will provide stability for the final bridge.

Use occlusal registration copings for accuracy of articulating the master model.

The try-in stage will reveal deficiencies in the fit and occlusion of the retainers and pontics.

Aesthetics must be approved by the patient; always use a trial cementation phase.

Always choose bridge designs that are simple.

22

Removable prosthodontics: Partial denture design

This chapter considers the first stages in the provision of partial dentures and the principles of their design. A step by step development of the design should be used to create the components for support and retention. Clinical experience and a detailed knowledge of the materials available will produce rational designs.

Diagnosis and treatment planning

Supplying a partial denture to a patient is usually the last phase of a course of restorative treatment. The decision to make a partial denture is made following a thorough history and examination and discussion with the patient.

The dental history should include details of previous denture wearing experience (if any), such as:

- Do you wear a partial denture?
- If so, do you find it satisfactory?
- How long have you worn it?
- If unsatisfactory, what are the complaints?

If the patient has never had a partial denture then it is helpful to ascertain if he or she would like one and, if so, why. These questions will help to clarify patient motivation and help in deciding first, whether to provide a denture and secondly, the type of denture that should be provided.

The examination of the mouth and oral tissues should include condition, location and number of remaining teeth, condition of the soft tissues, nature of the saddle areas, i.e. height, width and consistency of the residual ridges and an assessment of oral hygiene. The denture(s) should be inspected for fit, retention and stability, occlusal relationship, wear and cleanliness.

When all the information has been gathered and considered, a diagnosis can be reached and a treatment plan formulated. The plan will include a provisional partial denture design in order

that other dental treatment can be completed appropriately and the mouth prepared to receive the partial denture.

The design, therefore, must be decided before embarking on other restorative procedures, since it may affect the type and material of the other restorations to be placed. This will optimize the function of the denture and maintain the health of the mouth. Further information and investigation is necessary in order to consider the design of the appliance and this includes:

- Analysis of the occlusion
- Radiographs
- Model surveying

Study models serve a number of uses, of which the most important are:

- Examination of the occlusion
- Model surveying – analysis of path of insertion and withdrawal, location of undercuts
- Trial preparation of the teeth
- Construction of special trays
- Communicating with the patient and the laboratory technician

Examination of the occlusion

Although the occlusion can be assessed initially during an intraoral examination, the use of models permits a more detailed inspection and it is, of course, also possible to view the teeth from the lingual aspect. This enables tooth contact to be examined more easily to determine whether sufficient space exists for components of the partial denture design, e.g. occlusal rests. In many cases sufficient information can be gained by examining hand-held models. However, this reproduces the occlusion in a static state only. Therefore, for a more detailed analysis of occlusal function and articulation (movements of the mandible into and out of the position of maximum intercuspation), it is necessary to mount the models on a semi-adjustable articulator (Chapter 14).

Model surveying

Model surveying is performed in order to determine the *path of insertion* and removal of the denture and to locate undercuts on the dento-alveolar tissues suitable for its retention.

Trial preparation of the teeth

Earlier analysis of the occlusion and the model surveying might reveal the necessity for modification of the teeth, either to improve or eliminate occlusal interferences or to alter the shape of the crown of the tooth. For example, reduction of the height of contour on the proximal surface of a molar or premolar can produce a *guiding plane* parallel to the path of insertion in order to gain a more intimate contact between prosthesis and tooth. Such modifications can be rehearsed on the model before being performed in the mouth.

Construction of special trays

Special trays are essential for subsequent impression procedures to ensure accuracy and reproduction of detail and, where appropriate, proper tissue moulding of the borders.

Communication

Study models provide an excellent aid when discussing or explaining treatment to the patient and are an essential part of the prescription to the technician. An outline of the partial denture design can be drawn on the model to give a three dimensional appreciation in those cases where a drawing on paper could be open to misinterpretation.

Partial denture design

Designing the denture is a clinical responsibility, since the dentist is the only person with all the information concerning the condition of the mouth and teeth. Liaison with the dental technician is perfectly appropriate and the technician may have suggestions to make from his or her point of view. However, the denture remains the dentist's overall responsibility.

Partial dentures should be designed using basic principles in a logical step-by-step sequence. Before detail of the design is considered, four guidelines should be borne in mind:

- Simplicity
- Support from the teeth
- Relief of the gingival tissues
- Rigidity of the connectors

Simplicity

A partial denture is more likely to be tolerated by the patient if the design is kept as simple as possible. Components should be added for good reason only and to serve a definite function. The smallest number of clasps should be used compatible with retention and stability.

Support from the teeth

In the lower arch, with its reduced mucosal area available for support, it is especially important to take advantage of the remaining natural teeth for support.

Relief of the gingival tissues

Plaque is more likely to accumulate around teeth covered by a denture and the problem is greatly magnified in patients with poor oral hygiene. Where gingival coverage is unavoidable, the impression surface of the denture should be closely adapted to the underlying soft tissue so that this does not grow to fill the potential space.

Rigidity of the connectors

A thin flexible connector can be distorted easily during function or if gripped too firmly whilst cleaning.

Design stages

Provided a step-by-step sequence is followed, no important components will be omitted, the design will be functional and will satisfy the necessary criteria for clinical success. A number of choices are usually available when designing, and this means that it is possible to produce several different designs for the same patient. The final selection is based on many factors including knowledge of the

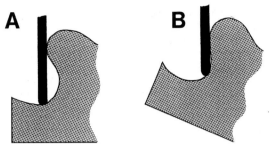

Fig. 22.1 Surveying an alveolar ridge. **A** The survey rod illustrates a path of insertion that is at right angles to the occlusal plane; the denture base would not enter the tissue undercut. **B** The surveyor is tilted to provide a path of insertion that allows the denture base direct access to the tissue undercut. In view of the likely displacing forces in function, this undercut area will now provide direct and possibly indirect retention

clinical condition of the mouth, shape and length of the edentulous saddles, the patient's motivation and previous dental experience, availability of technical support and the overall costs of the treatment to the patient.

Path of insertion/withdrawal

The *path of insertion/withdrawal* can be defined as the path followed by the denture from its first contact with the supporting tissues until it is fully seated. In effect this relates to the direction in which the patient will insert and remove the denture. There may be a single path, or multiple paths of insertion and it may or may not coincide with the path of displacement, i.e. the direction in which the denture tends to be displaced in function

(assumed for the purposes of design to be at right angles to the occlusal plane).

The path of insertion must allow the individual saddle areas to be seated but, in addition, varying the path may improve the ability to engage tooth undercuts with clasps (see below). It is therefore necessary to consider three areas of undercut in relation to the proposed denture at this stage:

- Alveolar bone undercut
- Undercut caused by the approximal surfaces of abutment teeth overhanging the saddles
- Buccal and lingual tooth undercut in relation to clasping

The path of insertion is chosen whilst surveying the model. Surveying is usually undertaken with the occlusal plane horizontal, but a tilt may allow hard or soft tissue undercuts to be engaged and therefore improve the fit of the denture to the tissues. An example of this would be when upper anterior teeth are missing and there is a labial boney undercut present. Tilting a model with the heel down may permit more efficient utilization of the labial undercut (*Fig 22.1*), always assuming that this does not compromise the insertion of the denture in other areas.

Many partial dentures have multiple saddles and the final path of insertion of the denture is likely to be a compromise between the ideal paths for each individual saddle together with the clasping sites. The approximal surfaces of abutment teeth may overhang the edentulous space and influence the path of insertion adversely (*Fig. 22.2A*). Here consideration should be given to modifying the approximal surface by grinding to produce *guiding planes* or, in severe cases of tilting, provision of a restoration with the correct contour (*Fig. 22.2B*). If undercuts remain in the approximal aspects, these

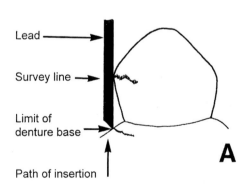

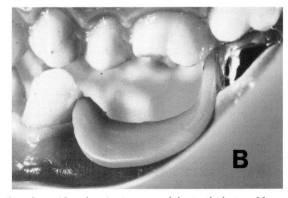

Fig. 22.2 Approximal undercut. **A** The survey line on an edentulous ridge showing an area of the tooth that could not be contacted by the denture base. This is a potential site for plaque accumulation. **B** Modification to the approximal surface will eliminate this undercut. In cases of tilting, a crown may be constructed to create a favourable relationship

will be blocked out on the master model to prevent the denture base from engaging them during processing and later at the fitting stage.

Having obtained the desired tilt, the path of insertion should be recorded on the model. This can be done either by 'tripoding' (marking the model at three widely-spaced points with the analysing rod fixed at the same vertical height) or by making vertical marks on the side of the base of the model in the anterior and posterior regions. Recording the path of insertion allows the model to be re-orientated to the same position during later stages.

Once the path of insertion has been chosen it is necessary to:

- Outline the saddles
- Define the support
- Provide direct retention
- Consider the provision of indirect retention
- Join the components with connectors

An integral and important component of these stages is the choice of materials.

Denture base materials

Partial dentures may be constructed from polymethyl methacrylate (acrylic resin) alone or, more commonly, in association with cast metal and/or wrought metal. The common alloys that may be used are cobalt–chromium, stainless steel and wrought and cast gold. Acrylic resin or ceramic may be used for the teeth.

Saddles Polymethyl methacrylate is used universally for replacing alveolar bone. Its ease of use and general physical properties are well suited to this. The only question mark over its use relates to the possibility of residual monomer within the material causing tissue reaction. This applies to both partial and complete dentures and is discussed in Chapter 28.

Clasps and connectors Whilst acrylic resin is cheap and simple to use, it is not an ideal material for partial denture connectors. It needs to be at least 2 mm thick for strength and therefore can be intrusive, particularly on the palate. Its plaque retaining ability is higher than the metal alloys and therefore its potential to initiate or aggravate periodontal disease is large. Notwithstanding these disadvantages, acrylic resin may be used successfully as a connector in the palate, provided the gingival tissues are not covered.

Cobalt-chromium alloys are the alternative for connectors whilst clasp materials are chosen according to the undercut that they are to engage.

It is generally accepted that a cobalt–chromium clasp should only engage 0.25 mm of undercut because this material has a high elastic modulus and will deform or fracture if a deeper undercut is engaged. Cast gold has a modulus of elasticity of approximately half that of cobalt–chromium and can, therefore, engage greater undercut (0.5 mm). A wrought structure, in the form of gold or stainless steel wire, has a lower modulus and good recovery and can be used in deeper undercuts (up to 0.75 mm).

Teeth Acrylic resin denture teeth have the advantages of being easy to adjust, chemically bonding to an acrylic resin denture base, and cheapness. Their disadvantages are having low wear resistance and the potential for becoming discoloured. Ceramic teeth, on the other hand, are more durable, retain their colour and are therefore more aesthetic in the long term. Their disadvantages are that they are more time consuming to adjust, both clinically and in the laboratory, and mechanical retention to the denture base must be provided.

Edentulous saddles

A classification of the edentulous saddles allows dentists and technicians to use a simple 'shorthand' description when referring to a particular case. The Kennedy classification, which follows, is probably the most widely accepted:

Class I   Bilateral edentulous areas (of any length) which lie posterior to the remaining teeth

Class II   A single edentulous area (of any length) which lies posterior to the remaining teeth

Class III   A single edentulous area (of any length) bounded by one or more teeth anteriorly and posteriorly

Class IV   A single edentulous area (of any length) which lies anteriorly to the remaining teeth

An early decision is required on which missing teeth (if any) need to be replaced. Guiding factors will include aesthetics, function, stability of the occlusion and wear of remaining teeth. The outline of the saddle(s) of the teeth to be replaced should be drawn on the design sheet.

Support
Support for the saddles can be provided by:

- Teeth
- Mucosa
- Teeth and mucosa in combination

As a general guide, permanent mucosa-borne dentures with no tooth support should be avoided in the mandible because of the danger of overloading limited support area.

A tooth-borne design is possible only when the saddles are bounded by natural teeth, i.e. in Kennedy classes III and IV. In these cases the load is transferred to the natural teeth through extensions of the partial denture positioned on appropriate areas of the teeth and named accordingly:

● Occlusal rests – molars and premolars
● Cingulum rests – upper canines and incisors
● Incisal rests – lower canines and incisors

In Kennedy classes I and II the support is provided by both teeth and mucosa. In these cases the saddle should cover as large an area as possible to distribute the load widely.

Direct retention

A *clasp*, or direct retainer, is the component that resists dislodgement of the partial denture along the path of withdrawal. It is a flexible metal arm that engages the undercut region on a natural tooth and forms part of a clasp unit, i.e.

● Retentive arm
● Reciprocating arm
● Occlusal rest

The reciprocating arm is used as a bracing component to prevent displacement of a tooth by a direct retainer in its active phase, i.e. when it is being inserted or withdrawn over the survey line. The retentive arm should always be used in combination with a rest to ensure a proper and constant position. The portion of the clasp arm above the survey line is thicker and provides bracing against lateral movement, whilst the portion below the survey line must flex to engage the undercut after insertion (*Fig. 22.3*).

The teeth chosen as potential retaining sites are examined with the analysing rod on the model surveyor and suitable undercuts and the survey lines marked with a lead marker. *Undercut gauges* can then be used to measure the depths of undercuts available in order to define the position

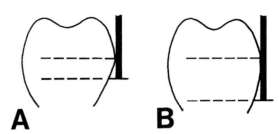

Fig. 22.4 An undercut gauge determines the position of the retentive part of a clasp arm within the tooth undercut. **A** The arm is nearer the survey line on a bulbous tooth. **B** The arm is more gingivally placed on a less bulbous tooth

of the retentive portion of the clasp arms in relation to the choice of material (see above). Three gauges are used, one for cobalt–chromium, one for cast gold and one for wrought gold. If the tooth surface is bulbous the clasp arm will be closer to the survey line, whilst if it is shallow the clasp will be more distant, i.e. the clasp arm is engaging a 'standard' degree of undercut for the chosen material (*Fig. 22.1*). On the other hand, if a retentive arm is placed in excessive undercut either the arm will be permanently deformed and no longer functional or it will fracture.

Although there are numerous designs of clasps, many linked with the names of their original protagonists, there are only two basic types (*Fig. 22.5*):

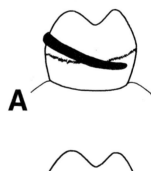

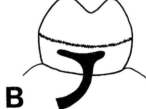

Fig. 22.5 The two basic types of clasp
A Occlusally approaching. This may engage undercut directly from the marginal ridge or from the opposite marginal ridge as an encircling clasp
B Gingivally approaching. This is able to engage a low undercut and also reduces tipping forces on the tooth if the denture base moves into the alveolar tissues

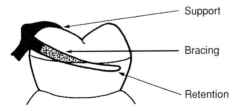

Fig. 22.3 Component parts of a clasp unit. The reciprocating arm will be on the opposite side of the tooth

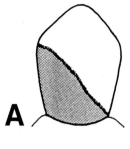

Fig. 22.6 The four basic survey lines with the undercut areas shaded

A Steep oblique. This is the most favourable line for an occlusally approaching clasp with the distance from the marginal ridge to the line permitting a good bracing component for the clasp arm

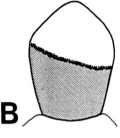

B Shallow oblique. This can be used for an occlusally approaching clasp but only the terminal third of the arm should be below the survey line

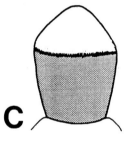

C Occlusal third. This is an unfavourable line for an occlusally approaching clasp because too great a length of the retentive arm will lie below the survey line. Alternatively the line is ideal for a gingivally approaching clasp.

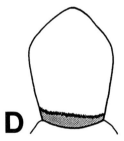

D Gingival third. This is an unfavourable line with no usable undercut available. The tooth contour could be changed by a buccal restoration that increases bulbosity

- Occlusally approaching: those which approach the undercut from the occlusal surface – *suprabulge clasps*
- Gingivally approaching: those which approach the undercut from the gingival surface - *infrabulge clasps*

The type of clasp used will be determined by:

- Depth of undercut
- Position of the survey line
- Prosthetic considerations

The depth of undercut that can be utilized has been discussed previously in relation to the choice of materials.

The position of the survey line will have an important influence on the choice of clasp type. There are broadly four types of survey line (*Fig. 22.6*).

- Steep oblique
- Shallow oblique
- Occlusal third
- Gingival third

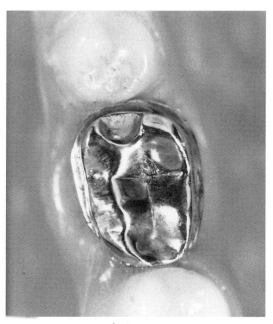

Fig. 22.7 A full crown denture abutment with a rest seat and clasp ledges. The clasps will be constructed within the normal tooth contours rather than adding bulbosity to the tooth

As was mentioned earlier, the survey line can be varied by changing the path of insertion. Whilst this can be superficially attractive in terms of the retentive arm, it must not be forgotten that the reciprocating arm and the denture base must also be capable of being inserted. For example, the low survey line may not allow placement of a clasp arm. It could be 'raised' by the tilting of the model towards this side to produce a higher line. However, the possible result would be to reduce undercut on the opposite side and also prevent seating of the denture base.

A low survey line can often be engaged more appropriately by a *gingivally approaching clasp* (*Fig. 22.5B*). This has the advantage that the arm is longer and more flexible and, because of its position, is often less visible and therefore aesthetically more acceptable to the patient. However, because of its length and relationship to the gingiva, it is more likely to cause food stagnation around the neck of the tooth.

If the survey line is very close to the gingival margin, there will not be space for the clasp arm (*Fig. 22.6D*). Here the contour of the tooth could be increased by a restoration, perhaps simply an acid-etch retained composite supplement.

The design of restorations that are needed for abutment teeth should include consideration of providing retentive contours, shoulders and ledges for clasps and denture bases and rest seats within

the overall contour (*Fig. 22.7*). This is why it is so important to decide upon the denture design before embarking upon restorations.

Indirect retention

Indirect retention is retention obtained by the extension of the partial denture base to provide the fulcrum of a class II lever. The retainer(s) providing direct retention lie(s) between the fulcrum and that part of the denture which is subject to the displacing force. In practice, indirect retainers assist clasps in resisting displacement of the partial denture in function by providing resistance to rotational dislodging forces. The main need is with tooth/mucosa borne (free end saddle) partial dentures, especially in the maxilla because of the constant additional effect of gravity tending to dislodge the saddles.

Indirect retention can be provided by, for example, an extension of the major connector on the palate, additional rests on the natural teeth and the use of a lingual plate instead of a lingual bar connector in the mandible.

Connectors

As the term suggests, connectors join the component parts of the partial denture and are the final stage in the design sequence. They can be classified as either *minor* or *major* connectors. The role of minor connectors is to link the rests and clasps to the major connector or denture base. They should be strong enough to withstand heavy occlusal loads and usually be positioned to lie in embrasures in order to be unobtrusive.

Major connectors join the saddles and should be rigid, so that the partial denture transfers forces to all the supporting structures on both sides of the arch and therefore functions as a single unit. The major connector should, ideally, lie at least 3 mm from the gingival margin in order to maintain health of the tissues.

In the mandible the major connectors can be classified into five categories:

- Lingual bar
- Sublingual bar
- Lingual plate
- Dental bar
- Buccal bar

Variations are, however, possible and include the combination of lingual bar and 'continuous clasp' (a misnomer since no part of the structure engages undercut – it functions as an indirect retainer). The lingual bar and lingual plate are the most commonly used. The lingual bar does not overlay the gingival margins and therefore does not promote plaque accumulation, but requires approximately

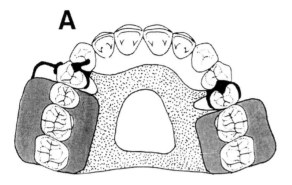

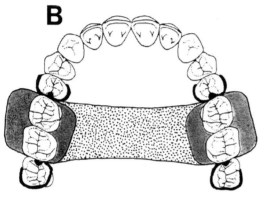

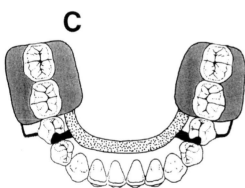

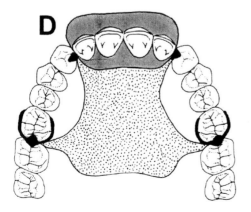

Fig. 22.8 Schematic partial denture designs with details of the components

A Upper bilateral free end saddle (Kennedy class I)

<u>Saddle areas</u>: 765|67, denture base and teeth in acrylic resin

<u>Tooth support</u>: Occlusal/cingulum rests 43|45

<u>Direct retention</u>: i) Gingivally approaching clasp 4| wrought gold – this has better aesthetics on the more anterior tooth

ii) occlusally approaching clasp unit |5 cobalt–chromium

<u>Indirect retention</u>: The posterior aspect of the denture will tend to drop about the fulcrum of the occlusal rests. Components anterior to this fulcrum will resist this displacement. These are rests 3|4 and the anterior aspect of the palatal ring

<u>Connector</u>: Palatal ring

<u>Framework material</u>: Cobalt–chromium

B Upper bilateral bounded saddle (Kennedy class III)

<u>Saddle areas</u>: 76|67, denture base and teeth in acrylic resin

<u>Tooth support</u>: Occlusal rests 85|58

<u>Direct retention</u>: i) Occlusally approaching clasp units 5|5, buccal arms engaging mesial undercut

ii) Occlusally approaching clasps 8|8 again engaging mesial undercuts but because the origin of the clasps is mesial as well the clasps must come from the distal aspects as encircling clasps

<u>Indirect retention</u>: None required in addition to that provided above

<u>Connector</u>: Posterior palatal bar

<u>Framework material</u>: Cobalt–chromium

C Lower bilateral free end saddle (Kennedy class I)

<u>Saddle areas</u>: 76|67 denture base and teeth in acrylic resin

<u>Tooth support</u>: Occlusal rests mesially 5̅|5

<u>Direct retention</u>: Gingivally approaching clasps 5̅|5, I-bars

<u>Connectors</u>: Major – lingual bar

Minor – to rests 5̅|5

<u>Framework material</u>: Cobalt–chromium

Occlusal forces on the denture will cause rotation around a fulcrum joining the mesial occlusal rests – see RPI (mesial rest, distal plate and I-bar clasp) system in text – and the gingivally approaching clasps will be disengaged. Unfavourable tipping forces will therefore not be applied to the abutments

D Upper anterior saddle (Kennedy class IV)

<u>Saddle areas</u>: 21|12 denture base and teeth in acrylic resin

<u>Tooth support</u>: Occlusal rests 76|67 and cingulum rests 3|3

<u>Direct retention</u>: Occlusally approaching clasp units 6|6

<u>Indirect retention</u>: The clasp units on 6|6 approach the mesial undercuts from the distal. Therefore when the denture tends to rotate around the fulcrum between the occlusal rests the clasp arms are engaged to prevent it. Distal extension of palatal plate

<u>Connector</u>: Palatal plate

<u>Framework material</u>: Cobalt–chromium

8 mm of height measured from the gingival margin to the depth of the sulcus i.e. 3 mm from the gingiva to the bar, at least 3 mm depth of bar, and a further 2 mm below the bar to the sulcus.

The lingual plate covers the lingual surface of the anterior teeth and the upper portion of the lingual aspect of the alveolar process. It provides excellent indirect retention and is generally well tolerated by patients but is likely to lead to an increase in plaque deposition and so is best avoided if there is evidence of susceptibility to periodontal disease.

The sublingual bar lies in the floor of the mouth and fills the entire depth and width of the lingual sulcus. It is an attempt to lessen tongue irritation. Since it is shorter than the lingual bar, and also thicker, it is more rigid. A very careful impression technique with functional moulding of the lingual sulcus is required, otherwise the bar will cause irritation of the tissues.

The dental bar is a modified 'continuous clasp' which lies on the lingual surface of the anterior teeth and is clear of the gingival margins. Although ideally positioned, since it can be used regardless of lingual alveolar ridge depth and there is no gingival coverage, it needs to be made sufficiently thick to be rigid and this can reduce its acceptability to the patient.

If the anterior teeth are markedly retroclined and it is impossible to develop a suitable lingual path of insertion, a buccal bar can be used. This is positioned in a similar relationship to the gingival margins and sulcus as the lingual bar. Since it has a wider arch than a lingual bar it is longer and therefore needs to be made thicker to maintain the rigidity. In practice it is rarely used.

In the maxilla there is greater flexibility in the design and type of major connector(s) that can be used. The main requirements are, as with lower connectors, that the structure is rigid, well tolerated by the patient and compatible with gingival health. The following designs are generally recognized:

- Palatal plate
- Anterior palatal bar
- Mid-palatal bar
- Posterior palatal bar
- Open ring (anterior and posterior palatal bar combination)
- Horseshoe, U-shaped

The term 'bar' can include connectors that are wider than the term suggests when compared to use in the lower arch. In these cases others have favoured the term 'strap'.

Indicative designs

Figure 22.8 illustrates four designs that incorporate features that have been discussed above. As with fixed prosthodontics there are no 'standard' designs, with clinical experience being a large factor in choice and there being little biomechanical evidence for many empirical principles.

The RPI case system

The RPI (mesial rest, distal plate and I-bar clasp) system was originally described in the 1960s and further developed in the 1970s although its usage is still limited. The concept attempts to distribute masticatory loads between the saddles and abutment teeth. For each saddle the occlusal rest is placed mesially (as *Fig. 22.8C*), since there is evidence that this gives more favourable and even load distribution. Guide planes mesially and distally are utilized by the minor connector joining the rest to the major connector and the distal plate. This plate lies on the 3–4 mm guide plane so that when the denture is fully seated, the plate contacts only the lower 1 mm of that surface (the portion over the gingiva is relieved).

The I-bar clasp tip is positioned on, or anterior to, the midpoint of the buccal surface and is braced by the guide plane contacts. The load on the saddle causes the denture to rotate about the occlusal rest and the distal plate and I-bar tend to disengage, preventing further stress being posed on the abutment tooth.

Partial denture design – Summary

The design of partial dentures is the responsibility of the dentist and not the technician.

All partial dentures should, wherever possible and particularly in the lower arch, utilize teeth for support to complement support provided by the alveolus.

Cast metal frameworks (direct and indirect retainers and connectors) are recommended for strength, durability, periodontal health and patient comfort in comparison with acrylic resin.

Whilst there are many options for inclusion in a denture design, the overriding consideration is to keep the structure as simple as possible.

23

Removable prosthodontics: Clinical procedures for partial dentures

> The clinical stages in the construction of a partial denture are described, together with their practical problems.

The stages in the construction of a partial denture are:

- Preliminary impressions
- Secondary (working) impressions
- Occlusal registration
- Try-in of metal framework
- Try-in of waxed dentures
- Fit
- Review

Preliminary impressions

An elastic impression material is required to reproduce the details of the natural teeth and tissue undercuts. Alginate is the material of choice but it requires support from an adequate stock tray made from either metal or plastic. Metal is more rigid, whilst the plastic type may be prone to deformation, depending on its design.

A suitable size should be chosen that encompasses all the teeth and extends into the labial and buccal sulci. In areas where there are several missing teeth, for example free end saddles in the lower arch, the tray should be modified by addition of impression compound (suitably moulded) to take up some of the excess space and also extend the tray into the sulcus. This will ensure that the alginate is adequately supported and hence used within its functional limits for maximum accuracy of reproduction. Although only one partial denture may be required, it is necessary to take impressions of both jaws in order to record the occlusion.

After trying-in, the impression trays should be dried and an even, thin layer of adhesive applied to aid retention of the impression material to the trays. The alginate should be mixed according to the manufacturer's instructions using water at room temperature and transferred immediately to the lower tray using a spatula. It is preferable to take the lower impression first since this is generally tolerated better and allows the patient to become accustomed to the procedure.

When taking the upper impression, two techniques are commonly described. In the first the posterior portion of the tray is seated first and then the anterior portion. This is intended to force the alginate upwards and forwards away from the sensitive posterior areas of the palate and fauces. For the second, the anterior portion is inserted with the lip held away from the tissues to aid inspection, and then the tray gradually pushed up posteriorly until a slight excess of material exudes from the border of the tray, at which point the tray is held firmly in position until the alginate sets.

When the surface of the alginate is no longer tacky, it is set and the impression tray can be removed from the mouth. Removal should be performed with a single firm motion, after breaking the seal between impression and tissues, by pulling the cheeks or lips away from the periphery of the tray. Alginate has poor mechanical properties and is likely to tear when removed from deep undercuts or in thin sections, particularly between teeth.

The impressions should be rinsed under running water to remove mucus and/or blood and spray disinfected with aqueous 0.5% chlorhexidine solution or immersed in 1% sodium hypochlorite solution for 10 min. Following decontamination, the impressions should be washed in running water and then sealed in a clear polythene that allows the laboratory technician to inspect them prior to casting the models.

These models may be used for the diagnostic stage (see Chapter 22) or may be constructed after preprosthetic restorative work has been done.

Secondary (working) impressions

All other dental treatment should usually be completed prior to the secondary impression stage. This might include:

- Extraction of unsavable teeth
- Scale and polish and oral hygiene instruction
- Restorations
- Other periodontal therapy
- Mouth preparation for the denture

The design for the partial denture may require preparation of the teeth for rest seats and/or modifying the shape of the teeth in other ways, e.g. grinding, to achieve the chosen path of insertion.

Special tray

A secondary impression is taken in a specially constructed spaced tray and is only necessary for the arch in which a denture will be constructed. The special tray is usually made of acrylic resin, thus allowing it to be easily modified by reduction or addition to the borders. The tray should be tried in the mouth and examined to ensure it is short of the tissue reflection by approximately 2 mm if alginate is to be used. This space allows the impression material to flow around the borders and be moulded by the tissues. There is no need to spend time accurately defining the border extension in those areas of the mouth not related to the fit of the denture; for example, with free end saddles the anterior labial sulcus depth is of no consequence. However, the areas immediately adjacent to the saddles require special attention.

The tray should be constructed with spacers contacting the teeth or tissues in at least three positions, avoiding teeth with rest seat preparations, to ensure correct relocation of the tray and an even thickness of impression material. In the case of a standard impression technique for a lower arch with free-end saddles, the spacers should contact the ridge towards the posterior aspect of the tray.

The most commonly used impression material for partially edentulous mouths is alginate. It is

sufficiently accurate, when supported by an evenly spaced tray, for the construction of cobalt-chromium frameworks. However, it does have some limitations:

- Tearing on removal from severe undercuts
- Poor dimensional stability due to syneresis
- Rapid setting reaction at higher temperatures – therefore the material in contact with the tissues sets first, which may give rise to stresses within the material if the tray is moved during setting

The likelihood of tearing can be reduced by blocking out approximal areas provided they are not essential to the overall impression. Soft carding wax is a suitable material since it is easy to apply and to remove. If it is necessary to reproduce severe undercuts, then an elastomeric impression material should be chosen, i.e. polyether, silicone or polysulphide. The polyethers are stiffer than other elastomers and therefore may be difficult to withdraw from severe undercuts. All three materials are expensive, relative to alginate, and therefore not frequently used in impressions requiring large quantities of material. They are, however, more dimensionally stable and should be considered when the impression cannot be cast within 30 minutes of removal from the mouth (see Chapter 17).

Free-end saddles

Opinions vary regarding the best impression technique for the lower arch with extensive free-end saddles. The single-stage elastic impression produces a cast which represents the hard and soft tissues at rest (mucostatic). It has been argued that a functional relationship should exist between the various supporting structures so that both the teeth and the mucosa are compressed equally. To achieve this and to control the load applied to both teeth and ridges there are two main approaches:

- Reduce the load
- Distribute the load between teeth and residual ridges

The load can be reduced by leaving a tooth off the saddles and/or using narrow teeth.

Distribution of load is more complex and includes such methods as stress breaking and various combinations of the position of rests and clasps. Mucocompressive impression techniques attempt to distribute the load by reproducing the tissues covering the ridge as they are under load.

Free-end saddle rock (downward movement of the saddle under load) can occur if the denture is constructed using a mucostatic impression when there is displaceable mucosa overlying the edentulous ridge. When load is applied to the occlusal surface of the artificial teeth, part of the force is transmitted through the denture base and displaces the underlying mucosa. The degree of movement of the saddle will depend on the load applied and the condition of the tissues underneath it.

Although it is possible to use a dual impression technique, comprising a first stage mucocompressive impression of the saddle areas with an overall alginate final impression, this is a cumbersome procedure. An easier and more effective way is to construct the metal framework on a cast from a mucostatic impression and then to obtain mucocompressive impressions of the saddle areas in order to modify these areas of the cast. This is known as the *altered cast technique*.

Procedure for the altered cast technique

1. Working impression in alginate taken in evenly spaced special tray
2. Construction of cobalt–chromium framework with the addition of close-fitting saddles
3. Clinical try-in of the metal framework
4. Border trimming of the saddles using greenstick tracing compound, or other suitable material
5. Zinc oxide–eugenol paste (or elastomer or impression wax) impression of the saddle areas ensuring that the metal framework is held firmly in position on the teeth whilst the material sets. No direct load is applied to the saddle areas; this ensures the fit of the framework is not disturbed
6. In the laboratory the free-end saddles are cut away from the original working cast and the denture then seated in place; the cast is made good by pouring gypsum into the saddle areas
7. The saddle areas are processed on to the metal framework using the altered working cast

This technique has the advantage that it should avoid free-end saddle rock occurring with a new denture. However, it requires additional clinical and laboratory stages which, it can be argued, are not always necessary. An alternative approach is to complete the construction of the partial denture on the original working cast and to assess the fit in the mouth.

Occlusal registration

There may be sufficient remaining natural teeth to allow the working models to be mounted on the articulator in centric occlusion simply by placing them together by hand. Their relationship should be checked against that of the natural teeth and, if they are in accord, guide lines can be marked across upper and lower teeth to inform the technician of this relationship.

If there are too few teeth to provide a stable and precise relationship but there are some natural teeth that contact and form an appropriate occlusal vertical dimension in centric occlusion, then an occlusal registration using shellac-based wax rims is required. One or two rims may be necessary, depending upon the number of teeth remaining. Here the rim(s) simply aid registration of the horizontal relationship around the existing teeth.

The wax rim(s) can be trimmed vertically until just out of contact either with each other or the opposing teeth and a layer of bite registration material placed on them. The patient is asked to close his or her back teeth together and the occlusion is registered.

If, however, the natural teeth do not give an indication of either the vertical or horizontal relationship, then the reference position for the construction of the dentures will be centric relation. The registration procedure resembles that used in the complete denture technique discussed in Chapter 24.

Sometimes it is more convenient to register the occlusion after the construction of the metal framework with wax rims attached to the framework, for example in cases of lower free-end saddles. This has the advantage that the framework will ensure proper location and support for the rims. However, if there are sections of the framework that have an occlusal relationship, e.g. the occlusal aspects of rest seats, then occlusal registration and articulation will be essential for the construction of the casting. If the metal framework is not constructed to an accurate occlusal record in the first place, much grinding may be necessary at try-in.

Try-in of the wax/metal partial denture

First check that the design constructed by the laboratory conforms to the prescription and that the fit on the model is satisfactory.

The try-in procedures will be determined by whether the try-in is wax or metal. If a wax try-in, then the artificial teeth will have been set up. The check procedure in this case should include:

- Fit and adaptation
- Retention and stability
- Occlusion
- Occlusal vertical dimension
- Tooth position and aesthetics

First examine the mouth and occlusion without the denture, as a reminder of the relationship. An appreciation of the retention and stability of the denture can be gained at this stage by checking the general fit of the base and adaptation to the supporting tissues. A comparison should be made of the occlusion with and without the denture in place to ensure that the natural teeth still come together – unless, of course, the partial denture(s) has been specifically designed to modify the horizontal and vertical occlusal relationships. Tooth position should be assessed in relation to both stability of the prosthesis and aesthetics. Finally, the dentist should check the shade of the artificial teeth against the natural teeth before allowing the patient to inspect them. The patient's opinion is obviously important but, if possible, try to persuade him/her to look at the mouth in a mirror at a realistic viewing distance, i.e. 2 or 3 feet away. Many patients hold a mirror very close to the face and mouth rather than from the distance others normally see them. When both dentist and patient are satisfied with the trial procedures the wax try-in can be returned to the laboratory.

For a metal try-in, first check the general fit by ensuring that the rests fit snugly into the prepared seats and that the denture can be inserted and removed with relative ease. It is most important to check that the metalwork does not interfere with the occlusion. For this reason it is common to inspect the metal framework before the addition of the artificial teeth or saddles. If the patient is to receive partial dentures in both upper and lower arches then the sequence is as follows:

● Check the occlusion of the natural teeth
● Seat one framework in the mouth and reassess the occlusion. If the natural teeth do not contact, reduce the metal accordingly
● Take out the first framework and seat the other and repeat the occlusal examination
● When satisfied that both frameworks are individually satisfactory, examine the occlusion with both in place. Once again adjust the metal accordingly.

NB, it is usually appropriate to limit grinding to the metal framework, but on occasions reduction of the opposing tooth structure may be warranted to gain sufficient space to accommodate a sufficient thickness of metal.

If the upper anterior teeth are to be backed with an extension of the metal framework to give them additional protection, then it is important that a wax trial of tooth position is assessed to establish the correct tooth position and hence the appropriate position of the metal backing.

When the metal try-in has been performed, teeth can be added, either in the laboratory or at the chairside (if small in number) and a further try-in completed. On this occasion occlusal discrepancies should, if the previous visit was performed adequately, be due only to the artificial teeth or wax and can be dealt with accordingly. When satisfied with the occlusion and aesthetics, the try-in is sent to the laboratory for processing.

Insertion of dentures

When the processed dentures are returned from the laboratory the acrylic resin components should be checked for surface imperfections such as sharp ridges or 'pimples'. The denture should then be inserted without undue pressure until firmly seated. Once again a check is made of the fit in relation to adaptation and the extension of the borders. The fitting surface can be checked using a pressure-indicating paste to ensure even contact over the entire surface.

If the partial denture has a metal framework, adaptation of the rests to the teeth and the general fit of the metalwork should be inspected as during the try-in visit. If the denture does not appear to be fully seated then, if the metal try-in was performed properly, it should be only the acrylic resin component that requires attention. Ensure that resin 'flash' has not extruded under the rests or the metal contact areas adjacent to the natural teeth.

If the design of the lower denture includes a free-end saddle, the denture should be examined for downward movement of the saddle under load. This is done by resting the fingers of one hand on the anterior framework while applying pressure to the saddle with the index finger of the other hand. If a free-end saddle rock is evident it will be determined by movement of the anterior framework away from the teeth. In this case the fitting surface of the free-end saddle(s) will require modification. This can be done using either a chairside or laboratory reline.

Chairside reline

A chairside reline can be completed using one of the self-curing resins marketed for use in the mouth (e.g. Tokuso Rebase). The technique is as follows:

1. Having checked for correct extension, the fitting surface of the saddles and the borders are cleaned and dried; they can be roughened if the resin is not 'fresh'
2. Bonding agent, if supplied, is painted sparingly on the area to be relined
3. By following the manufacturer's instructions, a mix of the resin is applied to the saddle areas and the denture inserted in the mouth
4. The framework is held firmly in place with no direct load being applied to the saddles
5. After 2 or 3 minutes the denture is removed whilst the resin is still rubbery, to check that it has not flowed into undercut areas and that there are no imperfections
6. Excess can be trimmed away with a sharp knife and the denture returned to the mouth for a further period to allow curing

7. When rigid, the borders are trimmed and polished
8. A final check is made of the occlusion.

Such a reline should last many months and has the advantage that it is completed with the patient present. A period without the denture is therefore avoided. It is also suitable for domiciliary visits.

Laboratory reline

A laboratory reline requires impressions of the saddles, which can be completed using zinc oxide–eugenol paste, elastomers or impression wax. It may be necessary to reduce undercuts to prevent fracture of the stone model when the denture is removed and also to grind a thickness from the fitting surface to make more space available for the impression material. As before, the fitting relationship of the metal framework to the natural teeth must be maintained by ensuring that the occlusal rests are correctly seated throughout the impression. Readjustment of the occlusion must be anticipated when the relined denture is fitted.

If a reline is a planned procedure at the fit stage of denture construction, sufficient space to accommodate the impression material can be predetermined by using metal foil 1 mm thick over the saddles prior to adding the acrylic resin in the laboratory.

Completion of the insertion stage

When the fit of the denture is considered satisfactory, it should be examined for an even and simultaneous occlusion and adjusted, if necessary, to allow free movement between centric occlusion and centric relation.

When satisfied with all aspects of the denture, the patient is shown how to insert and remove it from the mouth without damaging either the tissues or susceptible components such as clasps.

Finally, the patient should be given advice and guidance on denture wearing, especially if a first-time wearer, and instructions on cleaning both the denture and the natural teeth. Verbal communication should be reinforced by giving the patient a sheet of written instructions. Simple guidelines on cleaning are as follows:

> Unless your denture(s) and remaining natural teeth and gums are kept really clean, there will be an increasing amount of tooth decay and gum disease. To prevent this you should:
> - Clean your teeth and rinse your denture(s) after each meal
> - Pay particular attention to cleaning the teeth next to the denture
> - Avoid in-between meals snacks, especially sweet and sticky foods.
>
> When brushing your partial denture, handle it carefully to avoid bending or breaking any of the parts. The intricate design of a partial denture makes it susceptible to plaque build-up and a routine of brushing using a soft toothbrush and soap and water and soaking in a denture cleanser every night will ensure maximum cleanliness.

Review

A week after the insertion, the patient should be reviewed. Any problems to do with comfort and function should be discussed, and the denture supporting area examined for ulceration or erythema. It may be necessary to ease the denture in such areas.

The occlusion should be rechecked with articulating paper and adjusted if displacement of the denture bearing areas has resulted in uneven contact.

Continuing care should be arranged and the patient told about the importance of maintenance of the denture and surrounding tissues and the need for regular recall to check for caries and periodontal disease.

24

Removable prosthodontics: Complete dentures

Whilst the number of edentulous individuals is decreasing as more people retain their teeth into old age, the provision of complete dentures remains an important aspect of restorative dentistry. It is still much more of an art than a science and the skilled operator exercising a judgement based on experience and artistry will have greater success. This chapter considers the design and construction of complete dentures together with overdentures.

Introduction

When the natural teeth are lost there is a corresponding reduction in alveolar bone, resulting in loss of support for the perioral muscles and tissues. Complete dentures are necessary to restore and preserve the facial appearance and masticatory function and they play a major role in the physical and mental well-being of the individual. The loss of all the natural teeth and the construction of complete dentures can be considered as the final phase of restorative treatment and should, where possible, be the product of a planned transition from the natural dentition. This transition period would normally include a period when partial dentures are worn and would allow the individual to adapt to and master the techniques of wearing prostheses that should encourage ready adaptation to complete dentures.

Functional aspects of complete dentures

Retention

Retention may be defined as the resistance of a denture to dislodgement (usually directly away from the ridge) and in complete dentures depends on two interacting factors. These are:

- Muscular forces
- Physical forces.

Muscular control is very important for complete dentures, especially in the lower arch. If the shape of the polished surfaces of the denture is in harmony with the oral musculature, so that the muscles when functioning tend to seat the dentures rather than dislodge them, retention will be enhanced and the patient's acquisition and development of the necessary controlling skills will be easier.

Physical forces depend upon:

- Adhesion – the force of attraction between dissimilar molecules in close contact (acrylic resin–saliva–mucosa)
- Cohesion – the force of attraction between like molecules (saliva–saliva)

Both are influenced by the nature, quantity, surface tension and viscosity of saliva as well as accuracy of fit of the prosthesis. A thin saliva film provides the best retentive force. For optimum retention dentures must be correctly extended and closely adapted to the tissues.

The flanges of a denture must be adequately extended and correctly shaped to produce the border seal and to provide resistance to the ingress of air that would otherwise destroy the physical forces. The magnitude of physical retention is also related to the area covered by the denture, and it is therefore important to utilize the maximum available (*Fig 24.1*).

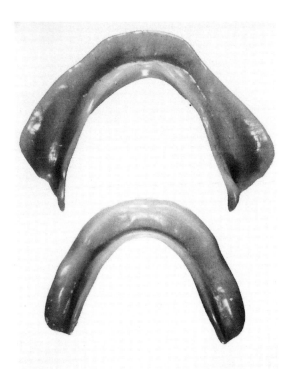

Fig 24.1 The fitting surface of two lower dentures. Lower picture shows a denture that is grossly underextended in both lingual and buccal sulci. Upper picture shows one that is correctly extended

Support

Support provides the resistance to the compressive forces of chewing, swallowing, clenching, etc. The pressure on the underlying mucosa and bone is reduced as the support area is increased, even though there is evidence that individuals with well supported dentures can chew with higher forces, so again the maximum possible area should be used. Close adaptation of the impression surface of the denture ensures an even distribution of load to the tissues.

Stability

This may be defined as the resistance of a denture to displacement (mainly in a lateral direction) by functional forces. The degree of stability depends upon the shape and consistency of the ridges and palate for an upper denture, and the relationship of the denture base to the underlying bone. Flat ridges readily allow lateral movement of the dentures. Maximum stability is gained when the ridges have pronounced contours and where there is little displaceable overlying soft tissue (*Fig 24.2*).

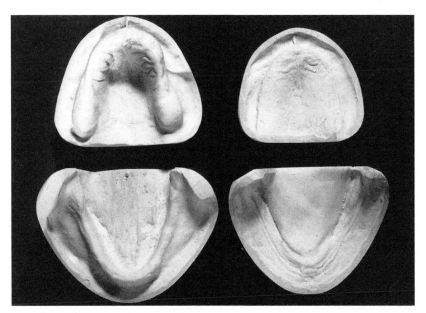

Fig. 24.2 Types of alveolar ridge. The models on the left show ridges that are pronounced and will give good support to the dentures, whilst those on the right show considerable resorption. A denture made for such a flat lower ridge will require considerable adaptation by the patient in order to stabilize and control it

Construction of complete dentures – clinical stages

The construction of complete dentures by conventional techniques involves the following clinical stages:
● Assessment of the patient, treatment planning and preliminary impressions
● Final impressions
● Recording jaw relationships and choice of artificial teeth
● Checking trial dentures
● Inserting and reviewing the dentures

Assessment of the patient

An assessment of the patient will include a past dental history and medical history taken in a calm and relaxed atmosphere. This background information is possibly more important with complete dentures than with any other aspect of dental treatment. A great deal can be ascertained about the individual's expectations and his or her motivation for seeking treatment that can have a direct bearing on the eventual success or otherwise of dentures. Sometimes, especially with those with no previous denture wearing experience, the level of expectation for both aesthetics and function from dentures can be unreasonably high.

The history of experience of wearing dentures is particularly valuable, since it is likely that the individual who has worn the same set of dentures successfully for a reasonable length of time will more readily adapt to new dentures than will the individual for whom a series of unsuccessful dentures has been made. Time spent at this early stage will help elicit whether it is the design and construction of previous dentures that is at fault, or if the personality and mental attitude of the patient are the over-riding factors. It will also help develop a closer rapport with the patient and help the dentist gain a greater understanding of the prosthetic requirements.

Medical history

A thorough medical history should include knowledge of any drugs being taken, since their relationship to certain oral symptoms is well recognized. It is also important to recognize that the elderly tend to suffer from multiple pathology and a patient may be taking several drugs. A complaint of a dry mouth may well be associated with atropinic or tricyclic drugs and can have important consequences for successful denture wearing. There are few medical conditions that contraindicate the construction of complete dentures, though several, e.g. stroke, Parkinsonism and debilitating disease may severely reduce the patient's adaptive capacity and chances of success.

Examination

An examination of the patient should include an extraoral inspection that effectively begins when the individual enters the room. Information on mobility, communication and general demeanour can be rapidly ascertained. Attention should be paid to the face, particularly lip posture at rest and during function, and possible habits associated with denture wearing such as lifting the lower denture with the tongue. The intraoral examination should include a thorough screening of all the tissues for pathology and a more detailed assessment of the denture-bearing tissues. The dentist has an important role in the early detection of oral neoplasia, particularly carcinoma. Palpation of the alveolar ridges will determine their consistency and elicit the presence of painful areas. Denture construction should be delayed if pathology is present, until such time as the oral tissues are returned to an appropriate healthy state.

The patient's dentures should be inspected first out of the mouth for cleanliness, general shape, tooth position and occlusal relationships and tooth wear. They can then be examined individually intraorally for fit, border extension, tooth position in relation to the tongue, cheeks and lips, and aesthetics before making a general assessment of stability and retention. With both dentures in place, horizontal and vertical occlusal relationships and freeway space can be determined. This examination will identify design features that can either be reproduced in the new dentures or modified to create improvements.

Other investigations that may be necessary include radiographs that may reveal the presence of retained roots and buried teeth, and other rarer pathology such as cysts, blood screening for deficiency states and smears or culture to confirm the presence of *Candida albicans*.

Preprosthetic preparation of the mouth

Extractions

Retained root fragments are the most common radiographic finding but, as with unerupted teeth, their removal should not be automatic. Surgical removal can involve the loss of a great deal of bone, which may already be in short supply, and could result in a reduction of the useful denture-bearing foundation. Therefore, removal of roots or teeth should normally be limited to those:

● Incompletely covered by bone
● Associated with periapical infection

- Showing signs of cystic change around the crown
- Associated with pain or discomfort

Modifications to the alveolar ridge

The success of complete dentures may be improved by surgical modification to the alveolar ridge. The procedures that might be used are:

- Reduction of bulbous maxillary tuberosity
- Smoothing of irregular bony prominences
- Trimming and smoothing of knife-edge ridge
- Ridge augmentation

Treatment plan and prognosis

Having considered all the available information it may well be that the dentist considers that he or she cannot improve upon the existing dentures. Also, if it has not been possible to determine the cause of a complaint it is unwise to offer to make new dentures, since faults (if they exist) may be perpetuated and the chances of success reduced. In either case, consideration should be given to referring the patient to a specialist. Certainly, in these circumstances, the first option on the treatment plan could be to explain matters carefully to the patient with suitable reassurance, but to offer no treatment.

Other treatments, depending on clinical findings, could include:

- Relining/rebasing or other adjustments to an existing denture
- Construction of new dentures using either a conventional or duplication technique

The prognosis for successful treatment is dependent on a number of factors including the patient's age, adaptability, demeanour, previous denture experience, and anatomy of the mouth.

Preliminary impressions

Preliminary impressions can be taken using either metal stock trays or plastic disposable trays. A high viscosity, irreversible hydrocolloid (alginate) or impression compound is the material of choice.

Coverage

Each impression should cover the entire denture-bearing area and should achieve the closest possible contact with the mucosa.

Extension

The upper impression should extend to the functional depth of the labial and buccal sulci,

including the tuberosities and hamular notches, and posteriorly to the junction of the hard and soft palate. The lower should extend to the functional depth of the lingual, labial and buccal sulci and cover the retromolar pads posteriorly. Only limited accuracy is needed at this stage since this will be an essential component of the final impression.

Final impressions

Special trays

Special trays are required to ensure that the final (secondary or working) impressions can be achieved with accuracy of detail and borders moulded to the functional width and depth of the sulci. Stock trays are manufactured to average sizes and therefore are likely to be less than ideal for any individual. Although modification of stock trays is possible, the resultant impression is still unlikely to be extended correctly.

Self-curing acrylic resin is most commonly used for special tray construction. It has the advantages of being relatively inexpensive, simple to shape and is rigid in modest thickness. The upper tray should have a small handle placed in the midline of the anterior region, sloping forward at an angle of 45°. This configuration avoids interference with the lip. On the lower, the handle is vertical and two finger rests are placed, one in each of the second premolar regions. This enables the index fingers to support the tray without interfering with the borders of the impression.

Special trays can be divided into two types: close-fitting or spaced.

Close fitting As the term implies, no spacing is used. Zinc oxide–eugenol paste is usually the material of choice in this type of tray, although other materials such as silicone perfecting pastes may be used. These materials are accurate in thin film but require adequate support, especially at the borders. Correct tray extension is therefore important and can best be achieved by checking that the borders are slightly short (1–2 mm) of the functional depth of the sulci, and then using greenstick tracing compound (or other suitable material) to establish the optimum extension. This technique will define not only the depth of the sulcus but also its width. This combination can be used for upper and lower impressions provided there are no opposing bony undercuts.

It has the advantage that the materials are stable when set and less susceptible to distortion than alginate. No adhesive is necessary for zinc oxide–eugenol but the tray must be clean and dry.

Spaced

Alginate and plaster of Paris impressions require spaced trays. The spacers ensure an even thickness of the impression material for maximum accuracy. Alginate is specifically indicated when opposing substantial undercuts exist that could prevent the withdrawal of a close-fitting tray and a non-elastic material.

The tray can be constructed with 'built-in' stops that contact the mucosa, or greenstick tracing compound can be added at the chairside. This should be completed before checking the border extension, since the stops will effectively lift the tray away from the tissues and it may then appear underextended.

The tray borders should only extend to within 1–2 mm of the full depth of the sulcus to leave room for the impression material to flow around them and fill the remaining space. This avoids the common error found with alginate impressions of displacing the tissues and thus overextension.

Adhesive specific to alginate is more efficient than depending solely on holes drilled in the trays for retention. No adhesive is required for plaster impressions but the tray must be clean and dry.

Objectives of final impressions

The objectives of the final impression are to define the support area for the denture to achieve optimum retention and stability.

Flabby upper ridge

The combination of a complete upper denture opposing natural lower anterior teeth may result in the destruction of the maxillary alveolar ridge opposite the natural teeth and its replacement with fibrous tissue. Conventional impression techniques will tend to displace this type of ridge, which needs to be recorded in its 'rest' position. To minimize displacement, a low viscosity alginate or plaster of Paris can be used. An alternative is to take a two-stage impression using a zinc oxide–eugenol paste in a close-fitting tray that covers only the firm part of the ridge and then filling in the anterior region with a fluid mix of plaster of Paris.

Jaw relationships

Jaw relationships are recorded using occlusal rims; these consist of a base and a rim. A variety of materials may be used for constructing the bases, but a rigid material such as shellac or acrylic resin is preferred, to avoid distortion. Rims are invariably made of wax, either preformed or fashioned from sheets.

Objectives of occlusal rims

Occlusal rims are used to transfer morphological information about the eventual polished surfaces and occlusal surfaces of the dentures from the patient to the laboratory, to enable the technician to proceed to the wax trial denture stage. In essence, they provide the technician with details of precisely where, in relation to the denture-bearing areas, the artificial teeth and supporting material should be located. Occlusal rims should record the following information:

- Aesthetics and arch form
- Jaw relationships

Aesthetics and arch form   The upper rim should be adjusted to the required incisal level with the appropriate lip support. This depends on the length of the lip and the age of the patient. The average visibilities of the central incisors to the upper lip line (at rest and without smiling) are often quoted as:

- Young person: 2 mm below lip
- Middle age: 1–1.5 mm below lip
- Old age: 0–2 mm above lip

However, there can be considerable individual variation and these measurements should therefore only be used as a guide.

The labial surfaces of the upper anterior teeth give support to the upper lip and provide facial contour. Frequently, the artificial incisors may be incorrectly sited in a more lingual position than their natural counterparts. The incisive papilla is an important landmark that can be used as a guide when trimming the labial face of the rim. Studies have shown that the incisal edges of the upper central incisor teeth lie approximately 8–10 mm anterior to the centre of the incisive papilla when the dental base relationship is class I. This structure is affected very little by resorption and remains fairly constant in position.

The upper rim should be trimmed parallel to the interpupillary line. The ala-tragal line (passing through the tragus of the ear near the external auditory meatus and the ala at the base of the nose) can be used as a guide in the anterioposterior plane. The centre line is marked on the labial face of the rim; this usually corresponds with the centre of the philtrum (*Fig. 24.3*).

Correct arch form is achieved by trimming the buccal and palatal surfaces so that the rim lies within the neutral zone, i.e. it lies between the opposing forces of the lips/cheeks and tongue, which ensures stability. The tongue should not be cramped and therefore the lower rim should be trimmed from the lingual aspect until the tongue can lie in its normal resting position without dislodging the rim.

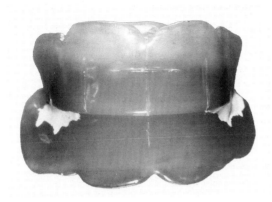

Fig. 24.3 Occlusal registration for complete dentures. Upper rim shows the registration of the occlusal plane, the intercanine distance, incisal length and tip position and midline. The rims are sealed in centric relation by plaster of Paris impression material

Registration of jaw relationships The objective is to record the jaw relationship at the chosen occlusal vertical dimension with the condyles in their most superior, posterior position (centric jaw relation/centric relation, Chapter 8). With complete dentures, centric occlusion is constructed to be coincident with centric relation.

The height of the lower occlusal rim must be adjusted so that, with the patient in the upright position and the mandible at rest, there is a space of approximately 3 mm between the rims. This separation is called the *freeway space* (interocclusal clearance). This is achieved by assessing the rest vertical dimension with the patient sitting upright with the head supported so that the tissues are in their normal relationships. Direct measurement is usually made with either a Willis gauge or marker dots (on the skin) and dividers. The weight of the lower denture (or occlusal rim) can affect the rest position of the mandible, and the lower rim should therefore be *in situ* during the assessment. The occlusal vertical dimension is then assessed with the two rims in contact and wax removed from the height of the lower until there is sufficient freeway space.

In the elderly it is usually wiser to accept a slightly larger than average freeway space, especially if old dentures with a reduced occlusal vertical dimension, resulting from a combination of alveolar resorption and tooth wear, have been worn for many years.

When the rims have been adjusted to their final shape and size, *centric jaw relation* can be recorded. This can be achieved using a variety of techniques but the objective is to ensure that the rims contact simultaneously on both sides and therefore that

there is even pressure. This can be ensured by removing 1–1.5 mm of wax from the posterior parts of the lower rim, leaving pillars of wax in the anterior areas to maintain the occlusal vertical dimension.

The patient is manipulated into the retruded arc of closure with both occlusal rims in the mouth. Locating lines can be scored through both rims in the premolar areas to serve as a guide. V-shaped notches are cut into the upper rim in the molar regions and it is then returned to the mouth. Mounds of a recording medium, such as plaster of Paris (Gypsogum), softened wax or a bite registration paste, are placed on the lower rim, that is then placed in the mouth. The patient is guided again into the retruded arc so that the rims contact evenly and the mandible is supported whilst the material sets. Both rims can then be removed from the mouth while sealed together (*Fig. 24.3*).

The guidelines are checked to ensure that they correspond, and finally sticky wax is run over the rims and recording medium to reinforce the areas prior to despatch to the laboratory for the fabrication of trial dentures.

Choice of teeth

The prescription to the technician should include the mould size and shade, together with the make and material to be used for the anterior and posterior teeth. Anatomical or non-anatomical (cuspless) posterior teeth should be considered, with non-anatomical usually being reserved for those with:

- Atrophic alveolar ridges
- The elderly
- Difficulty in consistently returning to the centric jaw relation (e.g. Parkinsonism)
- Existing dentures with very worn teeth that have permitted unrestricted jaw movements

The size, shape and arrangement of anterior teeth have a significant influence on facial appearance and the psychological importance of the face and teeth cannot be over exaggerated. The choice of tooth mould is difficult when no natural teeth or pre-extraction records are available. There is little evidence to support the much publicized theories of matching tooth mould to face form or that females have rounded teeth and males square, rugged teeth. In general, the size and mould of the artificial teeth should be chosen to fill the space available on the intercanine region of the upper occlusal rim.

Individuals often request small, light coloured teeth arranged symmetrically to create a youthful appearance but this can result in a typical 'denture wearer's look' not reflecting their biological age. There is, however, much that can be done to achieve a natural appearance, including setting the teeth irregularly and using darker shades to more appropriately match the patient's age.

Articulation

In the laboratory, the type of articulator appropriate to the chosen posterior teeth should be used. An average condylar path (average movement) or adjustable articulator is necessary for setting up cusped teeth to ensure a balanced articulation. This type of articulator simulates protrusive and lateral movements of the jaw and working and balancing side contacts can therefore be assessed.

A simple hinge articulator should only be used for setting up cuspless teeth using either metal templates of a sphero-ellipsoidal nature (Boyles plates) or the teeth set to a flat occlusal plane with posterior balancing ramps to maintain a three-point contact rather than full balanced articulation.

Trial dentures

The wax try-in denture should be returned to the clinic together with the articulator. This allows the clinician to assess the dentures on the articulator prior to examining them in the mouth. The assessment on the articulator should include tooth position, arch shape, extension of the wax work into the sulci and across the retromolar pads and the posterior aspect of the palate. It should also include the occlusion and general standard of the wax contouring and surface finish.

The objective of the intraoral inspection is to check the information recorded on the occlusal rims and to correct any errors before processing the dentures. The wax try-ins should therefore be checked for retention, ensuring that maximum coverage has been achieved, and that the borders are suitably extended. The jaw relationships can then be assessed first in the horizontal plane, and then the vertical dimension. With the patient sitting upright, the head supported and the mandible in the retruded position, the occlusion should be even and simultaneous without interference or deviation.

If the occlusion is obviously incorrect then, following an assessment of the occlusal vertical dimension and freeway space, the lower posterior teeth should be removed and the wax rim re-established prior to a new occlusal registration.

When the dentist is satisfied with all aspects of the try-in, the patient should inspect the trial dentures in front of a mirror. It may be helpful if the patient's partner also takes part in this exercise to ensure agreement on the appearance of the teeth.

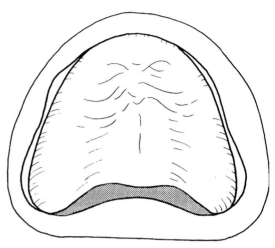

Fig. 24.4 Post dam outlined on model

Finally, the extension of the posterior border of the upper trial base is checked. This should normally be placed at the junction of the moving tissues of the soft palate and the fixed tissues anteriorly, and should extend laterally over the hamular notches. The Cupid's bow shape gives an effective seal and is achieved by carving into the surface of the working model using, for example, a Lecron carver. The shape is carved deeper at the posterior edge with a gradual taper anteriorly to account for the reduced thickness of the submucosa. This carving can be performed after the patient has left the surgery (*Fig 24.4*).

Processing

The procedures used to flask, pack and process heat-cured acrylic resin can result in dimensional changes and are commonly known as the *laboratory processing errors*. These can cause occlusal disharmony and an increase in the occlusal vertical dimension, which will need to be eliminated at the fitting stage. The most likely causes are:

- Dimensional change of the wax during flasking
- Excessive packing pressure, resulting in the teeth being forced into the plaster
- Incorrect alignment or badly fitting sections of the two halves of the metal flask
- Excessive flash either because the acrylic resin dough was too rubbery when packed or insufficient packing pressure was used
- Thermal and polymerizing changes in the acrylic resin

If the dentures have been processed using the split cast technique they can be remounted on the original articulator. Usually the incisal guidance pin will not be in contact with the incisal guidance table and equilibration of the artificial teeth will be necessary. This involves first correcting the centric occlusion at the defined occlusal vertical dimension and then developing balanced articulation.

Insertion of the dentures

Prior to inserting the processed dentures they should be inspected to ensure that the fitting (impression) surfaces are free of imperfections, such as acrylic resin pearls or sharp ridges. If present, these should be trimmed and smoothed. Excessive, opposing undercuts should have been assessed at an earlier stage and, if appropriate, blocked out prior to processing, but it may be necessary to remove minor undercuts to allow the dentures to be inserted.

The dentures should be individually assessed in the mouth for fit, stability and comfort before examining them in combination. If there are signs of discomfort, pressure disclosing pastes in spray form can be used to determine local areas of pressure that can then be trimmed and smoothed accordingly.

On closure, the teeth should meet evenly and simultaneously without interference or lateral deviation. Minor adjustments to the occlusion can be performed at the chairside using thin articulating paper to mark the teeth and appropriately sized burs or stones. The aim should be for a positive, even occlusion with evidence of some lateral and protrusive movement without interference. If a more major occlusal error is evident this should be corrected using laboratory facilities.

Check record

A thin layer of warmed, toughened wax is applied to the lower posterior teeth and the mandible closed in the retruded relationship, ensuring that closure of the mandible is stopped before tooth contact occurs to prevent premature contact and lateral or protrusive slide. This precentric record allows the technician to remount the dentures on the articulator and to carry out the necessary modifications to the occlusion.

When satisfied with all aspects of the dentures the patient is given information and guidance on wearing dentures and instructions on keeping them clean. Follow-up visits are made, as necessary, to ensure that the new dentures are comfortable and successful.

Duplication technique (copy dentures)

The duplication technique can be used to construct new complete (or partial) dentures if suitable existing dentures are available. The dentures are duplicated (copied) and these duplicates then form the framework for the new set. A variety of techniques is available, all have the same objective, with a number of the techniques being very similar, differing only in the materials used.

Existing dentures need to have been worn successfully to warrant duplication, although (rarely) the 'best of a bad bunch' can be chosen for a patient who has had many dentures constructed by a variety of dentists, in order to make controlled modifications without damaging the set that they prefer. The common indications for duplicating dentures are:

- The elderly, who may have a reduced adaptive capacity that restricts the use of conventional construction techniques
- Others with reduced adaptive capacity (e.g. stroke and Parkinsonism patients)
- Immediate dentures – to reproduce the original tooth position
- Dissatisfied patients – in order to modify the most acceptable dentures
- Special features – to copy the shape of an existing denture that may have unusual design features, such as flange plumping in cases of seventh nerve facial palsy
- Spare dentures – for those who require an extra set to avoid embarrassment

Advantages of the duplication technique include:

- Exact reproduction of tooth position and contour of the polished surfaces
- Ability to incorporate controlled modifications
- The minimization of problems of adaptation
- Clinical attendances are reduced

The most commonly used techniques can be performed at the chairside although laboratory methods are available. The objective of them all is to take impressions of the existing dentures in order to be able to pour duplicates in self-curing acrylic resin, which are then used to record the impressions of the mouth and jaw relationships. The duplicates (copies) are obtained at the chairside by taking impressions of both surfaces of each denture with alginate or silicone putty, either in pairs of disposable plastic trays or in a plastic soap dish that has had a window cut in the side to allow space for the sprues. The sprues, which are attached to the heels of the dentures, permit the duplicates to be poured using a fluid mix of self-curing acrylic resin. This is usually carried out in the laboratory under an extraction hood, for health and safety reasons.

The resin duplicates can be modified to correct under/over extension and used as 'special trays' in order to obtain final impressions, and also to record the jaw relationships by placing a suitable registration material between the teeth. The contours of the polished surfaces should be carefully guarded, unless there is reason for change, in order to preserve the overall shape of the final dentures. It should be appreciated that the self-cure duplicates are only used as templates for processing heat-cured resin dentures and are not incorporated into the final prostheses.

Immediate dentures

An immediate denture is one that is constructed prior to the extraction of the natural teeth and inserted into the mouth immediately after their removal.

The benefits to the patients are: they are never without teeth and therefore the soft tissue profile is maintained; the dentures assist mastication and hence nutrition; and adaptation is enhanced and the development of abnormal muscle behaviour is avoided by maintaining normal function. Benefits to the dentist include: use of the existing dentition for recording jaw relationships and for choosing shade and mould of artificial teeth; and tooth position can be reproduced and controlled modifications made as desired.

Disadvantages of immediate dentures include the extra clinical visits that are necessary for aftercare and eventual replacement of the dentures. It is not possible to check the aesthetics of the teeth to be replaced as there can be no try-in stage. If it is not possible to extract the teeth without resorting to surgical techniques, cast trimming to simulate the residual ridge may be unsatisfactory.

Due to the improvements in adult oral health it is now relatively uncommon to have to provide immediate dentures replacing most of the natural teeth. However, depending on the number of teeth remaining, various options for tooth replacement should be considered as follows:

1. Extract posterior teeth, allow the ridges to heal for at least three months and construct immediate dentures to replace the anterior teeth. The advantages of this are that the healed posterior ridges extend the life of the prostheses and it is an economic procedure, requiring the minimum number of patient visits. It may, however, allow the possibility of lateral tongue spread

2. The first procedure can be modified to: extract posterior teeth and allow the ridges to heal, construct partial dentures and then add the remaining teeth to these dentures as an immediate procedure. Alternatively, extract the posterior teeth and fit immediate partial dentures and then add the remaining teeth to these dentures as an immediate procedure

Both modifications attempt to bring about a successful transition to complete dentures; however, the number of extra visits may be unrealistic. Also, a high level of motivation is required to wear simple resin partial dentures replacing only posterior teeth.

3. Extract all the remaining anterior and posterior teeth and fit immediate dentures. This has the advantage of completing the extractions at one operation which may be important, for example, prior to cardiac surgery but can result in rapid loss of fit of the dentures caused by widespread alveolar resorption, which necessitates frequent maintenance visits

Whenever practicable, flanged immediate dentures should be used, since they give superior retention, increase the life of the dentures, add strength to the denture base, allow for repositioning of the artificial teeth, protect extraction sockets and aid healing. They can also be used when marked periodontal pocketing is present, which would preclude use of the open face (gum fitted) design, and they support the use of temporary lining materials, which is helpful during the maintenance phase.

Principles of overdentures

The term overdenture describes a prosthesis that derives support from one or more abutment teeth or roots by completely enclosing them beneath its fitting surface. Complete overdentures are more common than partials.

Rationale for overdentures

The maintenance of alveolar bone is probably the strongest argument for retention of teeth or roots as overdenture abutments:

● The mandibular ridge is particularly susceptible to postextraction change; maxillary and mandibular alveolar resorption rates are approximately in the ratio 1:4
● Clinical experience confirms that alveolar bone is maintained whilst healthy teeth or roots remain

- Retention of a number of abutments maintains a positive ridge form with a greater height and volume of bone. The denture is therefore more stable and retention should also be improved

The success or failure of a prosthesis is dependent upon integration of sensory feedback and motor response and the masticatory system relies on feedback from receptors in temporomandibular joints, ligaments, muscles, mucosa and periodontal tissues. The loss of teeth decreases the level of proprioceptive information.

Sensory feedback can be considered under two headings that relate to research studies:

- *Tactile sensitivity discrimination* (the discrimination of differences in thickness of objects placed between the teeth). Little difference has been reported between natural teeth, conventional complete dentures and overdentures; it is possible that muscle spindles play the major role
- *Minimal load thresholds* (the discrimination of varying levels of force). Overdentures give improved discriminatory ability at both higher and lower biting force levels. This may prevent excessive loads being applied and hence maintain loads directed to the alveolar bone within physiological limits

There may be some psychological benefit gained from an overdenture. By retaining some of the teeth it may prevent the feeling of total loss of natural teeth and perhaps make eventual transition to conventional complete dentures more acceptable. Masticatory performance is enhanced, since the overdenture wearer has a functional advantage over those with conventional dentures. There is scientific evidence that overdentures allow the food to be chewed more effectively.

Indications for overdentures

- Complete denture opposing natural teeth – prevents overloading of mucosa caused by high masticatory forces and retards rate of alveolar resorption, thus enhancing long-term success of the prosthesis
- Cleft palate and surgical defects – if the defect is extensive it may be impossible to provide a satisfactory conventional denture if teeth are lost
- Extreme wear of natural teeth – see Chapter 25
- Hypodontia – often substantial number of permanent teeth absent
- Poor prognosis for conventional complete dentures – degree of bone loss in edentulous areas and unfavourable muscle attachments may indicate potential problems

- Doubtful partial denture abutment – over-erupted or periodontally involved teeth may not be satisfactory as conventional partial denture abutments

Patient selection

Overdentures should be considered whenever loss of teeth is anticipated. There are few general health contraindications except for severe debilitating illness, mental handicap, history of bacterial endocarditis and some candidates for cardiac surgery. Youth or old age is not a contraindication in itself and overdentures should be constructed when clinically indicated. It is important to inform potential patients of the number of visits and time required since this will be greater than, for example, for a clearance and conventional dentures. The ability to attain and maintain a high standard of oral hygiene is essential.

Abutment selection

The choice of abutment is dictated by the number and location of remaining teeth. Bi-lateral abutments symmetrically located are ideal. Canines are the most often used teeth with premolars the next favourite (the second premolar being preferred in the maxilla since it is commonly single rooted). Maxillary incisors are satisfactory but mandibular incisors are the least acceptable and the use of molars may be limited by endodontic considerations. Approximating abutments are more difficult to clean and can make the maintenance of gingival health a problem.

Dental examination

The clinical examination should include charting of caries and defective restorations, assessment of gingival condition, periodontal pocket depth and tooth mobility and periapical radiographic survey of possible abutments and study models.

A high level of caries activity is undesirable since there is a possibility of recurrence in unprotected abutment teeth or adjacent to margins of copings. Root caries precludes the use of a tooth.

Teeth with a less than ideal periodontal condition may have to be accepted. However, the abutment should have minimal mobility and adequate bone support (half the root length surrounded by bone). An improved crown:root ratio, achieved by reduction of the clinical crown in the doming procedure, will enhance likely success. If positive retention, in the form of root face attachments, is envisaged the abutment tooth will be subjected to considerably greater forces. Substantial bone support for the root is therefore essential. Active gingival and periodontal disease should be eliminated prior to further treatment.

When considering endodontic therapy, radiographic evaluation is essential although root canal therapy may be unnecessary in cases of severe wear, when the root canal may be obliterated by secondary dentine. Single rooted teeth are preferred for ease of root filling and the possible use of the canal for post retention if copings on the abutments are envisaged.

Treatment plan

There are several methods of progressing to complete overdentures.

Immediate complete overdentures

The treatment sequence might include periodontal therapy and endodontics prior to preliminary and final impressions and recording the jaw relationship.

At the try-in of the trial set-up a decision is taken on the position of the artificial teeth to replace those being extracted or reduced as abutments, and on the provision of a flange. Similar criteria are used as for the normal immediate denture procedure, i.e. is the appearance of the natural teeth to be copied or is the position of the artificial teeth relative to their natural predecessors to be altered to modify the aesthetics? Although desirable, it may not be possible to use a full flange because of bony undercuts adjacent to the abutments.

On completion of the denture, the chosen teeth are prepared as overdenture abutments to produce a smooth dome shape with the highest point approximately 2 mm above gingival level. A glass ionomer restoration is placed in the entrance to the root canal. Other teeth are then extracted and the denture fitted.

At the first review visit, one day after the extractions, the root faces and restorations are polished. The overdenture is adapted to the abutments by adding self-curing acrylic resin to the depressions in the denture over the root faces. Excess resin is allowed to escape via small vent holes drilled through the denture base whilst the denture is retained in position by light occlusal pressure.

Further review appointments will be necessary during the socket healing and ridge remodelling period. After approximately six months the root face can be assessed for possible coverage with copings.

Conversion of existing partial denture to complete overdenture

Existing partial dentures can be utilized and converted to complete overdentures using either a laboratory based technique or a chairside method.

Laboratory method

1. Dome-shaped preparation of endodontically treated abutment teeth
2. Impression with partial denture *in situ* (plus impression of other arch and occlusal record)
3. In the laboratory – artificial teeth positioned over domed root faces and flange added
4. Converted dentures fitted

This method has the advantage that the converted denture has been made in the laboratory and the disadvantage that the patient will be without a denture during construction.

Chairside method

1. Endodontic treatment of abutment teeth
2. Impression with denture *in situ* (leave denture in impression)
3. Dome-shaped preparation of abutment teeth
4. Tooth coloured self-curing acrylic resin is placed in the abutment teeth indentations of the impression and the impression (with the denture still included) is positioned carefully in the mouth
5. When polymerization is complete, the flange is added with hard chairside reline material

This method has the advantage that the patient is not without the denture but has the disadvantages that a lengthy appointment is necessary and the additions may be weaker and more prone to fracture.

Treatment of abutment teeth

There are several ways in which abutment teeth can be used in association with overdentures:

● Domed with access sealed with glass ionomer cement
● Gold coping on root face with post
● Gold thimble on vital tooth
● Attachment fitted to the coping

The selection may often be a personal preference but the essential difference between the systems is the retention of the denture and the extent to which lateral forces are transmitted to the abutment teeth. The dome transmits the least force whilst the attachment transmits the most.

Domed root face

This is the simplest method. The teeth will normally be root filled and the access sealed with glass ionomer cement to provide a fluoride reservoir to assist the prevention of recurrent caries. The level of the dome in relation to the gingival tissue may vary according to the restorative state of the tooth. Whilst the ideal level is 2 mm above the soft tissue, pre-existing deep restorations may cause the removal of more tissue. In any event the root face should not be subgingival. If this occurs, a coping should be used.

Gold copings

Dome-shape   This will provide some protection to the root face from recurrent caries, together with some additional resistance to lateral displacement of the denture. It is the most common and usually uses the root canal for retention on a cast post; therefore endodontic treatment is necessary. The profile of the coping may be flat or raised as a stud (*Fig. 24.5*) and deficiencies caused by previous caries/restorations can be occluded. Placement of the copings should be delayed, if possible, for approximately six months after the overdenture is fitted to allow the gingivae to reach a realistic level

Thimble shape   This is designed to protect the dentine overlying a vital pulp. It offers more retention and stability to the denture, but greater stress is placed on the root and the extra height creates a less favourable crown:root ratio. Because of its size, it intrudes further into the denture base.

Attachments   These increase the retention of the denture greatly, but increased stresses are transmitted on insertion and removal of denture and during function. Therefore the abutment roots require excellent periodontal support. Good maintenance is essential and time-consuming, and the laboratory costs are greatly increased over simple castings.

They are very useful when the denture foundation is unfavourable, as in a cleft palate or a flat lower ridge or when displacing forces may be high, e.g. a complete overdenture opposed by natural teeth. In patients who cannot tolerate a conventional denture palate, attachments can overcome the loss of retention where palatal coverage has to be reduced.

There are two basic types of attachment:

- Stud attachments
- Bar attachments

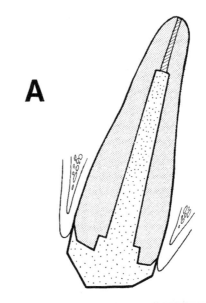
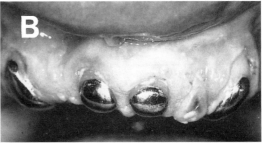
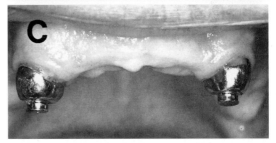

Fig. 24.5 Overdenture abutments – A Diagram of root face coping and post (the coping is shaped here to receive a stud rather than being domed); B Clinical case with gold copings on 31|13 and glass ionomer cement in |2; C Stud attachments on 3|3

The male portion of the stud attachment is usually on the root and the female portion in the denture (*Fig. 24.5C*). The space required is approximately midway between a dome-shape and thimble coping; space is also required in the denture base to accommodate the female portion. Examples of this type are the Rothermann Eccentric, Dalla Bonna 604 and the Kurer Press Stud system (see manufacturers' list, p. 281).

The bar attachment consists of a rigid bar attached to abutment teeth and a sleeve in the overdenture. The bar splints the abutments and distributes stress between them. Substantial loads can, however, be generated with this system. Plaque control is difficult and maintenance of attachments complicated. The Dolder bar and Ackerman bar are examples of this type (see manufacturers' list, p. 281).

Clinical appraisal

Good oral hygiene is the single most important factor that influences continued health of the supporting tissues. With inadequate oral hygiene, wearing overdentures can cause:

● Periodontal damage – either gingival hypertrophy or retraction of the gingival tissue with loss of bony support; there is a specially high risk if attachments are used
● Caries of the root face

Preventive measures and continuing care

Patients should be on a structured continuing care programme to provide regular inspection and maintenance of the denture and abutments.

Effective plaque control of the root faces is essential using a fluoride toothpaste. Topical fluoride gel may also be useful, both applied directly to the root face and into the depressions in the fitting surface of the denture that overly the abutments. The patient must also adopt an efficient denture cleansing programme using hypochlorite solution (see section below on 'keeping dentures clean').

Gingival recession is a possible problem and this may indicate reshaping of the dome preparation, modifying the fit of the dentures using self-curing acrylic resin chairside reline material and carrying out periodontal treatment as appropriate.

Recurrent caries of the root face may be removed, thus modifying its shape, or a gold coping might be provided.

Alveolar resorption occurs mainly distal to the abutments, following which stability of the denture will deteriorate. This will require correction, either with a conventional reline technique or a chairside reline material.

Advice for new denture wearers

A patient receiving new dentures should be given guidance as to the difficulties that may be encoun-tered and advice on a cleaning and maintenance regime. Since patients tend to forget verbal information given at the chairside, written instructions to take home and read at leisure are helpful. There are many denture cleansing agents on the market but the following guidelines are suggested.

Getting used to complete dentures

The best results from your new dentures can be achieved only with practice and patience. It may take several weeks for you to become fully accustomed to the dentures. Do not be discouraged by friends or relatives who tell you how easy it was for then.

To begin with, the dentures may cause an increase of saliva in your mouth. This should return to normal in a few days. Eat mainly soft foods for the first few days and don't take large bites.

Cut your food into small portions and try to chew with your back teeth on alternate sides. Some people with new dentures find that sucking boiled sweets helps them to get accustomed to the dentures.

When to wear your dentures

You may wear your dentures during the day and night for the first week to help you get used to them more quickly. From then on you should leave them out at night, in a container of water or recommended cleaning agent. Your mouth needs a rest if it is to remain healthy.

Keeping your dentures clean

Ensure that your dentures are kept really clean. Rinse them after each meal and brush all of the surfaces morning and night with a soft toothbrush and soap and water.

Use the commercially produced cleanser 'Dentural' regularly. Follow the instructions on the container carefully. If your denture has any metal components, the 'Dentural' will not cause any damage provided you use only the short (ten-minute) cleaning period. Rinse your dentures well after using 'Dentural'.

The comfort of your mouth

New dentures sometimes cause areas of soreness. These may be relieved by leaving the dentures out of your mouth for 24 hours. If the trouble persists, an adjustment will be necessary. However, if it has been necessary to leave the dentures out, ensure that they are worn for 12 hours immediately prior to visiting the dentist for an adjustment. This will help in locating the exact cause of the trouble.

PROBLEMS

25

Tooth surface loss

The loss of enamel and dentine caused by means other than caries and trauma has become more significant as teeth are retained for longer and people's dietary habits change.

The aetiology is often complex, as can be the treatment. Prevention of the condition by education and intervention by the dentist is important.

Tooth surface loss, also called *tooth wear*, refers to the interrelated effects of attrition, abrasion and erosion.

- *Attrition* is the loss of enamel and dentine resulting from tooth to tooth contact
- *Abrasion* involves an abrasive agent between or against the tooth surface
- *Erosion* involves a chemical agent

The principal causes or predisposing factors are:

- Developmental anomalies
- Malocclusion
- Posterior tooth loss
- Parafunctions and habits
- Restorative materials
- Diet
- Systemic disease
- Natural wear and tear

Aetiology and clinical features

Developmental anomalies

Localized enamel hypoplasia is never a serious problem since isolated zones of surface loss will not usually disturb occlusal stability.

However, the more difficult conditions are those of *amelogenesis imperfecta* and *dentinogenesis imperfecta*. These are part of a range of pathology, including osteogenesis imperfecta, that are manifestations of disturbances in the formation of calcified tissues. These disturbances are genetic in origin and are often seen as familial traits.

In amelogenesis imperfecta, the enamel matrix formation is disturbed, with normal calcification of what does form. The extent of the disorder varies from localized areas of pitting, to a very thin shell of enamel. The enamel is hard but may be deposited in fine lamellations as well as in normal prismatic structure in other areas.

The teeth are poor aesthetically and vulnerable to caries and attrition in affected areas.

Dentinogenesis imperfecta is uncommon and is due to defective odontoblastic activity. The dentine is soft, with the deeper layer having few tubules and incomplete calcification. Also, the pulp chamber becomes obliterated.

Clinically, the weak bond of the enamel to the dentine results in enamel loss, even though the enamel itself is usually normal. The colour of the teeth is abnormal, being brownish, and the roots may be stunted. Because of the obliteration of the root canals, apical infection may occur.

Malocclusion

Certain malocclusions, particularly involving the anterior teeth, may bring the teeth into abnormal functional contacts. Those that create the most problems are an edge to edge incisor relationship and an unfavourable Angle's class II division 2 incisor relationship. The latter case may involve close apposition of the palatal surfaces and tips of the upper incisors with the labial surfaces of the lower incisors. Also, gingival trauma may result from the deep overbite. Surface loss can be dramatic (*Fig. 25.1*) if the malocclusion remains untreated.

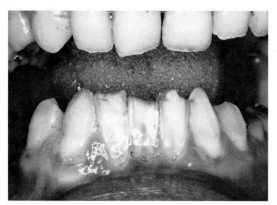

Fig. 25.1 Severe surface loss and periodontal trauma caused by a long standing Angle's class II division 2 malocclusion. Management of such a case would require prerestorative orthodontics

Posterior tooth loss

If several posterior teeth are lost, mastication is likely to be effected on the remaining anterior teeth. These teeth are not well suited to grinding movements and rapid surface loss can result. This type of problem is more common in geographic areas where the level of dental care and awareness has been inadequate, and is usually coupled with non-provision of, or refusal to wear, dentures.

Even with partial dentures present, there is a great tendency to use the natural teeth, and part of the education of the patient at the fitting stage of the dentures should be to stress the need to use them effectively.

Cases exhibit progressive loss of incisor and canine crown length and when this becomes unsightly the patient is prompted to seek treatment (*see Fig. 18.5*).

Parafunctions and habits

Bruxism (Chapter 26) is the most dangerous para-function, with enamel and dentine loss. Again, the incisor length loss is what prompts the request for treatment, but prevention, in the form of an occlusal splint, should be applied as soon as the surface loss is noted.

The exposed dentine may be sensitive, but since the attrition is usually coupled with secondary dentine formation and the retreat of the pulp, it is more often symptomless. The obliteration of the root canals by secondary dentine can lead to apical infection, and the routine use of apical radiographs in the diagnostic phase is important. Root canal

therapy would be indicated before the canals become obstructed.

Habits, such as nail biting, pipe smoking, hair grip opening and so on, can cause abnormal wear patterns, particularly of an isolated nature.

Toothbrush abrasion may be caused by incorrect brushing technique, seen particularly at the cervical margin of the buccal surfaces of the left side in a right-handed person (or vice versa). It is accompanied by gingival recession and loss of exposed cementum. There has been a suggestion that the occlusion may cause cervical stresses leading to dentine fatigue and breakdown rather than brushing.

Restorative materials

Conventional composites and unglazed dental ceramics can remove enamel quite successfully during normal function, with their effect greatly accelerated by parafunction. Again, correct treatment planning, or early intervention, is the best course.

Coarse particled composites should be avoided for large restorations. If a ceramic occlusal surface has been prescribed (in spite of the advice given in Chapter 14!) this should be reglazed following adjustments, rather than 'polished'.

The creep of dental amalgam (Chapter 9) represents a loss of occlusal stability due to surface deformation, and the upshot of this may be to put an extensively restored case into the same treatment planning group as surface loss cases.

Diet

High consumption of acidic food and drinks such as citrus fruits, cola and lemonade removes surface enamel; even wine is incriminated. Cola is a particular hazard as it contains phosphoric acid, citric acid and carbonic acid. The labial aspects are usually affected, unless drinking is via a straw, in which case the palatal aspects of the upper incisors may dissolve. The worst cases are 'diet freaks' who eat large amounts of citrus fruit and brush their teeth immediately afterwards. The acid removes the mineral and the brushing removes whatever matrix is left – thus accelerating the process. Another modern habit is to sip cans of fruit drinks throughout the day; this simply drips acid continuously on to the tooth surface. As with carbohydrate intake and caries, it is the frequency of exposure rather than the volume.

Prevention via dietary advice is the best approach, and patients could be advised to rinse with fresh water after eating fruit, rather than brushing. A reduction in intake of fruit and acidic

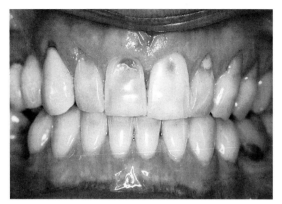

Fig. 25.2 Labial erosion of the upper incisors and canines with exposure of dentine. The patient was obsessed with a fresh fruit diet and tooth brushing. There is loss of much enamel with absence of lamellae, with the dentine showing through and consequent sensitivity

drinks should also be advised and particular effort be made in advising parents about their children's diet.

The surface enamel loses its lamellated appearance and will have a high amorphous gloss. Eventually, dentine will be exposed in the eroded areas, particularly bucco-cervically and occlusally. Because the erosion causes a more rapid enamel loss than that caused by attrition alone, secondary dentine does not form quickly enough to prevent sensitivity (*Fig.25.2*).

Systemic disease

Childhood diseases may interfere with the enamel mineralization of developing teeth and these may erupt with bands or localized zones of hypo-mineralization. These areas are weak and, if in functional relationship with opposing teeth, will be lost fairly rapidly. The zones or bands are chalky white and rough; they will be more prone to staining than the adjacent enamel.

In the adult, the most common systemic problem affecting the tooth surface is *gastric reflux*. Due to cardiac sphincter problems, gastric secretions are forced up the oesophagus and into the mouth. These secretions are highly demineralizing and the areas most commonly affected are the palatal surfaces of the upper teeth. Occlusal surface loss also occurs, leading to existing restorations being left above the level of the surrounding tooth. This is a classic feature of erosion in the absence of occlusal forces, where the affected tooth surface has no occlusal contact.

Prolonged vomiting may also create the same picture, and is one hazard of pregnancy. In addition, the disorders of bulimia and anorexia nervosa may be accompanied by vomiting.

Natural wear and tear

Teeth are kept longer by a population of increasing average age. It is therefore inevitable that teeth simply wear out.

Indications for treatment

Cases with tooth surface loss will require restorative treatment if there is:

● Associated pathology, e.g. caries, apical infection
● Sensitivity
● Loss of occlusal stability and function
● Deterioration in aesthetics

Principles of treatment

Where there is a clear external aetiological agent, this should be eliminated prior to restorative work. Elimination of habits, dietary advice for citric acid erosion, medical referral for gastric reflux and occlusal splints for bruxism fall under this heading.

Provision of partial dentures to provide posterior support prior to consideration of advanced restorations for worn anterior teeth is essential. A complicated treatment plan will fail if the patient does not wear the dentures!

The severe malocclusions mentioned above will require orthodontic correction or simply extractions. The correction of unfavourable relationships by crowns has limitations due to root position.

Patients with progressing anterior surface loss, particularly male, may only be concerned that the condition does not worsen. Timely provision of partial dentures coupled with glass ionomer cement restoration of incisal edge 'saucers' may well be sufficient in many cases.

Application of desensitizing agents for patients with dentine sensitivity of occlusal surfaces may not be successful. There seems to be a difference between the response of a relatively localized zone of cervical dentine and the larger area of occlusal exposed dentine. This is particularly true of acid erosion cases where the dentinal tubules will be opened by demineralization.

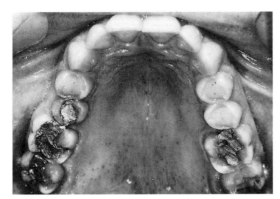

Fig. 25.3 Posterior surface loss in a young adult. The incisors were the only teeth relatively unaffected

Localized hypomineralized areas of enamel can be successfully restored with acid-etch retained composite. Larger areas with aesthetic problems will require veneers or crowns, and those with occlusal functional problems will require onlays or crowns.

In treatment planning the more extensive case, the decisions are influenced by the age of the patient and the number of missing teeth. In the younger adult patient with an intact dentition, the indications are likely to lead to multiple crowns and ultimately to a full mouth rehabilitation (*Fig. 25.3*).

In the older patient with many missing teeth, a transition from partial dentures to overdentures is the better course of action.

The grey area between the two extremes of decision-making depends on economic factors and the skill of the dentist. Complex treatment involving partial dentures, root canal therapy and crowns is quite possible, but patient assessment must be thorough.

Multiple crowns and full mouth rehabilitation

This very expensive and technically demanding line of treatment should not be embarked upon first without discussing the procedures and their implications with the patient, and secondly without the dentist having the necessary clinical training and skills to provide work of a high standard.

The sequence of treatment is as follows:

1. Stabilize active disease and surface loss aetiological agent
2. Establish excellent plaque control
3. Provide intermediate (precrown) restorations including dentures if necessary
4. Advanced preoperative phase
5. Patient discussion, education and agreement
6. Diagnostic splint
7. Determine anterior guidance
8. Restore anterior teeth
9. Restore posterior teeth

The first phase of treatment should result in a stabilized mouth with an adequate occlusion and basic restorations on healthy supporting tissues. The prognosis for each tooth needs to be reliable and teeth of dubious vitality should be root filled or, failing this, extracted. In any event, they should not be used as strategic teeth for a prosthesis if possible.

The posterior teeth should be restored with cores of good retention that can act to stabilize the teeth and the occlusion during the diagnostic period. Considerable difficulty will be experienced with dentinogenesis imperfecta, since the dentine may not be able to retain pins effectively. A combination of pins and dentine adhesive core material may work, but dentine fragility may make the teeth unrestorable.

Having established the basic foundation for advanced dentistry, accurate impressions are taken and a centric relation diagnostic mounting done (Chapter 14). A diagnostic waxing of the proposed occlusal scheme is carried out using the wax added technique to establish the tooth contours required for restorations and pontics (or denture teeth).

Where occlusal surfaces have been extensively lost, no occlusal reduction at the time of posterior preparations will be possible without loss of retention (*Fig. 25.4A*). The possible ways of dealing with this are:

- Crown lengthening
- Intrusion/overeruption
- Increasing the vertical dimension and intruding into the freeway space

Crown lengthening is appropriate when the surface loss is not extensive. If it is, then there will be danger to the underlying periodontium after surgery. Partial coverage occlusal splints may be used to cause intrusion of anterior teeth accompanied by overeruption of the posteriors. This overeruption exposes more tooth to the mouth and therefore increases clinical crown height.

Perhaps the most common technique is to increase the vertical dimension by constructing the new crown occlusal surfaces without tooth reduction. The amount of this intrusion fixes the occlusal plane level, and the incisor heights are increased to match. Cusp height and slopes, and the new curve of Spee, must match the proposed anterior guidance. It is wise to adopt the original shape of the curve of Spee.

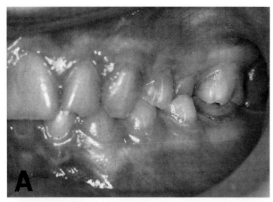

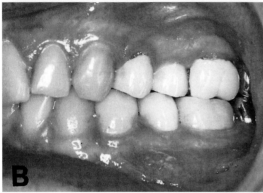

Fig. 25.4 The occlusion on the left side of the case shown in *Figure 25.3*. **A** Before treatment, showing the reduced crown heights. **B** After crowning, with an increase in vertical dimension

The lower incisor tip is the starting point for determining the new anterior guidance. Its new position should be in line with the long axis of the tooth to maintain it in muscle balance. The height of the tip, determined from the new occlusal plane, in turn dictates the position of the cingulum centric stops on the upper incisors. The remainder of the incisor crowns can be shaped empirically at this stage to provide overbite and overjet consistent with the dental base relationship.

Clinically though, the upper incisor tip position will be determined by aesthetics, speech and muscle activity. Tooth length and width need to be matched to facial characteristics, but speech is the most important determinant. Use of the 'F' and 'S' sounds is important to relate the upper incisal edges to the lower lip.

The provisional restorations should be constructed to the diagnostic scheme, and care taken to adjust them correctly at the fitting stage.

Upon completion of the diagnostic waxing, it should be duplicated into stone and remounted.

The incisal table should be customized to the new guidance.

The next part of the diagnostic phase is to construct an occlusal splint that represents the increase in vertical dimension required by the new scheme and incorporates the predicted anterior guidance.

A lower splint, constructed from heat cured, hard acrylic resin, retained by cribs, is the most unobtrusive design. Initially, this is made from the prewax diagnostic mounting, with the articulator opened by the amount shown by the diagnostic waxing; the occlusal surface should be smooth.

On fitting, the splint is adjusted to provide even contact on closure on the retruded arc into centric relation. Since centric occlusion is being remodelled, it is now necessary to adopt centric relation as the reference position. The new centric occlusion position will be made coincident with centric relation at the new vertical dimension.

The patient should be manipulated onto the retruded arc of closure (Chapter 14) and the splint marked with articulating paper at the retruded contact position. These markings should be indented to provide locating fossae for the new occlusal position.

The splint should be worn for about eight weeks, full time, to assess tolerance of the intrusion into the freeway space. After this has been successful, the preparations may be commenced.

The sequence should be:

1. Preparation of the twelve anterior teeth with the splint cut back to provide posterior support. Impressions and centric record
2. Provisional restorations in accordance with the diagnostic waxing
3. Trial cementation of the anterior crowns – speech, aesthetics and guidance checked and adjusted
4. Posterior preparations with splint now discarded. Impressions and centric record
5. Provisional restorations in accordance with the diagnostic waxing. Check for conformity of cusp slopes and height to the anterior guidance
6. Trial cementation of posterior restorations
7. Permanent cementation after review(s) and adjustment

The centric record for both stages 1 and 4 is a centric relation record taken at the new vertical dimension. Because of the use of the arbitrary hinge axis the articulator cannot simply be opened to the new vertical dimension. A recording splint is required, whose thickness is equal to the height of the diagnostic splint and which locates accurately on the unprepared posteriors for stage 1 or the restored anteriors for stage 4. In this way, the

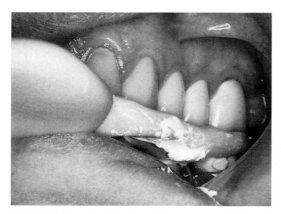

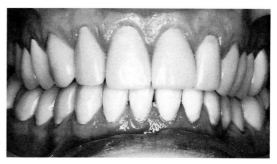

Fig. 25.6 Completed reconstruction of the case shown in *Figure 25.5* with 28 full crowns

Fig. 25.5 Occlusal registration splint in a case where the lower posterior teeth are being restored to an increased vertical dimension. The splint locates the mandible to the new vertical dimension on the retruded arc of closure, and the preparations are registered with a zinc oxide–eugenol cement

The maintenance of the final restorations requires periodic inspection by the dentist, but more important is the continued high standard of oral hygiene by the patient. The patient must be capable of preserving the restorations and be aware of the importance of his/her role (*Fig.25.4B* and *25.6*).

mandible is guided into centric relation by the recording device and the preparation positions can be recorded by a zinc oxide–eugenol wash (*Fig. 25.5*).

The new restorations are constructed and adjusted with centric occlusion = centric relation, but there is some evidence that bony remodelling occurs to eventually re-establish a new centric relation position, posterior to the new centric occlusion.

Overdentures

These are technically less demanding and more cost effective in comparison with the provision of multiple crowns. They are the treatment of choice for the older patient with a number of missing teeth in addition to surface loss. The principles of treatment are described in Chapter 24.

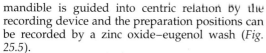

Tooth surface loss – Summary

There are immense variations between individual patients in their requirements, and in the ways in which treatment can be provided. This chapter has given a basic outline of the technical procedures involved, and their complexity, in providing multiple crowns, but the dentist is advised to approach these cases with caution.

Providing multiple crowns is not a single crown procedure repeated many times, and too often patients are asked to adapt to ill conceived occlusal schemes with poorly constructed restorations.

To be successful, the work must be painstakingly planned and executed, and a high reliance placed on the patient's ability to maintain the restorations in a plaque- and caries-free state.

Prevention of surface loss is essential by recognizing that it is occurring and by providing the appropriate interceptive treatment.

26

Temporomandibular dysfunction

This topic is the most controversial aspect of occlusion. The number of therapies proposed to treat the condition probably reflects the lack of a fundamental scientific understanding of its aetiology and pathology. Much confusion is caused by the inclusion of several different conditions under the one heading.

In spite of this, there is a body of moderate opinion that is in basic agreement; this chapter presents this mainstream approach.

General features

Pathology in the temporomandibular joints (TMJs) and muscles of mastication together with disturbance of their neural control may lead to incoordination or restriction of mandibular movement, and pain.

Whilst the principal outcome of this is pain in the muscles of mastication, which may be reported as headache or even toothache, the underlying pathologies that give rise to this are complex and varied.

The primary cause may be within the joints themselves, leading to movement problems or, more commonly, a relatively simple but poorly understood muscle problem.

The most straightforward aspect of this wide range of pathology is that affecting the TMJs. This includes:

- Derangement of the joint
- Inflammation of the joint
- Degenerative disease
- Extrinsic trauma
- Growth disorders

Detailed description of the last four conditions is outside the scope of this book and the reader is referred to texts on oral pathology and surgery for this. However, the conditions must be included in the differential diagnosis of temporomandibular dysfunction.

Derangement of the joint has already been mentioned in Chapter 8 and may involve the articular disc being out of phase with the condylar head or simply trapped permanently out of place. This is considered further below.

The muscle problem, *temporomandibular dysfunction syndrome* also termed *muscle dysfunction syndrome*, or *temporomandibular joint/muscle dysfunction syndrome*, is characterized by one or more of the following, independent of other oral pathology:

- Incoordination of mandibular movement
- Pain in the muscles of mastication
- Restriction of movement

The disorder may or may not be accompanied by joint derangement or may have been preceded by painless clicking of the TMJ.

It is important to note the proviso that the condition is independent of other oral pathology. i.e. it is a primary condition (see below).

Aetiology

The neuromuscular control of mandibular movement is extremely complex and was outlined in Chapter 8. There are various irregularities of tooth relationships, some caused by dentists, that were discussed in Chapters 8, 14 and 18. These include precentric prematurities, working and non-working interferences, tilting, overeruption, missing teeth, malocclusions and, sometimes, faulty restorations.

There is a central nervous system function, referred to as the 'adaptive capacity', that is able to compensate for hard tissue irregularities by controlling muscle function. This CNS centre is able to control mandibular movement to take account of all the irregularities mentioned above. Probably the most important oral function affected is swallowing, which involves the learnt position of centric occlusion.

The closure of the mandible into centric occlusion is performed on a preferred arc of closure that avoids any precentric prematurities. Being able to reach centric occlusion without touching interferences is partly learnt and partly reflex behaviour and, in the normal subject, is easily reproduced. Further, man has the capacity to adapt to and use many extremes of malocclusion quite successfully for functional purposes. Indeed, this adaptation can be quite rapid in the presence of, say a newly restored occlusal surface, whose 'strangeness' disappears after a few days.

However, several things may interfere with muscle and joint coordination which may have more lasting effects:

- Trauma, such as prolonged opening, wide yawning, or tough foods
- Pernicious habits such as nail biting
- Parafunctional clenching or grinding – *bruxism*.
- 'Correction' of gross malocclusion by posture
- Extensive restorations or dentures of incorrect occlusal contour
- Independent oral pathology
- Emotional stress – anxiety, worry, major life event
- Psychiatric illness

The effects of trauma as an aetiological agent are very basic and can be understood clearly. Nail biting requires the mandible to be advanced to edge-to-edge incisal contact and maintained in that position for nibbling. The masticatory apparatus is not well suited to this function, and fatigue and spasm may develop in the lateral pterygoid and masseter muscles. Bruxism consists of continued parafunctional movements, which again cause the muscles to tire.

The moderate-to-gross class II division I malocclusion causes problems in the achievement of a conventional oral seal and also, to compensate for the aesthetic problems of a chinless profile, subjects often posture forward continuously. This again fatigues the muscles.

A faulty occlusal surface may induce an abnormal pattern of chewing, either because of avoidance, or because of awareness of a problem, and incoordination results. It is assumed that the adaptive capacity is exceeded in these cases.

Independent oral pathology is a major heading in the differential diagnosis of temporomandibular dysfunction. The true syndrome occurs in the absence of such pathology, but sometimes the syndrome is induced by other disorders. These include carious teeth, pulpal conditions, apical pathology, split roots – the list is very long. The aetiology is simply based on avoiding a painful or uncomfortable contact during function or parafunction.

Neuromuscular coordination is lost because a new pattern of movement is being attempted, and joint clicking and muscle tenderness may be the results. Treatment to remove the pathology will usually induce the temporomandibular dysfunction to resolve, with no active occlusal therapy.

Emotional stress, worry, anxiety-based and psychiatric disorders are considered to be major factors in the aetiology. These factors are recognized to be of importance in other conditions such as duodenal ulcer, low back pain and migraine, and temporomandibular dysfunction falls into the group of psychosomatic pathology. Why some people get ulcers while others get facial pain is not clear, but it would seem that susceptible patients are at risk of certain conditions.

The influence of psychological factors would appear to be the interference with central functions. Again, the neural control of mastication is affected, leading to incoordination. Psychological problems are complex and it is not for dental surgeons to play the amateur psychiatrist! However, some understanding is necessary.

Surveys have indicated that 40% of the population may have temporomandibular dysfunction during their lives. Classically, there is an acute episode in late teens that clears quickly, followed by a more chronic recurrence in middle age. Women and men are affected equally but in many clinical studies there are as many as seven times more women than men attending for treatment. This finding is likely to be influenced by the fact that women seek medical advice more frequently than men.

Clinical features

The principal symptoms are masticatory muscle pain or spasm that builds to a peak of pain that then declines over a period of several months or even years. The disorder has no physical signs and is solely reported by the patient on the basis of symptoms. Whilst palpation of the muscles will result in reported tenderness and there may be limitation of opening, all of these are reliant on the patient's response.

Pain around the face and head will cause patients concern and may be exaggerated by focused attention, misconception and fear. An account of the pain picture based on the information seen in *Figure 2.1* may be valuable for diagnosis. As was mentioned above, the condition affects susceptible patients and such patients may be treatment seekers, exaggerating their symptoms for attention. Superimposition of anxiety may reduce the pain threshold of the individual.

The acute muscle symptoms may have been preceded by locking of the mandible or be accompanied by clicking in the TMJs. Other TMJ pathology may provoke muscle pain but this, although the same as that of temporomandibular dysfunction, is a secondary aspect of another primary pathology.

The classic TMJ click occurs on opening and/or closing with tooth separation of about 1–2 mm that is caused by the articular disc becoming displaced from the head of the condyle and then catching up either from posterior or anterior. The disc can become permanently displaced but this may be found in the absence of any symptoms at all. The click can be felt by palpation of the joints or heard via a stethoscope.

Failure of the relocation of the disc–condylar complex during opening can result in locking of the mandible at mid-opening. The disc is trapped anteriorly on or beyond the eminence. This again can be painless and patients may become used to relieving the problem themselves. However, once locking is accompanied by pain, the patient will seek treatment.

If treatment is not sought and the condition does not resolve, then progress of the disorder may continue with painful function, permanent displacement of the disc and eventually osteo-arthritis. However, locking will usually have disappeared to be replaced by the pain from the joint in all functional positions.

Diagnosis of disc displacement is notoriously difficult to confirm, since conventional radiographs are often normal. To demonstrate the pathology, an arthrogram or computerized tomography (CT) scan is required.

The joint derangement may occur alone, but in patients seeking treatment it usually occurs in parallel with muscle pain and headache.

Muscle pain, spasm or tenderness plus limitation of opening can occur without joint disturbance, but the reverse is unlikely.

Bilateral palpation of each pair of masticatory muscles in turn is required to build up a picture of the severity of the disorder, but subjectively this can be done by careful questioning. The extent of sleep loss, inability to chew and pain on opening will all contribute to an understanding of the extent of the problem; this in turn will give a guide to the possible success of treatment.

Management

This is perhaps one of the most controversial areas of dentistry and the multitude of treatments used probably reflect the difficulty of accurate diagnosis and the low level of understanding of the disorder pathology.

The other complicating factor in the assessment of treatment methods is the self-limiting nature of the disease. There is definitely a peak of pain and dysfunction and then resolution, and much treatment is likely to be applied in the declining phase of the disease, thereby showing favourable results.

Broadly, conservative treatment may be categorized as follows:

- Reassurance and explanation of the condition
- Basic physiotherapy
- Occlusal therapy
- Systemic therapy

Of these, probably the third and fourth are mutually exclusive, with individual practitioners having a strong preference for using one or the other. A balanced view would be that there is a place for all of these possibilities in the treatment of the condition, but the difficulty is to define the exact type of patient and syndrome which would benefit from each therapy.

There is some evidence to suggest that personality type or psychological morbidity have a bearing on the success of treatment. Some patients may be treatment seekers and would not be satisfied with reassurance only. Others with a high psychological morbidity might be better treated with systemic antidepressants rather than local occlusal therapy.

There is a high level of placebo response reported in several studies and the confidence of the operator in his favoured therapy also influences the outcome.

Reassurance and explanation

This is of fundamental importance, particularly in those patients who are in severe pain, may have lost sleep and find it difficult to eat. They need a simple explanation of the condition that will allay their fears that their condition is serious or even sinister.

An explanation based on the analogy of the pulled muscle or sprained ankle seems readily acceptable to most patients. The particular muscles involved can be demonstrated, and headache from the temporals or neckache from the sterno-mastoid or posterior belly of the digastric is easily explained. Clicking of the TMJs can also be compared with common clicking in other joints.

The relationship of the condition to anxiety or stress can be discussed, particularly if the patient admits to clenching or grinding during the day.

Basic physiotherapy

The role of basic physiotherapy is to rest the affected muscles, ease spasm by the application of moist heat or cold (as in sports injury therapy) and, with the use of appliances, again to rest or support the affected parts.

Patients should be advised to avoid wide opening, to let their jaw 'hang loose' to relax the muscles, and take a soft diet. An insulated hot water bottle is probably the most readily available way of applying heat to the muscles, though there are commercially available 'heat packs'.

Having relieved muscle spasm, the jaws should be gently and steadily restored to normal function, either by positive exercise or by increasing the normality of the diet.

The exercises could be called neuromuscular retraining and one of the more popular is making symmetrical opening and closing movements from a central starting position. However, if these cause pain or fatigue they should be restricted. Indeed, the use of exercises before the pain has been relieved by rest can be positively harmful.

The most common physiotherapeutic appliance is the occlusal splint, which is considered below.

Occlusal therapy

This may consist of:

- Occlusal splint
- Occlusal equilibration
- Provision of restorations

Occlusal splint

The purpose of the splint is to rest the masticatory muscles and allow the musculature to place the mandible into whatever position is desired without being influenced by the teeth. The precision of centric occlusion requires the mandible to always reach this position for swallowing, and this may not be the most 'comfortable' position for the muscles with their neuromuscular incoordination. The splint should introduce freedom of movement and also balance and stability to the mandible in its closed position.

A further function is to increase the muscle length, which thereby reduces the power that can be generated by the muscles.

A large number of designs have been advocated and these include upper splints, lower splints, soft splints, hard splints, part occlusal coverage splints, total occlusal coverage splints, smooth splints, indented splints. The reader who would like to pursue this myriad of techniques is referred to the bibliography to complete his or her confusion!

All designs seem to have moderate to good success rates and because of the particular history of temporomandibular dysfunction, Solberg has suggested that the occlusal splint is the 'gold plated placebo'. The confidence of the operator in his or her splint could be very important in inducing a positive response from the patient. There are very high placebo responses in many studies, some of the order of 45%. Suggestion and cognitive awareness complement the placebo effect. Cognitive awareness in this context is the reminder of there being something to be avoided by the presence of the splint.

This writer has his own favourite, which works in his hands, and describes this in detail below, together with his justification for using it.

The type and features are as follows:

- Lower – this is less obtrusive than an upper and seems better tolerated
- Hard — accurate adjustment is possible together with exact stability on closure
- Smooth – allows freedom for the musculature to take the mandible to a range of stable positions
- Canine guided – posterior teeth are discluded and non-working interferences are eliminated

Again, the explanation of the function of the splint to the patient is crucial to its success.

The splint is basically acrylic and can be made either in the laboratory on an articulated mounting of a precentric record, or from a vacuum formed plate that has cold-curing acrylic added at the chairside. The former is expensive of laboratory time and the latter is expensive of chairside time. The final features of each should be the same:

- The base must be stable on the lower teeth, be retentive and not rock
- The supporting cusps of the upper premolars and molars should meet the splint with even contact on flat plateaux in any position from centric relation to centric occlusion and slightly anterior to that (long centric) (*Fig. 26.1A*). This freedom of movement and evenness of contact should extend about 1 mm in each lateral direction. The patient should be able to slide smoothly on the splint by about 1 mm radius from centric occlusion
- There should be no incisal contact in long centric. This allows freedom in the arc of closure (*Fig. 26.1B*)
- Canine guidance should be incorporated by a raised plane anteriorly, providing posterior disclusion

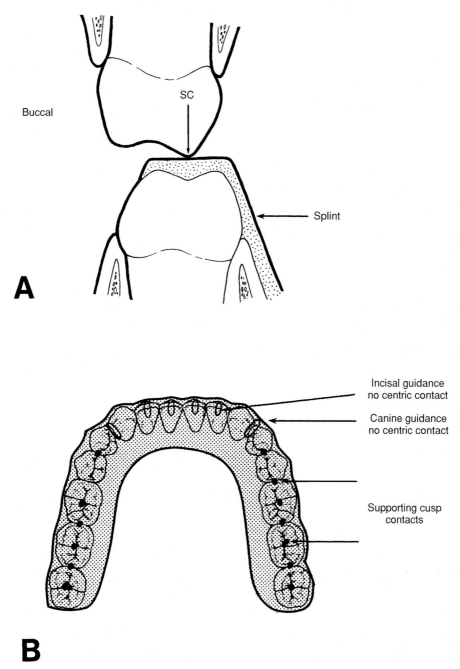

Fig. 26.1 A Transverse section of a splint in the molar region. The upper supporting cusp meets the splint on a flat plateau. **B** Ideal occlusal contacts shown diagramatically

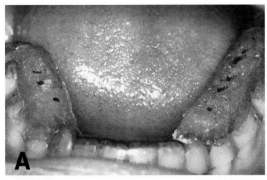

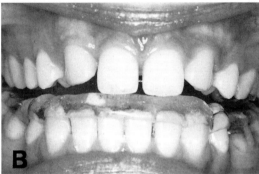

Fig. 26.2 A Articulating paper markings on a completed splint, showing the centric stop contacts. This splint is thicker than usual to disclude a deep anterior overbite. **B** Anterior guide provides posterior disclusion on forward movement

- Incisal guidance is provided in the same way, giving posterior disclusion in protrusion (*Fig. 26.2B*)

The occlusal contacts should be checked carefully with articulating paper and shimstock (*Fig. 26.2A*).

The splint should be worn full-time, particularly during eating and only removed for cleaning. It should be reviewed at one week and the occlusal contacts checked again, and then at four–six weekly intervals.

The resolution of the muscle pain is likely, provided it is not severe and long standing, within two-three months. The superimposition of an internal derangement of the joint may require consideration after the muscular pain has diminished (see below).

Following relief of symptoms, a decision must be made as to whether the splint can be discarded or whether some occlusal treatment is required.

Initially, the splint should be reduced to night wearing only for four weeks to judge response. If pain does not recur, then the splint can be left out

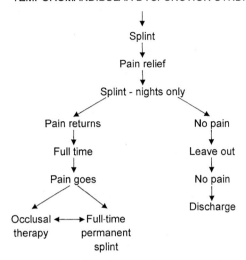

TEMPOROMANDIBULAR DYSFUNCTION SYNDROME

↓

Splint

↓

Pain relief

↓

Splint - nights only

Pain returns   No pain

↓   ↓

Full time   Leave out

↓   ↓

Pain goes   No pain

↓

Discharge

Occlusal ←——→ Full-time
therapy   permanent
              splint

Fig. 26.3 Flow chart showing the progress of temporomandibular dysfunction with treatment

altogether, followed again by review. The decision about long-term therapy can then be made with confidence (*Fig. 26.3*).

Bruxism may also be treated by such a splint, though the splint should be heat cured for strength, and an upper one is usually more durable. Nights-only wearing is quite successful as this is when most parafunction occurs. The bruxist will almost certainly continue nights-only wearing for some considerable time.

Occlusal equilibration

This was discussed in Chapter 14. In relation to temporomandibular dysfunction, some authorities recommend equilibration as a preventive measure as well as a treatment method. This author does not share these views, and cautions against irreversible surface modification for a condition that is often self-resolving. Indeed, the occlusal disharmonies will have been present for some years prior to the commencement of the syndrome, and in many patients once the muscular pain has been resolved and whatever has predisposed them to the condition has been resolved, they return to adapting to the disharmonies.

Certainly, extensive equilibration should never be used as the primary treatment, since the musculature will be provoked by the periods of opening required for the therapy and centric relation is not likely to be reproducible with muscle pain and incoordination present.

If the pain is resolved by the use of the splint, then some workers consider this to be diagnostic of occlusal disharmonies being a primary aetiological agent. The complexity of the disorder, though, does not lend itself to such simple assumptions. A comparative study of equilibration *versus* feigned equilibration showed better resolution in the latter group!

Correction of major occlusal disharmonies is possibly of long-term value. This would include orthodontic correction of instanding incisors, or the extraction of overerupted wisdom teeth. There is some evidence to support the correction of a lateral deviation on closure into centric occlusion.

However, the presence of postero-anterior slides from centric relation to centric occlusion on closure is so common that these really cannot be classed as aetiological agents in their own right. It may be that they become significant when the syndrome has developed, and their reversible elimination by a splint helps the syndrome to resolve. But after this, they appear to return to their previous level of insignificance.

Provision of restorations

An incorrect occlusal surface can clearly initiate avoidance and then temporomandibular dysfunction. In these cases the syndrome is secondary to the primary agent, the poor restoration, whose correction would be likely to eliminate the syndrome.

This approach can be used in mild cases, but in others the syndrome must be resolved first, before restorative therapy is commenced. This is again related to the likelihood of provoking the muscles by treatment and the difficulty in obtaining reproducible occlusal contact positions whilst the syndrome is present. The occlusal splint is without doubt appropriate here and is almost certain to succeed. Following this, re-restoration can be started.

Simple restoration replacement should be straightforward, but more extensive restorations can present difficulties. Alongside this, one can consider the problems of providing restorative therapy in general for resolved temporomandibular dysfunction patients. The dangers are that the provision of prolonged treatment could restart the syndrome by fatiguing the muscles, and then that the new restorations could also restart it. The patient must also understand these dangers so that the operator is not held liable for the recurrence of the disorder.

Restorative therapy should be kept to the minimum possible and performed over short visits. An intraoral prop should be used to give a firm platform on which to stabilize the muscles. If there is any sign of the syndrome during the treatment, the treatment should be suspended immediately. It may be necessary to reimplement the splint therapy and restabilize the condition.

Systemic therapy

Some systemic therapy may be used to accompany the occlusal splint. This could be analgesics (soluble aspirin or non-steroidal anti-inflammatory drugs can be very effective), or muscle relaxants. The most common muscle relaxant for temporomandibular dysfunction is diazepam but this should be used only for two or three days and then in very low doses, about 4 mg at night. The tranquillizer effect and the possibility of dependence is then very low.

The major use of systemic therapy is to counteract the central aetiological agents of stress and anxiety by prescribing antidepressants. The proponents of this approach argue that occlusal disharmonies may be present but they always have been, and that what has happened is a neuromuscular problem induced by interference with neural pathways. Various antidepressants have been used and good success rates have been reported. However, these are not substantially better than the rates for splint therapy.

The average dental surgeon, if he believes in this approach, should make the diagnosis and then refer the case to a medical practitioner for prescription. Whilst lower doses of antidepressants are effective, possibly by virtue of their action in reducing muscle tone, the side-effects of the therapy must be monitored and appropriate training is necessary to do this.

Other therapies

Outside the mainstream of conventional and reasonably well substantiated therapy are other approaches. These are based on empirical theories and observations and may be related to chiropractic and osteopathy. A relationship of the occlusion to the biomechanics and balance of the vertebral column has been proposed, particularly to the skull position. Treatment aims here appear to be directed at correcting occlusal anomalies to reposition the skull and vertebral column. This is claimed to relieve headache and low back pain. The occlusal therapy may be accompanied by therapy from a cranial osteopath.

None of this has any scientific substantiation and it must be remembered that these patients are susceptible individuals, perhaps with subclinical psychiatric problems, who may be vulnerable to suggestion.

Internal derangement of the TMJ

The articular disc may simply be out of phase with the condylar movement or may be permanently displaced. In addition, there may be derangement of the articular surfaces, either from trauma or from chronic inflammation.

The simplest form of derangement is the click caused by the out of phase disc catching up with the condyle and, if this is painless, no treatment is usually necessary. If the clicking is accompanied by muscle pain, and this is stabilized first, then the result may be a painless click. Again, no active treatment for the residual click is necessary. The only problem is that the elastic fibres posterior to the disc, which bring it back from protrusion, can become stretched, leaving a prolapsed disc.

However, if the joint pain persists after splint therapy, together with limitation of opening and joint sounds, then further treatment will be necessary. This is also true of locking, which can occur without clicking. Further treatment must be done upon the basis of an accurate diagnosis, and to do this arthrograms of the TMJs are necessary. These reveal whether the disc is displaced or whether there are arthritic or other changes in the joint. A spin-off from arthrography is that adhesions may be broken down by the interference with the joint.

This may be done intentionally during arthroscopy. Some success in curing locking has been reported.

Simple conservative therapy has some success in releasing the displaced disc back to its normal position. This is done with a repositioning splint, which is very similar to the muscle stabilizing splint described earlier, but has positive tooth guiding planes for closure. The path of closure is anterior to that normally employed, and the maximum contact position is forward also. Thus the condyles are advanced and pulled downwards in the fossae. The splint should be made from a wax record which reproduces the position of the mandible on closure just before the click occurs. The splint must be worn continuously and should not be used in the presence of muscle pain, which will be made worse by the abnormal forward posture.

Success rates for repositioning splint therapy are variable and this type of therapy should be reserved for those cases which have remained insoluble from the muscle stabilisation splint.

The internal derangements resulting from trauma or osteoarthritic change require surgical management.

Temporomandibular dysfunction – Summary

The condition remains a controversial area because of the difficulties of defining and diagnosing the syndrome and the large number of treatments, including placebo, that have reasonable success rates.

Simple, reversible, non-invasive therapies are recommended as the first option, with the more difficult procedures and systemic drug therapy held in reserve for those who do not respond to the first approach.

There is clearly a small group of patients who show little response to all forms of treatment, and who eventually get better by themselves!

27

Management of failure in the restored dentition: Fixed restorations

We all have failures! But it is essential to learn from them and not make the same mistake again. This book has tried to give a practical, common-sense approach to many aspects of restorative dentistry, and to follow its advice, the author believes, would reduce the incidence of failures. The management of failures is a major challenge because of the damage already done. This chapter and the next deal with problems associated with fixed restorations and dentures.

Failure of restorations may be caused by the dentist, the patient, continuing pathology, inadequacies in materials and a combination of all four!

The dentist may be responsible for:

- Treatment planning errors
- Technical errors

The treatment plan must be tailored to fit the patient and be based on an accurate diagnosis of the pathologies present (Chapter 4). It must also fit the dentist's skills and facilities. For instance, a treatment plan based on the skills and experience of a specialist and his or her supporting team is likely to be quite beyond the reach of the average general practitioner.

Poor treatment planning, then, is a major problem, often compounded by technical errors. Simple plans made up of easy stages are always best, no matter how skilled the operator. Unreasonable demands on technical expertise that does not exist, and patient motivation and awareness that is half-hearted, are recipes for disaster!

It would be a boring world if everything was perfect, and thankfully a lot of less than perfect dentistry requires no treatment other than regular observation. The questions to be answered in the affirmative before embarking on re-restoration are:

- Is there any active pathology in the area of the problem?
- Are there any symptoms?
- Is there an aesthetic problem that disturbs the patient?
- Is there a functional problem?

If the answer is 'Yes' to any of these, then action is required, but there are many examples of imperfection where nothing should be done.

Examples for masterly inactivity

Ditched, corroded amalgam restoration

Do not replace such a restoration unless there is evidence of recurrent caries, either clinically or radiographically, or there are symptoms of microleakage (see *Fig. 3.3*).

Under- or over-filled root canal

Do not interfere unless there are clinical or radiographic signs of an enlarging apical area, or symptoms. If you do decide to interfere, be certain that there is some glimmer of hope that you can do better! Is the canal apical to the short filling obstructed, for example?

Intracoronal restorations

'Cracked tooth syndrome'

This condition can cause considerable difficulty in diagnosis. There is a hairline, vertical fracture extending from the base of a large cavity, either to the root furcation, or down the root as well. The patient complains of vague symptoms, perhaps mainly on biting, that are often poorly localized. Radiographs usually show no abnormality. If infection supervenes, then the affected tooth may be tender, but again there are usually no radiographic signs.

The affected tooth usually has a large mesio-occlusodistal amalgam present, again possibly with no apparent defects. Removal of the amalgam will reveal a deep occlusal floor and a flat plastic should be turned gently within the cavity to attempt to open the buccal wall from the lingual. A crack in the floor may then be revealed.

The prognosis for the tooth is poor, though symptoms may be relieved by placing an acid-etched composite restoration. The cusps will be held together, thus preventing the flexure stimulating the periodontium. However, the fracture line is vulnerable to infection, which may occur at time.

Dentine pins

Pins in the periodontal ligament or pulp are a complication that can be unavoidable, due to the blind nature of their insertion. The misplacement of the pin-hole should be diagnosed as soon as it has been drilled, either because the resistance to cutting was suddenly lost, or because blood appeared in the hole.

The hole should not be used, but filled with calcium hydroxide. However, if a pin has been inadvertently placed in such a hole, then pulpal or periodontal infection can occur. Treatment of the pulpal infection might require root canal therapy, whilst the periodontal infection may require raising a flap, cutting the excess pin away and smoothing it flush with the root.

If the pin is superficial, then a crown preparation could cover it as a method of sealing. If the pin is inaccessible, then extraction may be the only solution.

Beware of interpreting the two-dimensional radiograph incorrectly. A correctly placed pin may be superimposed on the pulp shadow.

Post crowns

These are particularly vulnerable to operator error during preparation. The root morphology is unknown and unseen, and it is easy to be misled by an apparently large root face which, in fact, tapers dramatically in the alveolus.

The side of the post hole may be perforated during preparation, or the root may be weakened leading to vertical fracture during preparation, cementation or later function. Posts may fracture in the canal.

Lateral perforation

Large, parallel sided posts are prone to this complication and particular teeth are also vulnerable. The upper lateral incisor, being small and angulated distally and palatally, is a particular trap, as are roots with mesial and distal concavities (see below).

Teeth that can be either two-rooted or single rooted, such as upper premolars, also give rise to problems, simply because the root morphology is unseen.

Perhaps the best advice is to avoid posts in teeth which are known to be variable in morphology, and construct pinned cores instead (see Chapter 11).

The differential diagnosis for a post crowned tooth that is giving problems must always include the possibility of a perforation, and a second radiographic view can be helpful (*Fig. 27.1*). This will also show the position of the perforation as labial or palatal by parallax.

The management of the lateral perforation depends upon its site and size, and the restorability and prognosis of the tooth as a whole. A carious, short rooted tooth is better extracted, rather than embarking upon difficult treatment. Also, if a perforation can be positively diagnosed as palatally placed, then the tooth should be extracted.

Having decided upon trying to save the tooth, the first decision is whether to remove the offending post, or leave it *in situ*. A small rooted tooth may not survive the stress involved in withdrawing a post, and a threaded post can stress the root excessively on being unscrewed.

If the post can be removed (or if the perforation has been observed at preparation), then the post hole should be re-established in the correct line (*Fig. 27.2*), an impression taken and the new post fitted at the time of surgical exposure of the perforation.

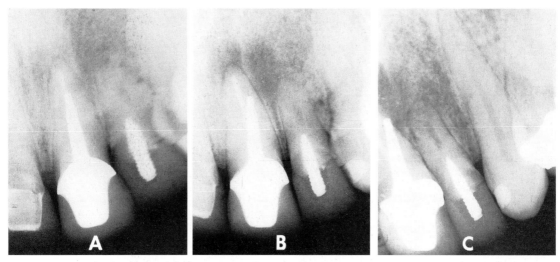

Fig. 27.1 Periapical radiographs of the 1̲2 region. **A** Suggests that the post is in the correct line of the canal. **B** Taken to show the 2̲, reveals the post off-line. **C**, Taken for the 3̲, reveals a palatal perforation of 1̲. Unfortunately, the original diagnosis had been made using **A** only, and the patient had been treated for temporomandibular dysfunction. The central incisor was later extracted

The perforation should be isolated so that cement does not enter the bone, and the post cemented with polycarboxylate cement. An acrylic provisional crown should be placed as well. The perforation should be cleaned and retention provided around it by a small round bur. Amalgam is then placed to seal the perforation (*Fig 27.2*). This procedure may be complicated by the wedge shaped nature of the perforation, which may be long in the long axis of the tooth and whose walls can be very thin.

If the original post cannot be removed, then surgical repair may be attempted by removing the post material that is outside the root profile, and cutting a channel around its end. This is then sealed with amalgam.

A small perforation, noticed at the time of preparation, may be packed with calcium hydroxide from within the canal, the post made in the correct line, cemented as usual, and periodically reviewed radiographically.

Two cautionary tales

Diagnostic disaster 1.

The case illustrated in *Figure 27.3* had a post crown constructed on the upper left lateral incisor some eight years previously. The tooth gave problems subsequently, and an apicectomy was performed. This did not resolve the problem and the patient, having moved home, consulted a new practitioner.

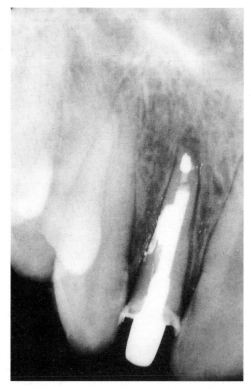

Fig. 27.2 A post crown with a lateral perforation has been removed, and the canal re-established in the correct line. A new post was constructed and cemented at apical surgery. The perforation has been repaired with amalgam, and a retrograde root filling placed

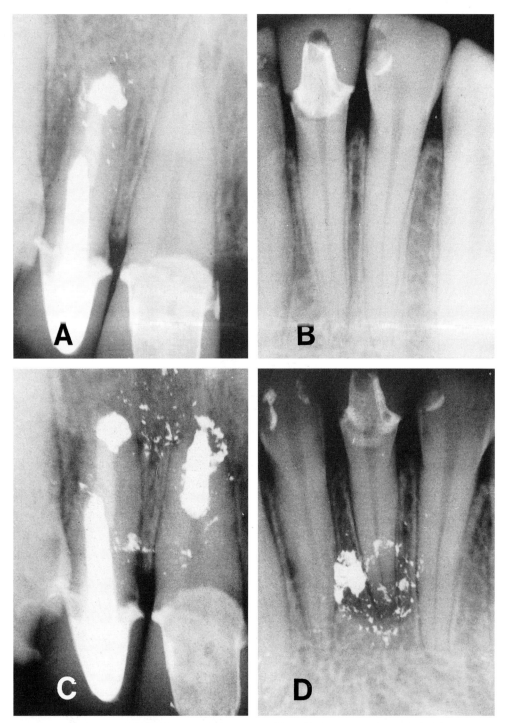

Fig. 27.3 A The post crown on the lateral incisor had given trouble since fitting, and the tooth had been apicected twice previously, with no benefit. There is no apical pathology present on the crowned 1⌋. **B** The lower central incisor had a badly fitting crown on it, but no apical pathology. The practitioner prescribed a further apicectomy for 2⌋, and because of negative pulp tests on 1⌋ and ⌊1, apicectomies were prescribed for these as well. **C** and **D** Results of the apical surgery. **C** The upper lateral incisor continued to be painful. **D** The operator failed to identify the apex of ⌊1 and has deposited amalgam in bone. The tooth was subsequently found to be vital

The new practitioner said that the previous apicectomy had failed, and the operation should be repeated. He provided the root seal shown in *Figure 27.3A*.

The tooth still gave trouble, and a further house move brought the patient yet another adviser. The hospital practitioner who saw her advised that the second apicectomy had failed, and that the operation should be repeated. He also tested the vitality of the crowned central incisor and the crowned lower

incisor (*Fig. 27.3B*) with ice and concluded that they were non-vital (ceramic is a good insulator!). He advised that both these teeth should be apicected also, in spite of the absence of any apical pathology.

After a nine-month wait, the three apicectomies were done by a further practitioner, as a day case. He provided the surgical results shown in *Figures 27.3C and D*.

The upper lateral still did not recover, and the patient was seen by the author. Surgical

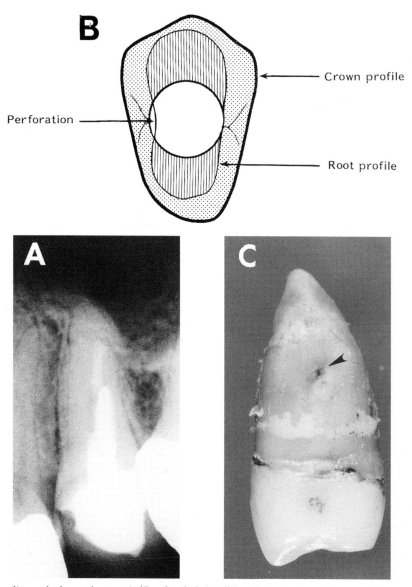

Fig. 27.4 A The radiograph shows the post in ⌊5 to be slightly off line, but not dramatically so. However, the root profile of single rooted upper premolars tends to have concavities (**B**), which cannot be seen. The large crown profile gives a false sense of security, but a perforation has occurred (**C**, arrowed)

investigation of the strong possibility of a lateral perforation by the off-line post was done, a perforation found and repaired, and the tooth settled. The lower incisor turned out to be vital, was root filled and post crowned, and the large mass of misplaced amalgam left under review.

The patient pressed a successful claim for damages, and all teeth were still present and symptomless four years later.

Diagnostic disaster 2

The upper second premolar illustrated in *Figure 27.4* had given trouble since the post crown had been fitted. Acute inflammation developed such that the whole quadrant was painful, with all the teeth being tender.

The patient attended a Sunday morning emergency service and, for some reason, the dentist diagnosed acute apical infection of the two perfectly sound incisors of the upper left side. These were 'opened to drain' and the patient attended hospital the next day.

The vital pulps, still present in the incisors, were extirpated and the teeth root filled later. The patient elected to have the perforated premolar extracted. No legal action resulted.

This case illustrates firstly, the danger of making posts on roots with unseen concavities, and secondly, the need to have the fullest information available before a committed diagnosis is made. In the face of seven tender teeth in a quadrant and no radiographs, the prescription of analgesics and antibiotics is a safer course of action.

Vertical fracture

Complete vertical fracture is often the consequence of a blow or jar to a post crown which knocks it out. Short, or ill fitting, posts are particularly vulnerable. Diagnosis may not be obvious, but root integrity must be checked before recementing the crown. A small flat plastic instrument should be inserted into the post hole, and turned gently to open any fracture line (*Fig 27.5*). Excessive force is not necessary and should be avoided. In the event of a vertical fracture, the tooth is unsavable.

Incomplete fracture is very difficult to diagnose. It is an occasional finding during apical surgery, and all roots with posts should be inspected carefully at the time of surgery. The crack, or cracks, may have been caused by over zealous preparation with large twist drills, or by a later blow. They can remain stable for some time, but in some cases tissue fluid leaks through and initiates corrosion, either of the post or of a metallic root

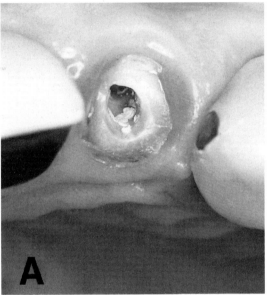

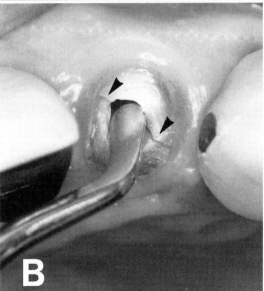

Fig. 27.5 Check for root fracture when a post crown has been lost. **A** The root face appears normal. **B** The flat plastic is twisted gently in the canal and the fracture (arrowed) has opened

filling. The corrosion products open the fracture line, infection supervenes, and the tooth gives symptoms. The tooth is unsavable, but diagnosis may not be made until surgery is attempted, at which time a stained root is revealed (*Fig 27.6*).

Vertical fractures may also be caused by tapered, threaded posts upon insertion. These are dangerous and should not be used.

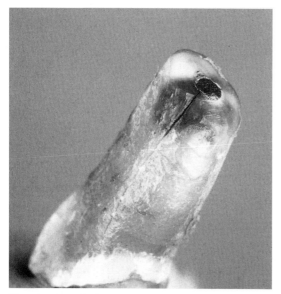

Fig. 27.6 A partly fractured root. Tissue fluid has reached the metal post, and corrosion has resulted. This was found at apicectomy and the tooth was later extracted

Fractured post

This is a particular complication of cast posts or small posts of all types. A blow, or a jar during eating, shears the post at a casting defect. The root should be checked for vertical fracture and, if intact, removal of the fragment performed.

A special kit (Masserann, Micro-Mega – see manufacturers' list, p. 281) is recommended (*Fig. 27.7*). This is a series of cutting tubes (trepans) designed to cut an annulus around the fragment, thus releasing it. Direct and straight access is required to the fragment and the choice of diameter of trepan used is important. It should be only fractionally larger than the fragment, so that the minimum of dentine is removed. Assuming that the root filling remains intact, the tooth can then be re-restored.

Fixed prosthodontics

High standards of treatment planning and construction, coupled with the joint efforts of the patient and the dentist in a continuing care programme ought to result in bridgework that has a minimum life expectancy of 10 years. Faults in treatment planning (such as the use of dubious teeth as abutments), faults in construction (such as poorly fitting margins), or inadequate oral hygiene by the patient may all reduce this dramatically.

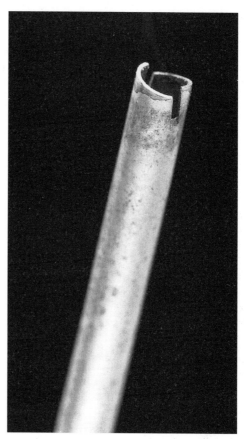

Fig. 27.7 A Masserann trepan. The cutting tube removes cement or dentine from around the object in the canal, which is thereby released

Possible sources of failure are:

- Cementation failure
- Recurrent caries
- Non-vitality and apical pathology
- Periodontal disease
- Incorrect occlusion
- Fractured ceramic
- Wear and tear

Cementation failure

This may be due to poor stability of preparations, differential biomechanical loading of abutments, or fatigue of the cement. In multi-retainer conventional bridgework, it can be very difficult to diagnose, since it may be partial, with the crown apparently still secure. The patient may report vague symptoms that will relate initially to dentine stimulation by microleakage and then to carious

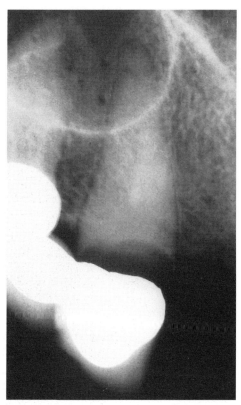

Fig. 27.8 Cementation failure. Radiograph of a bridge retainer whose connection with the bridge has been destroyed by slow caries. The pulp has disappeared also

attack. These symptoms may not be specific to one tooth and, in a multiple unit restoration, this can be perplexing.

Radiographs do not reveal anything at the early stage, unless there is a deficient crown margin. Applying displacing pressure to the restoration may reveal looseness or tell-tale bubbles at the cervical margin. This can be helpful in single crowns or on one side of a pontic, but multiple retainers may be supporting the failed one. Unfortunately, the diagnosis can be made with confidence only when the crown is fully unseated, by which time caries could have destroyed most of the preparation! (*Fig. 27.8*).

All this points to choosing luting agents of the highest possible resistance to dissolution and fitting bridges with the best possible marginal adaptation and retention.

Once cementation failure has been diagnosed on a bridge, the whole restoration must be removed without damage (see below), the integrity of the abutments checked and the bridge recemented if the abutments are satisfactory.

Recurrent caries

This is potentially serious, as once the preparation dentine is reached, caries can spread rapidly. It is revealed at routine maintenance visits, either by clinical or radiographic observation. Provided it is limited to the immediate area of the margin, the caries can be removed and the area restored with glass ionomer cement. A more extensive zone of caries, and particularly any that runs some way out of sight under a retainer, will necessitate the removal of the crown.

It is interesting to note how patients' habits and diet may change. A stable mouth with low caries rate at the time of treatment planning may exhibit increased caries activity if the patient changes to a high refined carbohydrate diet. This may be provoked by stress – (e.g. sugary tea as a stress relief mechanism), or changes in working pattern (e.g. sucking sweets as a way of passing long journeys). These factors need to be considered within the continuing care programme.

Non-vitality and apical pathology

Teeth that have suffered carious attack and are then subjected to pins and core placement followed by crown preparation will have had their pulps considerably insulted. It is not surprising that a small proportion of crowns and bridge retainers become non-vital, often without symptoms. Teeth that have been traumatized may also succumb. Symptomless non-vitality is difficult to diagnose without apical pathology to reveal it. Hence the need for radiographic review of the apices of crowned teeth, as well as those that have been root filled.

The management of such cases is by root filling the tooth through an access cavity in the crown. If this is impossible then apical surgery should be considered and failing this, the tooth should be extracted after sectioning it from the bridge.

Periodontal disease

Assuming that the bridge was made on a sound periodontium, i.e. one that was stable and free of inflammation, then prevention is better than cure! Whilst every patient should be instructed to use Superfloss at least twice a day, it is quite surprising to note how this slips to twice a week. The result of lack of diligence in plaque removal is marginal inflammation, particularly in the embrasure areas. Regular reinforcement of oral hygiene instruction with periodic visits to the hygienist will always be necessary.

Periodontal breakdown accounts for a surprisingly small number of bridge failures. This reflects operation of the biofeedback occlusal load modification mechanism, as well as the resilience of the periodontal ligament. Rotational forces are potentially the most damaging and these may be caused by an incorrect occlusion, usually on a cantilever design in lateral excursions.

Breakdown may be manifested by pain on biting, tenderness to percussion and mobility. Group function should be established by equilibration of the bridge or the bridge remade to a fixed–fixed design.

Incorrect occlusion

This may give the patient the feeling that the teeth do not meet evenly, or worse, induce temporomandibular dysfunction. Changes in overjet may make the patient feel as though the teeth are 'cramped'.

The occlusion should be examined first with articulating paper and shimstock, as described in Chapter 14. If the discrepancies are seen clearly and are not large, simple equilibration can be successful. Where there is any doubt about the errors, a diagnostic centric relation mounting should be done to permit clear examination of the occlusal contacts.

A trial equilibration can be carried out on the articulation and, if successful, repeated on the patient. If the discrepancies are too large, then the bridge will require remaking (see below).

If the bridge appears to have induced temporomandibular dysfunction, then this condition must be stabilized first and under no circumstances should there be any irreversible adjustments made to the bridge. It is possible that the dysfunction was coincidental with the bridge fitting, and not actually caused by it. Once the dysfunction has been resolved (Chapter 26), a detailed examination of the bridge can be made with a view to accurate diagnosis.

Fractured ceramic

The most likely causes of this are incorrect metal subframe design, so that the ceramic is not supported, or insufficient occlusal clearance leading to the ceramic being too thin.

Small areas may be repaired using a proprietary silane coupling agent and a composite resin. The disadvantage of this is that the composite is less durable than the ceramic and may deteriorate in time. Replacing the lost material with a ceramic veneer is a useful technique if a standard veneer preparation can be done on the fractured component (*Fig 27.9*).

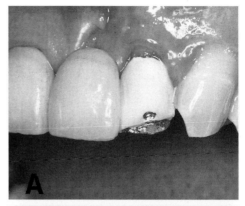

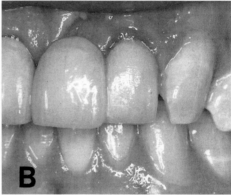

Fig. 27.9 A The incisal edge of the bridge retainer on ⌐2 had fractured. A veneer preparation has been done on the remaining crown. **B** A ceramic veneer has been cemented with dual affinity resin-retained bridge cement

Wear and tear

Long-term durability of bridge components is variable, even without the supervention of the pathology mentioned above. The most vulnerable aspect of a well made bridge is the ceramic. The material absorbs water and undergoes static fatigue as well as losing surface stain and becoming lighter. Before the advent of shoulder ceramic, a dark line at the gingival margin was an inevitable consequence of gingival recession.

Changes in colour that affect aesthetics can be improved only by replacing the whole prosthesis.

Management of the failed bridge

A bridge may be a candidate for replacement if:

● There is recurrent caries
● There is cementation failure

- One or more abutments show active pulpal or apical pathology
- One or more retainers show bad marginal adaptation
- The aesthetics are unacceptable
- The function is unacceptable

Limited recurrent caries might be amenable to local excavation and restoration, and a single pulpally involved tooth in an otherwise acceptable bridge could be root filled through the retainer.

In other cases, particularly where several of the replacement criteria are fulfilled, removal of the bridge is the only satisfactory solution. Because the basic condition of the abutments is hidden by the retainers, the patient must be clearly informed that no guarantees can be given about the eventual re-restoration. They must understand that if the abutment teeth prove unsatisfactory, a partial denture could be the end result.

The sequence for management is:

1. Preoperative diagnostic mounting
2. Construct provisional replacement, usually a partial denture
3. Remove the bridge
4. Section bridge into individual retainers for use as provisional crowns; fit denture
5. Inspect and assess each abutment tooth – vitality, restorability, prognosis
6. Stabilise abutment teeth as appropriate – e.g. root canal treatment, pinned cores
7. Plan new bridge (or alternative replacement)
8. Construct new bridge

Perhaps the most difficult stage is the removal of the old bridge. Since it may be desirable to use the retainers as individual provisional crowns, removal should create the least damage possible. There is, of course, the very real danger of damaging the abutment teeth as well.

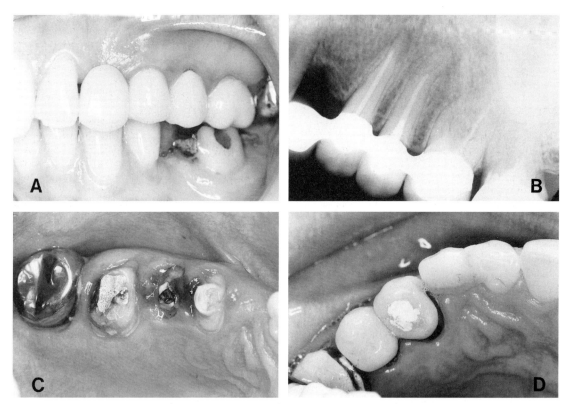

Fig. 27.10 A This bridge replacing ⌊3 is cantilevered from ⌊456, which is probably one retainer too many. **B** The radiograph shows that the premolar crowns have poor margins and short root fillings. There is an apical area on the ⌊4, and a second root which has not been filled. The buccal root canals of ⌊6 have not been filled. **C** The underlying teeth showing recurrent caries and inadequate preparations on the premolars. **D** The bridge has been sectioned into individual provisional crowns to allow the root canal therapy to be redone, and a denture tooth has been acid-etched to the ⌊2. Following the root therapy, the bridge was remade from ⌊45, with the ⌊6 being restored with a separate crown

Gentle prising, by placing a Mitchell's trimmer or chisel at each retainer margin in turn, should be tried first. Then, if no movement results, mechanical shock can be applied to each retainer in an attempt to break the lute seal. Ultrasonic scalers can be successful, but the hammer blows of proprietary crown removers are more common. These are particularly unpleasant for the patient, and can fracture teeth underneath the bridge if not used with extreme care. Again, if no movement is seen after a few minutes the last resort is to cut each retainer with the air turbine. This technique, whilst destroying the bridge, at least means that the abutments escape with minimal damage.

A vertical cut should be made on the buccal aspect of each retainer, through the metal/ceramic only, using the appearance of the luting agent as a guide to depth. Special burs are available to do this. Care should be taken not to cut dentine, since this leaves grooves that may dictate an unfavourable path of insertion for the new bridge. A cut across the occlusal surface may also be necessary for the retainer to be released.

To construct the provisional restorations, temporary crown forms may be used or, alternatively, the preoperative mounting can be used as the template for resin-based provisionals (*Fig. 27.10*).

The obsessive patient

This is a failure, or series of failures waiting to happen! Feinmann and Harris have coined the term 'oral dysaesthesia' for patients who have an unnatural concern about their dentitions. The term 'phantom bite' is also used.

Dentists and plastic surgeons are very vulnerable to the demands of perfection-seeking individuals and in dentistry, whilst reasons for treatment can sometimes be found, no organic disorder will usually be found to underlie the request for treatment. (This is the third time this warning has been written in this book – it bears repeating!)

Such patients may complain about the aesthetics of their teeth or the arrangement of their 'bite'. In the writer's experience, many are women in their thirties, with apparently stable family backgrounds.

Other patients, particularly in the older age groups, complain of pain for which no organic pathology can be found. Some also give impossible pathologies as their diagnosis, e.g. a patient

believed that microleakage around a crown lead to air entering the nervous system and causing paralysis of the left side at night!

The dentist can easily be tempted by the history to undertake replacement of the dubious amalgam, provide crowns or even extract perfectly healthy teeth. Unless a pathological process is diagnosed, *no operative treatment should be performed*. This will be doomed to failure, and the patient will continue to demand more and more until the dentist calls a halt. The patient will then leave in a distressed state.

Recognition of the problem is the key to avoiding it. Beware of the patient who asks numerous technical questions, offers a history of unsatisfactory care elsewhere or who is overbearingly demanding about the standards of care required.

Medico-legal aspects of failures

Every patient with a failed restoration is a potential litigant, but fortunately the vast majority of patients are loyal to their professional advisers. By discussing possible problems as they are foreseen during treatment, the patient is taken into the dentist's confidence, and if the worst happens the patient is expecting it too! The patient then sympathizes with the dentist.

The ability of the dentist to communicate effectively is a major factor in avoiding litigation. When discussing failures with the patient, it is important to put the problem in the context of the general difficulty of the technical aspects of dentistry. Explanations about the variation in tooth form, technique sensitive materials and so on, often gain the patient's sympathy and understanding.

However, this is not to suggest that deceiving the patient is appropriate. It is very necessary to explain exactly what is wrong and what needs to be done to put it right, without apportioning blame. If the patient continues to express dissatisfaction with previous care, it is best to be non-committal and supportive of the previous dentist if at all possible.

The courts do not expect every dentist to have specialist skills and to be successful in every case. They require that the treatment provided is of a reasonable standard appropriate to the dentist's training and experience, and has been delivered in a careful manner.

Management of failure in the restored dentition: Dentures

Management of denture problems

Although the possibilities for complaints about dentures are numerous, the more common denture problems are:

- Pain/discomfort
- Looseness/loss of fit
- Inability to chew efficiently
- Appearance
- Speech
- Retching
- Broken dentures
- The burning mouth

Pain/discomfort

Important information necessary for diagnosis and treatment planning includes site, duration and aggravating/relieving factors.

Pain/discomfort may be related to:

- Extension of the borders
- Condition of the fitting (impression) surface
- Extension of the base
- Anatomy of the denture-bearing tissue
- Occlusal errors
- Occlusal vertical dimension

Overextension of the border usually causes localized pain and is most common in the early period following the provision of a new denture. It may be possible to detect the offending area by looking for deflection of the tissues in the sulci when the denture is inserted; otherwise, pressure indicating paste or spray can be used.

The fitting surface of a new denture should be examined for sharp ridges or acrylic resin pearls which, if present, should be trimmed and

smoothed. Undercuts may need to be reduced or eliminated to allow the dentures to be inserted atraumatically. With the passage of time and alveolar resorption, the adaptation of the fitting surface to the tissues may deteriorate and result in localized pressure spots. These can be identified with pressure indicating paste/spray and relieved but other treatment, e.g. relining, might also be considered.

In the lower arch, a complaint of generalized discomfort may result from an underextended base transmitting high pressure to the reduced area of supporting tissue. The remedy is to correctly extend the base and, of course, to optimize other design factors such as occlusion and occlusal vertical dimension.

Localised pain may be caused by anatomic features such as a narrow, sharp mandibular ridge and gross alveolar atrophy resulting in the superficial positioning of the mental foramen. The complaint is normally of sharp pain on pressure and, if the mental nerve is involved, of a shooting pain along its distribution into the lower lip.

If the occlusion is not even and simultaneous then excessive pressure will be transmitted to the underlying tissues on the side of the premature contacts. A locked occlusion will not permit lateral excursions without resulting in movement (dragging) of the entire denture base over the tissues (commonly the lower). This can be more obvious when new dentures with anatomic teeth replace an old set with a very worn occlusion which permitted unrestricted lateral movements.

Errors in the occlusal vertical dimension can lead to symptoms from the denture bearing tissues or the masticatory apparatus. Lack of freeway space may cause excessive loading of the tissues and resultant generalized discomfort. It might also lead to pain in the muscles of mastication. Excessive freeway space is unlikely to result in painful ridges but may cause symptoms in the musculature.

Looseness/loss of fit

A most important factor in looseness of a denture is the time scale. If the complaint is made at the insertion stage of a new denture, the dentist should first be satisfied that the design features and standard of technology are adequate, i.e. border and base extension, adaptation of the base to the tissues, posterior palatal seal, etc. The patient should then be reassured that all is well and that his or her muscular control of the denture(s) with habituation will enhance denture wearing. On occasions the patient may be advised to use a denture fixative to give added confidence in this early phase.

Inevitably the alveolar ridges will resorb with time, with the mandible losing ridge height and width at approximately four times the rate of the maxilla, and the denture base will no longer 'fit' the tissues. It may, however, be some time before the patient complains of looseness, because during the period of gradual ridge loss he or she has learnt control of the dentures. Indeed, some patients can control and manipulate old dentures that, in the view of the dentist, are well past their useful life.

If the looseness can be attributed to the fitting surface of the denture whilst other design factors are satisfactory, a reline/rebase can correct the deficiency.

Inability to chew efficiently

The complaint of lack of chewing efficiency may be due to worn teeth on an old denture or the use of non-anatomic teeth on a new denture. Excessive grinding of new teeth to correct occlusal errors will also spoil the shape of the teeth and limit their capacity to reduce foodstuffs.

Occasionally, patients may find difficulty chewing if the occlusal vertical dimension is outside their tolerance limit. A poor occlusion, for example when the number of teeth contacting is reduced, may also contribute to chewing difficulties.

Aesthetics

A complaint of poor appearance relating to dentures usually occurs either immediately the dentures are fitted, or following gradual deterioration of the condition of the dentures, some years later. If the wax trial stage has been correctly carried out, the patient should have had adequate time to examine and approve the appearance and therefore the finished dentures should be satisfactory. It is possible, though unlikely, that the teeth have moved or other errors have occurred during the flasking and processing procedures. Occasionally,

the dissatisfaction arises because the patient receives an unfavourable comment about his or her new teeth from a relative or friend. Whatever the reason, a patient unhappy with the appearance of the teeth is unlikely to persevere with the dentures.

Factors which may detract from the appearance include:

- Unsatisfactory tooth shade, contour or size
- Labio/lingual tooth position leading to incorrect lip support
- Too much/too little length of crown visible – lip coverage
- Poor contour of gingival margins
- Errors in the occlusal vertical dimension

New dentures can greatly enhance the appearance, but there are limitations and some patients' expectations may be unrealistic. For example, they cannot reverse the ageing process and they cannot eradicate the normal lines and creases in the skin.

Old dentures may have poor aesthetics because of worn or stained teeth and because of loss of lip support as the dentures 'settle' in the mouth following long-term alveolar resorption. Bleaching due to over enthusiastic or incorrect use of cleaning agents will also deleteriously affect both the denture base resin and the teeth.

Speech

A new denture may cause a change in the speech patterns although, with adaptation, this usually disappears within a few days. If persistent, it is probably because the shape of the polished surfaces and/or tooth position on the dentures has been changed beyond the adaptive capacity of the individual. In this case, the shape should be compared to the previous denture and, if necessary, consideration given to repositioning the incisors and/or modifying the palatal contours accordingly. The most common complaints relate to the 's' sound, which is dependent on the correct relationship of the tip of the tongue and the palatal aspect of the upper anterior teeth.

Retching

A few patients have great difficulty coping with a foreign body in the mouth, resulting in retching. Some, those with extreme difficulties, may retch even when an examination mirror is placed between the lips. Most, however, can tolerate instrumentation or a denture in the mouth for varying lengths of time. In the extreme cases there are strong psychological overtones which cannot be overcome simply; however, in others, the design and fit of dentures is the predisposing factor.

The most common cause of retching related to dentures is posterior overextension of the upper or lower denture. The soft palate and posterior areas of the tongue are sensitive to contact, causing the protective retching reaction. Thickness of the bases is also relevant as besides encroaching on the tissues, it may also lead to tongue cramping. Occasionally, a normally extended or underextended poorly fitting upper denture will cause retching when it drops and contacts the posterior region of the tongue. The management (modification) of the dentures will depend on the diagnosis and may well include guidance on wearing dentures, as well as reassurance.

Recurrent fracture of dentures

There are two mechanisms to describe the way dentures can break:

● Impact fracture
● Fatigue fracture

An impact fracture occurs due to a high, short-acting force impacting on the denture, such as can occur if the denture is dropped on to a hard surface. This type of fracture can occur at any time in the life of a denture. A fatigue fracture is the result of numerous, relatively low magnitude, repeated forces being applied that eventually cause a small crack, commonly in the midline, which then progresses by crack propagation to ultimate failure. Failure by this mechanism is common after a period of wear of several years.

Midline fatigue fracture is usually associated with one or a number of the following:

● Median diastema
● Large fraenal notch
● Absence of labial flange
● Wedging action of very worn occlusion
● Inherent weakness following previous repair

It will occur more readily in those with the ability to chew or clench using heavy masticatory loads and in those with bruxism.

The majority of midline fractures can be avoided by the application of established prosthodontic principles during denture construction, for example: even and adequate bulk of denture base material cured to achieve optimum polymerization and free of porosity; relief of incompressible tissue in the centre of the hard palate; addition of labial flange to increase rigidity of denture base; even and balanced occlusion to reduce wedging effect and locking of occlusion. Reduction of stress concentrators such as notches and diastema to a minimum would also help prevent these fractures. If notches are to be incorporated, a rounded notch is preferred to a sharp one. Consideration should be given to the use of either a high impact acrylic resin denture base material or a metal (cobalt–chromium) base.

Burning mouth

A complaint of burning or tingling associated with the oral tissues or lips is referred to as the burning mouth syndrome. It is most common in women who are over 50 years of age. Diagnosis is by a process of elimination since there are numerous potential causative factors. A detailed history and examination will lead to a provisional diagnosis in most cases but it can be very difficult, even with the aid of special tests, to reach a definitive diagnosis in a few cases. Timing and mode of onset should help define if the complaint is related to the provision of a new prosthesis.

Local factors such as denture design (e.g. incorrect occlusal vertical dimension, excessive loading of the supporting tissues, tooth position causing lip/tongue irritation, etc.) should be assessed and eliminated. Excessive residual monomer content (more than 1%) due to incomplete curing of the polymethyl methacrylate can lead to chemical irritation with a new or recently relined/rebased denture. This can be confirmed only by chemical analysis of the denture base using, for example, gas chromatography, but if suspected the practitioner could request the laboratory to re-process the denture. Other contributory factors include denture induced stomatitis, a dry mouth (note the variety of causes, including pharmacotherapy) and smoking.

Systemic factors include deficiencies that are only evident following blood screening tests for iron, folic acid and the vitamin B complex. Investigations might include: serum iron, serum folate, serum vitamin B_{12}, red cell folate, as well as the haemoglobin. Anxiety and depression (and their associated pharmacotherapy) should be borne in mind. Close liaison with the general medical practitioner is obviously important.

Denture relines

A reline can be described as the addition of material to the existing fitting surface of a denture base. It is evident, therefore, that the reline procedure can utilize a permanent or temporary material, which could be either hard or soft and which could be applied at the chairside or in the laboratory.

A reline is normally prescribed to improve the fit of an existing denture when the looseness is related to the fitting (impression) surface of the denture. This usually occurs due to alveolar resorption and is therefore time dependent. In this situation the denture should be examined to ensure that it is otherwise satisfactory, i.e. the occlusion, occlusal vertical dimension and aesthetics. Deficiencies in the border extension should be corrected using tracing stick impression compound and undercuts removed from the base before the wash impression is taken. Normally, the aim is to record maximum surface detail without disturbing either the vertical dimension or the occlusion, and therefore an impression material such as zinc oxide–eugenol paste or silicone, which can be used in thin section, is ideal. When recording the impression the borders should be moulded and then the denture brought into occlusion with the opposing natural teeth or denture whilst the material sets. This avoids disturbing the occlusion.

This clinical procedure is the same for both laboratory performed hard and soft relines (and for a rebase which involves removal and replacement of a significant proportion of the old base material).

A soft lining may be added as a reline procedure for a patient with a history of mucosal discomfort and chronic soreness, provided other predisposing factors have been eliminated. To be effective a permanent soft lining should be 2–3 mm thick. The lining acts to absorb part of the force of occlusion, releasing the stored energy as elastic recoil. It also assists in producing an even distribution of functional load over the entire denture-bearing area, avoiding local concentrations of stress. It should, therefore, increase a patient's ability to use a denture comfortably.

The most effective material is heat polymerized silicone, since this has good elastic properties and remains soft. An adhesive is required to ensure an adequate bond to the polymethyl methacrylate denture base material. Plasticized acrylic resin is an alternative, but is less soft than silicone and hardens as the plasticizer leaches out. It does, however, bond chemically to the denture base.

Autopolymerizing silicones and plasticised acrylic resin soft linings are available, but their properties do not compare favourably with those of the heat polymerized materials. They can, however, be used at the chairside and are suitable for domiciliary visits if laboratory support is not available.

Temporary soft linings (tissue conditioners) remain soft for a limited period only (days to weeks) and can be used when it is necessary to give the supporting tissues an opportunity to recover before fabricating a new denture or permanently relining an existing one. They may also be used as functional impression materials, for immediate denture maintenance, cleft palate speech aids and immediate surgical splints. The powder is a higher methacrylate, e.g. polyethylmethacrylate, or co-polymers, while the liquid is usually a mixture of ethyl alcohol as solvent and dibutyl phthalate as plasticizer. The alcohol and ester are solvents for the polymer beads, swelling them and allowing the plasticizer to diffuse in, and rapidly forming a gel through a physical process. Although initially very soft and fluid, leaching and evaporation of the compounds leads to hardening of the material in the mouth.

Repairs

The material most commonly employed in the construction of dentures is polymethyl methacrylate. Despite its popularity, the material, although adequate in satisfying aesthetic demands, is far from ideal in fulfilling the mechanical requirements of such appliances. This is reflected in the unresolved problem of denture fracture and the accompanying costs to effect repair.

The causes of denture fracture have been discussed above. Although repair of a broken denture should be carried out in the laboratory to achieve maximum strength, the patient and denture should be examined first in the clinic. This examination should elicit the cause of the fracture, health of the oral tissues and the suitability of the denture.

If relatively new and otherwise satisfactory, the denture should be sent for a standard repair. However, if the denture is also loose it may be necessary and appropriate to carry out a reline (or rebase) at the same time as the repair, since this will both strengthen the base and improve the fit.

The component parts should be assembled and if there is any doubt about their relocation, sticky wax should be used to hold them together so that the denture can be tried in the mouth. This same procedure is necessary before a reline impression, although it may be necessary to reinforce across the fracture line using pieces of wire, old burs or even matchsticks.

If the denture is inherently weak due to the design, e.g. no anterior flange on an upper complete denture or a small lower complete denture with a soft lining, then consideration should be given to modifying the denture by adding a flange or incorporating a cast lingual metal plate. The construction of a new denture should be considered.

Fractured metal components may be more difficult to repair. It is not always possible to solder new clasps to a cobalt–chromium denture framework. It may be necessary to construct a new clasp and retain it within the acrylic resin saddle region.

Causes of denture intolerance

An inability to cope with dentures can be due either to factors related to the design and construction of the dentures or attributed directly to the patient. A close examination and assessment of the dentures should always be made before putting the blame for failure elsewhere.

There are many possible causes of denture intolerance and often a diagnosis is reached only by a process of elimination. It is important, therefore, to follow an orderly pattern in the examination of denture and patient. This should always be proceeded by a history of the complaint(s) relating it to previous denture experience and the age and general health of the patient.

Design faults

Many complaints of intolerance can be related to extension of the bases, the occlusal vertical dimension or the relationship of the denture to the neutral zone. Overextension or excessive thickness of the borders is poorly tolerated and, on occasions, can lead to a complaint of retching. It can, of course, also cause discomfort and looseness. The complaint of retching is usually related to the posterior lingual extension of the lower denture and the posterior palatal extension of the upper.

Patients are less likely to cope with dentures with reduced (or negative) freeway space than if there is excessive freeway space. With reduced freeway space they may complain of the dentures feeling too big for their mouth, teeth clattering or meeting too early, generalized discomfort of the denture-bearing tissues or pain in the muscles of mastication.

A denture that does not conform with the neutral zone is likely to be displaced in function, with the patient complaining of looseness.

Design faults leading to poor aesthetics will, with a discerning patient, lead to rejection of a denture since good appearance is probably the strongest motivating factor for denture wear.

Adaptive capacity

The capacity of an individual to adapt to change may be determined by a number of factors including age and general health. Chronological age is less relevant than biological age since a sprightly, mentally active older person is more likely to be adaptive than a biologically old younger individual.

Adaptive capacity will also depend on general health and is reduced in chronic or debilitating conditions. The after-effects of cerebrovascular accidents can severely handicap adaptation, leading to considerable difficulties with dentures.

Even a normally adaptable individual can have difficulty meeting the demands of excessive changes in design if a new denture differs markedly from the old. For example, an individual who has worn the same under-extended dentures for more than 20 years and has become accustomed to the gradual loss of occlusal vertical dimension, with resultant gross overclosure due to wear of the teeth and alveolar resorption is perhaps unlikely to adapt to the sudden change to 'text book' dentures fully extended and with the average 3 mm of freeway space.

Personality and mental attitude

Most patients cope well with complete dentures even when the dentures are perhaps less than ideal. There are, however, some who are fussy and demanding with a high level of expectation. These individuals can usually be satisfied provided adequate time and appropriate expertise is devoted to them. Unfortunately, there are a few who are obsessive and often illogical in their attitude to denture treatment who cannot be satisfied. These individuals may seek treatment from a number of different practitioners but continue to find fault with all the prostheses and place the blame on anyone or anything other than themselves.

Lack of motivation

As has already been stated, most edentulous patients are strongly motivated to wear dentures to maintain or improve their appearance. Many, of course, also gain from the improvement in masticatory function. However, there are those who can cope with their diet perfectly adequately without teeth and who are not unduly concerned with their appearance. These individuals may be put under pressure from relatives or health workers to have dentures. In some cases they have been without teeth or dentures for years and it is unlikely that they will put sufficient effort into wearing dentures to give much chance of success.

Chronic alcohol abuse

Patients with a known history of alcoholism often do not tolerate dentures well. They may complain of retching whenever the dentures are inserted and may not persevere in order to learn control of the dentures. This link between retching and alcoholism may be due to the condition of gastritis which is common.

Soft tissue pathology related to wearing dentures

Traumatic ulceration

This is the most common pathology resulting from wearing dentures. This can occur during the first few days when new dentures are worn, usually because of areas of overextension, traumatic contact (in relation to undercuts) or irritation from sharp or rough areas of the fitting (impression) surface. Ulceration can also occur when a denture becomes loose and ill-fitting. When the source of irritation is removed the ulcer should heal within a few days. If it persists the area should be further inspected and, if necessary, biopsied.

Denture-induced stomatitis

This occurs mainly in the maxilla and is more common in females. It is a chronic irritation of the denture-bearing tissues, causing the mucosa to appear bright red. Most patients are unaware of its presence since it is normally asymptomatic. A number of factors are believed to contribute to the condition:

- *Candida albicans*
- Denture wearing habits
- Fit of the denture
- Excess residual monomer
- General health

Candida albicans

Poor oral and denture hygiene allows plaque and food deposits to accumulate, with an associated overgrowth of the mycelial and yeast forms of the fungus on both the tissues and denture base.

Denture wearing habits

When dirty dentures are worn day and night the tissues are in constant contact with the infected denture bases and the condition is aggravated.

Fit of the denture

Mechanical trauma from rough or ill-fitting dentures tends to irritate the tissues and make them more susceptible to candidal infection.

Excess residual monomer

It is possible that the residual monomer will chemically irritate the tissues and increase their susceptibility to infection.

General health

Systemic factors such as deficiencies of the vitamin B complex, iron and folic acid, and immunological defects should be borne in mind, especially in those resistant to normal treatment regimes.

Treatment

The treatment of the condition can be summarized under three headings:

- Improved oral hygiene
- Modifications to the fit of the denture
- Antifungal therapy

Advice should be given on denture hygiene and cleaning (see Chapter 24) and the patient requested to leave the dentures out during the night. A hypochlorite solution is probably the most effective cleaner for plaque removal and for sterilization of the denture base. A poorly fitting denture can be modified using a hard or soft lining material at the chairside (see section on denture relines). Antifungal therapy is directed locally using nystatin tablets (500 000 units) or amphotericin B lozenges (10 mg) dissolved in the mouth four times a day for up to two weeks or by the use of miconazole oral gel (25 mg/ml), that can be smeared on the fitting surface of the denture.

Other conditions

Angular stomatitis is an inflammatory, and sometimes erosive, condition which occurs in the folds at the corners of the mouth. It is usually seen in association with denture-induced stomatitis, and the presence of *Candida albicans* should therefore be suspected. Secondary bacterial infection can occur; also, *Staphylococcus aureus* is claimed to be a causative organism of the lesion even in the absence of *Candida albicans*. Inadequate lip support or insufficient occlusal vertical dimension from the dentures may lead to the development of folds at the corners of the mouth that, due to saliva moistening them, can be susceptible to infection. Initial treatment is based on that prescribed for denture-induced stomatitis; miconazole oral gel is probably the most effective agent since it is both antifungal and antibacterial. Modifications may be required to the dentures to improve lip support and occlusal vertical dimension. If the lesion is resistant to therapy, the possibility of an underlying associated deficiency (e.g. iron, or vitamin B or C) should be investigated.

Papillary hyperplasia of the palate is an inflammatory lesion which presents as multiple small nodules of granulation tissue. It usually occurs in the central portion of the palate and can correspond to the area underlying a relief chamber. Causative factors include chronic irritation from the denture and a superimposed denture-induced stomatitis. Again, treatment is first aimed at improving the oral hygiene and reducing irritation. Surgical treatment is probably only required in extensive cases or if there is doubt about its benign nature.

Denture-induced hyperplasia is an overgrowth of granulation tissue usually associated with the borders of ill-fitting dentures. Trauma from the borders causes recurrent ulceration and healing, with resultant growth of fibrous tissue. This can present as a fold or multiple folds of tissue and is more common in the lower jaw, associated with the buccal and labial borders. Treatment is aimed first at eliminating the source of irritation by substantially reducing the border of the denture, or by persuading the patient not to wear the denture (not always acceptable). Temporary lining of the denture may also be appropriate in order to improve the fit and stability. Since there is an inflammatory component to this pathological process, these measures should allow a regression in size of the lesion due to resolution of the inflammatory process. The resultant lesion may then be sufficiently small to allow routine prosthetic treatment to be continued. However, more extensive lesions, which would interfere with the construction of dentures, may require surgical excision.

Oral carcinoma

Whilst this pathology is not related to denture wearing it is important to remember the role of the dentist in identifying early lesions of the oral mucosa and lips. Discomfort, ulceration and/or loose dentures might relate to a soft tissue lesion. As was stated above, any ulceration that does not heal quickly should be investigated further.

Regular recall of complete denture wearers is not routine. After the first review the patient, if satisfied, is discharged. To be able to make an early diagnosis of silent lesions, a yearly examination should be arranged.

Bibliography

Below are listed some current textbooks on the individual principal subjects of restorative dentistry together with selected papers. Some of the papers are of considerable historical significance, whilst others deal with the 'state of the art'.

The patient

Medical history

Texts

Barnes I, Walls A, 1994. *Gerodontology.* Wright, Oxford.
British National Formulary 1997. British Medical Association, London.
Grundy M C, 1993. *An Illustrated Guide to Dental Care for the Medically Compromised Patient.* Wolfe, London.
Lewis M A O, Lamey P-J, 1993. *Clinical Oral Medicine.* Wright, Oxford.

Paper

British Dental Association, 1996. Infection control in dentistry. Advice Sheet A12. BDA, London.

Radiography and radiology

Text

Whaites E, 1996. *Essentials of Dental Radiography and Radiology,* 2nd edn. Churchill Livingstone, Edinburgh.

Guidance and legislation

HMSO, 1988. *The Ionising Radiation (Protection of Persons Undergoing Medical Examination or Treatment) Regulations.* Her Majesty's Stationery Office, London.
NRPB, 1994. Guidelines on radiology standards in primary dental care. National Radiological Protection Board, Vol 5, No 3.

Paper

Hutchinson I L, Hopper C, Coonar H S, 1990. Neoplasia masquerading as periapical infection. *British Dental Journal* **168**: 288–294.

Anaesthesia, analgesia and sedation

Texts

Hill C M, Morris P J, 1991. *General anaesthesia and sedation in dentistry.* Wright, Oxford.
Roberts G J, Rosenbaum N L, 1991. *A Colour Atlas of Dental Analgesia and Sedation.* Wolfe Medical, London.

Paper

Royal College of Surgeons of England, 1993. Guidelines for sedation by non-anaesthetists. RCS, London.

Trauma

Andreassen J O, Andreassen F M, 1994. *Textbook and Colour Atlas of Traumatic Injuries of the Teeth.* Munksgaard, Copenhagen.

The restoration and its environment

Oral biology and pathology

Texts

Berkovitz B K B, Holland G R, Moxham B J, 1992. *A Colour Atlas and Text of Oral Anatomy, Histology and Embryology,* 2nd edn. Wolfe, London.
Kidd E A M, Joyston-Bechal S, 1997. *Essentials of Dental Caries: the Disease and its Management,* 2nd edn. Oxford University Press, Oxford.
Thylstrup A, Fejerskov O, 1994. *Textbook of Clinical Cariology,* 2nd edn. Munksgaard, Copenhagen.

Periodontology

Text

Lindhe J, 1989. *Textbook of Clinical Periodontology*, 2nd edn. Munksgaard, Copenhagen.

Papers

Greene J C, Vermillion J R, 1964. The simplified oral hygiene index. *Journal of the American Dental Association* **68**: 7–10.

Hassell T M (ed.), 1993. *Periodontal Tissues – Structure and Function. Periodontology 2000*, Vol 3. Munksgaard, Copenhagen.

Lang N P, Karring, T (Eds), 1994. *Proc 1st European Workshop on Periodontology*. Quintessence Publishing, London.

Lang N P, Karring T (Eds), 1997. *Proc 2nd European Workshop on Periodontology*. Quintessence Publishing, London.

World Workshop in Periodontics, 1996. Vol 1, No 1. American Academy of Periodontology, Chicago.

Occlusion

Texts

Ash M M, Ramfjord S, 1995. *Occlusion*, 4th edn. Saunders, Philadelphia.

Kleinberg I, 1991. *Occlusion: Principles and Assessment*. Wright, Oxford.

Papers

Alexander P C, 1965. The periodontium and the canine function theory. *Journal of Prosthetic Dentistry* **18**: 571–577.

Bennett N G, 1908. A contribution to the study of the movement of the mandible. *Transactions of the Royal Society of Medicine* **1**: 77–84.

Beyron H L, 1969. Optimal occlusion. *Dental Clinics of North America* **13**: 537–542.

Celenza F V, 1973. The centric position: replacement and character. *Journal of Prosthetic Dentistry* **30**: 591–595.

Chasens A I, 1990. Controversies in occlusion. *Dental Clinics of North America* **34**: 111–123.

D'Amico A, 1961. Functional occlusion of the natural teeth of man. *Journal of Prosthetic Dentistry* **11**: 899–915.

Denbo J, 1990. Malocclusion. *Dental Clinics of North America* **34**: 103–109.

Jent T, Lundquist S, Hedegard B, 1982. Group function or canine protection. *Journal of Prosthetic Dentistry* **18**: 719–720.

Lauritzen A G, Bodner G H, 1961. Variations in location of arbitrary and true hinge axis points. *Journal of Prosthetic Dentistry* **11**: 224–229.

Lindhe J, Nyman S, 1977. The role of occlusion in periodontal disease and the biologic rationale for splinting in the treatment of periodontitis. *Oral Science Review* **10**: 11–17.

Posselt U, 1957. Movement areas of the mandible. *Journal of Prosthetic Dentistry* **7**: 375–379.

Schuyler S H, 1969. Freedom in centric. *Dental Clinics of North America* **13**: 681–685.

Stuart C E, Stallard H, 1960. Principles involved in restoring occlusion to natural teeth. *Journal of Prosthetic Dentistry* **10**: 304–313.

Restorative dental biomaterials

Texts

Anusavice K J, 1996. *Phillips' Science of Dental Materials*, 10th edn. W B Saunders, Philadelphia.

Craig R J, 1996. *Restorative Dental Materials*. Mosby, St Louis.

Van Noort R, 1994. *Introduction to Dental Materials*. Mosby, St Louis.

Papers

Eley B M, 1997. The future of dental amalgam: a review of the literature. Parts 1–7. *British Dental Journal*, 183.

Jacobsen P H, 1987. Biological and clinical testing of materials. *Journal of Dentistry* **15**: 266–268.

Jacobsen P H, 1988. Design and analysis of clinical trials. *Journal of Dentistry* **16**: 215–218.

Osborne J *et al.* 1978. Clinical performance and physical properties of twelve amalgam alloys. *Journal of Dental Research* **57**: 963–988.

Sarkar N F, 1978. Creep, corrosion and marginal fracture of dental amalgams. *Journal of Oral Rehabilitation* **5**: 413–423.

Clinical management and techniques

Intracoronal restorations

Texts

Kidd E A M, Smith B G N, 1996. *Pickard's Manual of Operative Dentistry*, 7th edn. Oxford University Press, Oxford.

Roulet J-F, Herder S, 1991. *Bonded Ceramic Inlays*. Quintessence, Chicago.

Papers

Burke F J T, Qualtrough A J E, 1993. Aesthetic inlays: composite or ceramic. *British Dental Journal* **176**: 53–59.

Jacobsen P H, Rees J S, 1992. Luting agents for ceramic and polymeric inlays and onlays. *International Dental Journal* **42**: 145–149.

Rees J S, Jacobsen P H, 1996. Restoration of teeth with composite resin 1: Direct-placement composite. *Dental Update* **23**: 406–410.

Rees J S, Jacobsen P H, 1996. Restoration of teeth with composite resin 2: Indirect-placement composite. *Dental Update* **24**: 25–30.

Management of deep caries

Brannstrom M, Isaacson G, Johnson G, 1976. Effect of calcium hydroxide and fluorides on human dentine. *Acta Odontologica Scandinavica.* **34**: 59–66.

Kidd E A M, Joyston-Bechal S, Beighton D, 1993. The use of a caries detector dye during cavity preparation: a microbiological assessment. *British Dental Journal* **174**: 245–248.

Oligushi K, Fusayama T, 1975. Electron microscope structure of the two layers of carious dentine. *Journal of Dental Research* **54**: 1019–1026.

Outhwaite W C, Garman T A, Pashley D H, 1979. Pins *v* slot retention in extensive amalgam restorations. *Journal of Prosthetic Dentistry* **41**: 396–400.

Endodontics

Texts

Cohen S, Burns R C, 1994. *Pathways of the Pulp*, 6th edn. Mosby, St. Louis.

Pitt-Ford T R, 1997. *Harty's Endodontics in Clinical Practice*, 4th ed. Wright, Oxford.

Wein F S, 1996. *Endodontic Therapy*, 5th edn. Mosby, St. Louis.

Papers

Saunders W P, Saunders, E M, 1994. Coronal leakage as a cause of failure in root canal therapy: a review. *Endodontics and Dental Traumatology* **10**: 105–108.

Zakariasen K L, Scott D A, Jensen J R, 1984. Endodontic recall radiographs: how reliable is our interpretation of endodontic success or failure and what factors affect our reliability? *Oral Surgery* **57**: 343–347.

Crowns

Harty F J, Leggett L J, 1972. Post crown technique using a nickel–cobalt–chromium post. *British Dental Journal* **132**: 394–397.

Jorgensen K D, 1955. The relationship between retention and convergence angle in cemented veneer crowns. *Acta Odontologica Scandinavica* **13**: 35–40.

Miller A W, 1982. Post and core systems: which one is best? *Journal of Prosthetic Dentistry* **48**: 27–38.

Wall G J, Cipra D L, 1992. Alternative crown systems. Is the metal ceramic crown the restoration of choice? *Dental Clinics of North Ameria* **36**: 765–769.

Colour and aesthetics

Texts

Chiche G J, Pinault A, 1994. *Aesthetics of Anterior Fixed Prosthodontics*. Quintessence, Chicago.

Muia P, 1993. *Esthetic Restorations. Improved Dentist Laboratory Communication.* Quintessence, Chicago.

Paper

Dunne S M, Millar B J, 1993. A longitudinal study of the clinical performance of porcelain veneers. *British Dental Journal* **175**: 317–321.

Bridgework

Texts

Rosenstiel S F, Land M F, Fujimoto J, 1994. *Contemporary Fixed Prosthodontics*, 2nd edn. Mosby, St Louis.

Shillingburg H T, Hobo S, Whitsett L D, 1981. *Fundamentals of Fixed Prosthodontics*, 2nd edn. Quintessence, Chicago.

Papers

Ante I H, 1926. The fundamental principles of abutments. *Michigan State University Society Bulletin* **8**: 24–28.

Becker C M, Kaldahl W B, 1981. Current theories of crown contour, margin placement and pontic design. *Journal of Prosthetic Dentistry* **45**: 268–275.

Eshleman J R, Janus C E, Jones C R, 1988. Tooth preparation designs for resin bonded fixed partial dentures related to enamel thickness. *Journal of Prosthetic Dentistry* **60**: 18–22.

Kayser A F, 1989. The shortened dental arch: A therapeutic concept in reduced dentition and certain high-risk groups. *International Journal of Periodontics and Restorative Dentistry* **9**: 427–449.

Livaditis G J, Thompson V P, 1982. Etched castings: an improved retentive mechanism for resin-bonded retainers. *Journal of Prosthetic Dentistry* **47**: 52–57.

Nyman S, Ericsson I, 1982. Capacity of reduced periodontal tissues to support fixed bridgework. *Journal of Clinical Periodontology* **9**: 409–412.

Rochette A L, 1973. Attachment of a splint to enamel of lower anterior teeth. *Journal of Prosthetic Dentistry* **30**: 418–422.

Removable prosthodontics

Bates J F, Huggett R, Stafford G D, 1991. *Removable Denture Construction*, 3rd edn. Wright, London.

Implants

Hobkirk J A, Watson R M, Albrektsson T, 1995. *Color Atlas and Text of Dental and Maxillofacial Implantology*. Mosby-Wolfe, London.

Problems

Tooth surface loss

Robb N D, Smith B G N, Geidrys-Leeper E, 1995. The distribution of erosion in the dentitions of patients with eating disorders. *British Dental Journal* **178**: 171–175.

Smith B G N, Knight J K, 1984. A comparison of patterns of tooth wear with aetiological factors. *British Dental Journal* **157**: 16–19.

Temporomandibular dysfunction

Feinmann C, Harris M, 1984. Psychogenic facial pain. *British Dental Journal* **156**: 165–170, 205–209

Gray R J M, Davies, S J., Quayle, A A, 1996. *Temporomandibular Disorders: A Clinical Approach*. British Dental Association, London.

Greene C S, Laskin D M, 1972. Splint therapy for myofacial pain dysfunction syndrome: a comparative study. *Journal of the American Dental Association* **84**: 624–628.

Solberg W K, 1986. *Temporomandibular Disorders*. British Dental Association, London.

Failures in the restored dentition

Text

Grant A A, Heath J R, McCord J F, 1994. *Complete Prosthodontics: Problems, Diagnosis and Management*. Wolfe, London.

Papers

Cheung G S P, Dimmer A, Mellor R, Gale M, 1990. A clinical evaluation of conventional bridgework. *Journal of Oral Rehabilitation* **17**: 131–136.

Crougers N H J, Kayser A S, 1992. An analysis of multiple failures of resin bonded bridges. *Journal of Dentistry* **20**: 348–351.

Karlsson S, 1986. A clinical evaluation of fixed bridges 10 years following insertion. *Journal of Oral Rehabilitation* **13**: 423–429.

Randow K, Glantz P-O, Zoger B, 1986. Technical failures and some related clinical complications in extensive fixed prosthodontics. *Acta Odontologica Scandinavica* **44**: 241–247.

And finally, *you*

Glyn Jones J C (ed.), 1994. *Self-assessment picture tests in dentistry - Operative Dentistry*. Wolfe, London.

Good luck!

Manufacturers of equipment cited in the text

Articulators and face-bows (Chapter 14)

Dentatus ARH articulator: *AB Dentatus, Stockholm, Sweden.*
Denar MkIIA articulator and Denar Slidematic face-bow: *Denar Corporation, Anaheim, California, USA.*

Precision retainers (Chapters 20, 21 and 24)

Ackermann Bar, Dalla Bona 604, Dolder Bar, Mini-Dalbo, Rothermann Eccentric Ring: *Cendres and Metaux, Biel-Bienne, Switzerland.*
Kurer Press Stud: *Prestige Dental, Bradford, UK.*

Crown and bridge removal (Chapters 21 and 27)

Beavers Jet carbide burs: *Beavers Dental, Ontario, Canada.*
Masserann kit: *Micro-Mega, Geneva, Switzerland.*

Index